Charlotte Rowe

GRAY'S *Dissection Guide for* Human Anatomy

GRAY'S Dissection Guide for Human Anatomy

SECOND EDITION

David A. Morton, PhD
Department of Neurobiology and Anatomy
University of Utah School of Medicine
Salt Lake City, Utah

Kerry D. Peterson, LFP
Director, Body Donor Program
Department of Neurobiology and Anatomy
University of Utah School of Medicine
Salt Lake City, Utah

Kurt H. Albertine, PhD
Professor of Pediatrics, Medicine,
and Neurobiology and Anatomy (Adjunct)
Course Director, Human Gross Anatomy
Assistant Dean of Faculty Administration

Editor-in-Chief, The Anatomical Record
Departments of Pediatrics, Medicine,
and Neurobiology and Anatomy
University of Utah School of Medicine
Salt Lake City, Utah

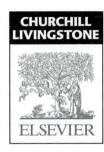

CHURCHILL LIVINGSTONE
ELSEVIER

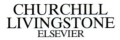

1600 John F. Kennedy Blvd.
Ste. 1800
Philadelphia, PA 19103-2899

GRAY'S DISSECTION GUIDE FOR HUMAN ANATOMY   ISBN-13: 978-0-443-06951-2
SECOND EDITION   ISBN-10: 0-443-06951-4

Copyright © 2007, 2004 by Churchill Livingstone, an imprint of Elsevier Inc.

All rights reserved. No part of this publication may be reproduced or transmitted in any form or by any means, electronic or mechanical, including photocopying, recording, or any information storage and retrieval system, without permission in writing from the publisher. Although for mechanical reasons all pages of this publication are removable, only those pages imprinted with an Elsevier Inc. copyright notice are intended for removal. Permissions may be sought directly from Elsevier's Health Sciences Rights Department in Philadelphia, PA, USA: phone: (+1) 215 239 3804, fax: (+1) 215 239 3805, e-mail: healthpermissions@elsevier.com. You may also complete your request on-line via the Elsevier homepage (http://elsevier.com), by selecting "Customer Support" and then "Obtaining Permissions."

Notice

Knowledge and best practice in this field are constantly changing. As new research and experience broaden our knowledge, changes in practice, treatment, and drug therapy may become necessary or appropriate. Readers are advised to check the most current information provided (i) on procedures featured or (ii) by the manufacturer of each product to be administered, to verify the recommended dose or formula, the method and duration of administration, and contraindications. It is the responsibility of the practitioners, relying on their own experience and knowledge of the patients, to make diagnoses, to determine dosages and the best treatment for each individual patient, and to take all appropriate safety precautions. To the fullest extent of the law, neither the Publisher nor the Authors assume any liability for any injury and/or damage to persons or property arising out of or related to any use of the material contained in this book.

The Publisher

Library of Congress Cataloging-in-Publication Data

Morton, David A.
   Gray's dissection guide for human anatomy / David A. Morton, Kerry D. Peterson, Kurt H. Albertine — 2nd ed.
      p. cm
   Rev. ed. of: Dissection guide for human anatomy / David A. Morton. 2004.
   ISBN 0-443-06951-4
1. Human dissection Laboratory manuals.   I. Title: Gray's dissection guide for human anatomy.   II. Peterson Kerry D.
III. Albertine Kurt H. Gray's dissection guide for human anatomy.   IV. Title.
   QM34.M59 2007
   611—dc22   2006040749

Acquisitions Editor: Inta Ozols
Developmental Editor: Katie DeFrancesco
Project Manager: Mary Stermel
Marketing Manager: John Gore

Printed in China

Last digit is the print number: 9 8 7 6 5 4 3 2 1

Acknowledgments

I express my appreciation to Tom Parks, Kerry Peterson, and Kurt Albertine, for the opportunity to participate in the creation of this dissection guide. I am grateful to my parents (Gordon and Gabriella Morton), who taught me to appreciate the miracle of the human body. I also thank my brothers (Gord, Joe, and Mike), my sister (Daniela), my in-laws, the Templeman family, Brian, and Bo, for their constant encouragement. I could not have completed this project without the support of my wonderful wife, Celine, and our children (Jared, Ireland, Gabriel, and Max), who are an inspiration in my life. This project has been one of the highlights of my career.

DAVID A. MORTON, PHD

I express my sincere thanks to the body donors and their families, who have taught me more about life than about anatomy. I am grateful to colleagues and students who have fostered my love for anatomy and its teaching. Foremost, I thank my wife (T.G.), for her unending support of my pursuits.

KERRY D. PETERSON, LFP

To health profession students who use this guide: Gross anatomy is learned through the dissecting of the human body. This conviction, coupled with sage advice from my gross anatomy professor, Dr. Sigfried Zitzlsperger — who wrote in the *Gray's Anatomy* textbook he gave me many years ago, "Don't forget the many hours in the gross lab. That is where you learned your anatomy and that's where you should return to refresh your knowledge" — stimulated me to direct this composition. My hope is that our road map to human dissection facilitates learning in today's climate of compressed medical curricula.

On a personal note, I too extend sincere thanks to Dr. Parks (Chairman of Neurobiology and Anatomy), for his undaunted support; to the body donors and their families (who are the real teachers of human anatomy and generosity); and to Kerry Peterson, for his expert direction of our body donor program, for his superlative teaching, and for his sense of humor. Thanks also go to the Dean's Office, particularly to Dr. Betsy Allen, Dr. Larry Reimer, and former dean Dr. Sam Shomaker, who provided institutional support and encouragement for our gross anatomy course. I am honored to have helped direct David Morton through this project, and I am proud to call him my colleague. I also appreciate the invaluable input provided by three classes of medical and dental students (graduating classes of 2004 to 2006). Their constructive criticism and ideas improved the guide from their perspective, which is to dissect efficiently and to learn what is expected. Last, I thank my wife (L.L.) for sticking by me despite the paucity of hours that I spend with her and our two children. To you, I dedicate my small part in this book.

KURT H. ALBERTINE, PHD

Preface to the Second Edition

With the second edition of *Gray's Dissection Guide for Human Anatomy* came a number of important changes, the principal stimulus for which was the publication of the first edition of *Gray's Anatomy for Students* (GAFS) in 2005, a year after the publication of the first edition of our dissection guide. The publication of GAFS provided the opportunity to coordinate the second edition of our dissection guide with that textbook. We did so through use of the same nomenclature *(Termina Anatomica)*, through balance of content, and through shared illustrations. Indeed, some of the illustrations from GAFS adorn the pages of our second edition, adding new graphic content and improving the delivery of information. In addition, not only have we cross-referenced our dissection guide to content in GAFS; we have also cross-referenced it to the fourth edition of *Netter's Atlas of Human Anatomy* (NAHA) and to the *Atlas of Clinical Gross Anatomy* (ACGA). Thus, for every dissection step, students are pointed to additional expert knowledge provided by GAFS, NAHA, and ACGA. For ease and convenience, the cross-references are positioned at the upper right of each page. This rich cross-referencing style adds to the original intent of our dissection guide: to focus on instructions that guide efficient dissection.

Another important modification in the second edition is expansion of the original four units into six. This was accomplished by dividing Unit 1 (Back and Thorax) into two units (Unit 1: Back; Unit 2: Thorax) and by dividing Unit 4 (Limbs) into two units (Unit 5: Upper Limb; Unit 6: Lower Limb). In the first edition of our dissection guide, the limb dissections provided a systemic anatomy approach. In this second edition, the approach for the limb dissections is regional, to maintain consistency throughout the guide. These organizational changes are intended to add flexibility to the dissection guide for use in human gross anatomy courses that follow an order of dissection that differs from the order followed at the University of Utah, the organizational template used for the first edition.

A third area of modification in the second edition is the addition of an osteology lab at the beginning of each unit.

A fourth area of modification in the second edition is the revision and correction of content. This important task was facilitated by the invaluable advice of a dozen expert anatomists. These experts also encouraged us to preserve the black-and-white illustrations, using color highlights to improve visual appeal.

The changes to the second edition prompted our editor to suggest the new title, *Gray's Dissection Guide for Human Anatomy*, a name that we feel honored to use. Accompanying this revision is a brilliant new cover.

Crafting the second edition of *Gray's Dissection Guide for Human Anatomy* has been an exciting endeavor whose successful completion can be attributed in no small part to contributions by numerous anatomists and by the staff at Elsevier. To all of you, we offer a heartfelt thank-you!

DAVID A. MORTON, PhD
KERRY D. PETERSON, LFP
KURT H. ALBERTINE, PhD

Preface to the First Edition

The key idea behind the writing of *Gray's Dissection Guide for Human Anatomy* was to produce a guide for efficient dissection of the entire human body in the reduced time that is allocated today to basic science courses in medical schools. The object was not to produce a textbook or atlas of human gross anatomy. Our goals, therefore, were (1) to make the guide practical and easy to follow for medical, dental, and graduate students so that they could finish each dissection during the assigned laboratory period and (2) to provide students with clear expectations of the anatomic structures to be dissected and learned.

Accomplishing both goals required selecting a format that served each one. We settled on a horizontal format that allowed us to position the text and corresponding illustration(s) on the same page. Thus, each page is divided in half by a vertical bar, with text positioned on the left and the corresponding illustration(s) on the right. The book is spiral bound to display two pages simultaneously and to make the book rest stably on the book racks that are attached to dissection tables. In addition, boldface type is used for the names of anatomic structures the first time a structure is identified in the text. This design alerts students that the named structure is to be dissected and identified.

The illustrations are simple black-and-white line drawings with occasional use of color. This illustration style focuses the reader's attention on a specific dissection task. Labels, which are kept to a minimum, are used to identify the anatomic structures to be dissected. Blue dashed lines highlight where cuts are to be made with a scalpel or saw.

Gray's Dissection Guide for Human Anatomy is organized into six regional units.
Unit 1: Back
Unit 2: Thorax
Unit 3: Abdomen, Pelvis, and Perineum
Unit 4: Head and Neck
Unit 5: Upper Limb
Unit 6: Lower Limb

For each laboratory dissection, the guide begins with an overview that identifies the structures to be dissected. The pages that follow contain the text and illustrations that direct the dissection. Each unit ends with a comprehensive listing that identifies all the structures that were dissected and that are therefore to be learned. *Terminologia Anatomica* (copyright ©1998; with permission from the Federative Committee on Anatomical Terminology) was used for anatomic nomenclature.

Because course hours for the study of gross anatomy are fewer today than they were in the past, rather than make the tables all-inclusive, we chose to select carefully—based on our practical experience—which anatomic structures in each region to include. We recognize that our guide is a distillation of the total body of gross anatomic information, and we hope that students who desire further information will invite their course instructors to elaborate and will engage in independent research through such authoritative textbooks of human anatomy as the 39th edition of *Gray's Anatomy* (Elsevier).

It is important to note that some of the dissection approaches require cuts that destroy continuity of structures. Such cuts are made to improve access to and/or visibility of anatomic structures. To minimize the impact of these cuts, we recommend that one or more cadavers per dissection room be spared so that structural continuity is preserved. Students should confer with their instructors to determine whether instructions to cut a structure are to be modified or skipped.

Key:
m. — muscle
mm. — muscles
n. — nerve
nn. — nerves
a. — artery
aa. — arteries
v. — vein
vv. — veins
r. — right
l. — left
CN — cranial nerve

Contents

UNIT 1
Back 1

Lab 1: Osteology of the Back *3*
Lab 2: Superficial Back *10*
Lab 3: Deep Back, Vertebral Column, and Suboccipital Region *23*
Lab 4: Spinal Cord *37*
Unit 1 Back Overview *44*

UNIT 2
Thorax 47

Lab 5: Osteology of the Thorax *49*
Lab 6: Anterior Chest Wall and Breast *55*
Lab 7: Thoracic Situs and Lungs *73*
Lab 8: Heart *84*
Lab 9: Mediastina *102*
Unit 2 Thorax Overview *113*

UNIT 3
Abdomen, Pelvis, and Perineum 115

Lab 10: Osteology of the Abdomen, Pelvis, and Perineum *117*
Lab 11: Anterior Abdominal Wall and Inguinal Canal *129*
Lab 12: Peritoneum and Foregut *147*
Lab 13: Midgut and Hindgut *170*
Lab 14: Posterior Abdominal Wall *183*
Lab 15: Gluteal Region and Ischioanal Fossa *196*
Lab 16: Urogenital Triangle *203*
Lab 17: Pelvis and Reproductive Systems *226*
Unit 3 Abdomen, Pelvis, and Perineum Overview *245*

UNIT 4
Head and Neck 251

Lab 18: Osteology of the Head and Neck *253*
Lab 19: Posterior Triangle of the Neck *267*
Lab 20: Anterior and Visceral Triangles of the Neck *278*
Lab 21: Scalp, Calvarium, Meninges, and Brain *300*
Lab 22: Base of the Skull and Cranial Nerves *317*
Lab 23: Orbit *329*
Lab 24: Superficial Face *338*
Lab 25: Deep Face and Pharynx *358*
Lab 26: Nasal Cavity, Palate, and Oral Cavity *373*
Lab 27: Larynx *393*
Lab 28: Ear *403*
Unit 4 Head and Neck Overview *411*

UNIT 5
Upper Limb 419

Lab 29: Osteology of the Upper Limb *425*
Lab 30: Superficial Structures of the Upper Limb, Shoulder, and Axilla *435*

Lab 31: **Arm** *454*
Lab 32: **Forearm** *466*
Lab 33: **Hand** *477*
Lab 34: **Joints of the Upper Limb** *490*
Unit 5 *Upper Limb Overview* *498*

UNIT 6
Lower Limb 501

Lab 35: **Osteology of the Lower Limb** *507*
Lab 36: **Superficial Structures of the Lower Limb and Gluteal Region** *516*

Lab 37: **Thigh** *524*
Lab 38: **Leg** *537*
Lab 39: **Foot** *546*
Lab 40: **Joints of the Lower Limb** *554*
Unit 6 *Lower Limb Overview* *562*

Index 565

Unit 1
Back

The purpose of this unit is to learn the anatomic structure of the back through dissection.

Lab 1 Osteology of the Back 3

Lab 2 Superficial Back 10

Lab 3 Deep Back, Vertebral Column, and Suboccipital Region 23

Lab 4 Spinal Cord 37

Unit 1 Back Overview 44

Osteology of the Back

Lab 1

Prior to dissection, you should familiarize yourself with the following osteologic structures:

OSTEOLOGY

Occipital Bone
- External occipital protuberance
- Superior nuchal line
- Inferior nuchal line

Temporal Bone
- Mastoid process

Vertebral Column (33 Vertebrae)
- Cervical vertebrae (7)
  - Atlas (C1)
  - Axis (C2)
- Thoracic vertebrae (12)
- Lumbar vertebrae (5)
- Sacrum (5 fused vertebrae)
- Coccyx (4 fused vertebrae)

Vertebral Structures
- Spinous process
- Transverse process
- Transverse foramen (cervical vertebrae only)
- Lamina
- Pedicles
- Vertebral body
- Vertebral arch
- Superior articular process
- Inferior articular process
- Vertebral foramen
- Intervertebral foramina (notches)
- Intervertebral disc

Ilium
- Iliac crest
- Posterior superior iliac spine

Ribs
- Head
- Neck
- Tubercle
- Angle
- Costal groove

Clavicle

Scapula
- Spine
- Acromion
- Lateral and medial margins
- Superior and inferior angles

Lab 1 Dissection Overview

The purpose of this laboratory session is to learn the osteology of the back through dissection. You will do so through the following suggested sequence:

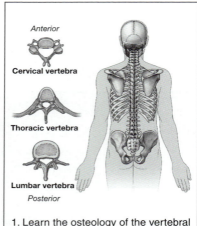

1. Learn the osteology of the vertebral column.

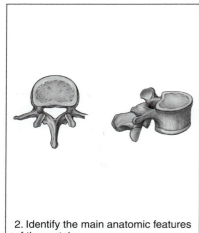

2. Identify the main anatomic features of the vertebrae.

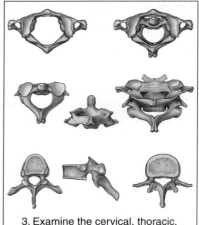

3. Examine the cervical, thoracic, lumbar, sacral, and coccygeal vertebrae.

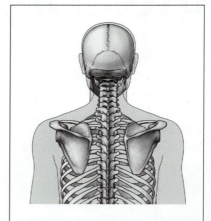

4. Examine how underlying osteologic structures create visual and palpable surface landmarks.

Vertebral Column

- The vertebral column consists of 33 vertebrae. The superior 24 vertebrae (cervical, thoracic, and lumbar) form a flexible, bony tube. The vertebral column not only serves as the axis for the body but also protects the spinal cord.

- Using a skeleton in your laboratory, identify the following **(Figure 1-1)**:

  - **Cervical vertebrae** — the superior 7 vertebrae of the skeleton (between the thorax and skull). Identify the superior 2 cervical vertebrae:
    - **Atlas (C1)** — articulates with the occipital bone to form the atlanto-occipital joint
    - **Axis (C2)** — articulates with the atlas
  - **Thoracic vertebrae** — the middle 12 vertebrae of the skeleton. Identify the 12 pairs of ribs that articulate with the thoracic vertebrae, forming the rib cage
  - **Lumbar vertebrae** — the 5 mobil vertebrae inferior to the thoracic vertebrae and superior to the sacrum
  - **Sacrum** — these 5 fused vertebrae articulate with the pelvic bones
  - **Coccyx** — 4 fused vertebrae that form the vestigial tailbone

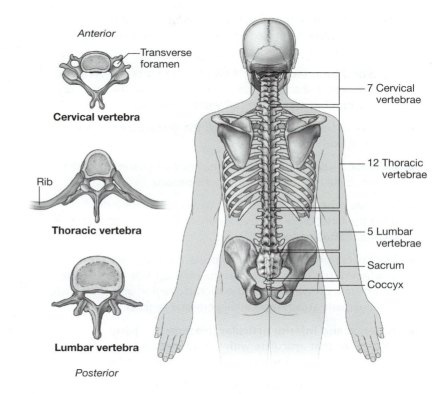

Figure 1-1 Vertebral column. (From Drake R, Vogl W, Mitchell A: Gray's Anatomy for Students. Philadelphia: Elsevier, 2005, Fig. 2.15)

Typical Vertebrae

- Using a thoracic vertebra, identify the following structures of a typical vertebra **(Figure 1-2A** and **1-2B)**:

  - **Vertebral body** — weightbearing part of the vertebra; it is linked to adjacent vertebral bodies by **intervertebral discs** and ligaments. The size of vertebral bodies increases inferiorly as the amount of weight supported increases

  - **Vertebral arch** — forms the lateral and posterior parts of the vertebral foramen; formed by the right and left pedicles and laminae

  - **Vertebral foramen** — the hole in the center of the vertebra through which the spinal cord courses. The combination of all vertebral foramina form the **vertebral canal**

  - **Pedicle** — bony pillars that attach the vertebral arch to the vertebral body

  - **Laminae** — flat plates of bone that extend posteriorly from each pedicle to meet at the spinous process

  - **Spinous process** — projects posteriorly and inferiorly from the junction of the two laminae; site for muscle and ligament attachment

  - **Transverse process** — extends posterolaterally from the junction of the pedicle and lamina on each side and is a site for articulation with ribs in the thoracic region and for muscle and ligament attachment in all vertebral regions

  - **Superior and inferior articular processes** — bony projections that articulate with the inferior and superior articular processes, respectively, of adjacent vertebrae

  - **Intervertebral foramen** — foramina formed on each side between adjacent parts of articulating vertebrae; allow structures such as spinal nerves and blood vessels to pass in and out of the vertebral canal

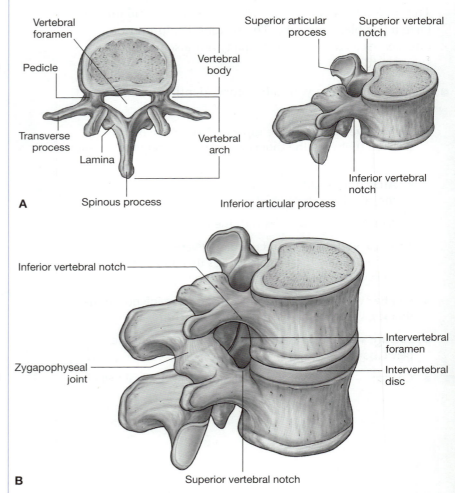

Figure 1-2 **A**, Typical vertebra. **B**, Intervertebral foramina. (From Drake R, Vogl W, Mitchell A: Gray's Anatomy for Students. Philadelphia: Elsevier, 2005, Figs. 2.20, 2.23)

Cervical, Thoracic, and Lumbar Vertebrae

- Examine the cervical, thoracic, and lumbar vertebrae **(Figure 1-3)**:
  - **Cervical vertebrae**
    - **Atlas vertebra (C1)** — articulates with the occipital condyles of the skull and lacks a vertebral body; forms the atlanto-occipital joint, allowing the head to nod up and down on the vertebral column
    - **Axis vertebra (C2)** — a bony projection from the axis vertebral body called the dens (odontoid process) projects superiorly to articulate with the atlas; the dens acts as a pivot that allows the atlas and attached head to rotate on the axis, side to side
    - **Vertebral body** — short in height and square shaped when viewed from above
    - **Vertebral foramen** — triangular in shape
    - **Spinous process** — short and bifid
    - **Transverse foramen** — each transverse process is trough shaped and perforated by a round transverse foramen
  - **Thoracic vertebrae** — the 12 thoracic vertebrae are all characterized by their articulation with ribs
  - **Lumbar vertebrae** — the 5 lumbar vertebrae are distinguished from vertebrae in other regions by their larger size

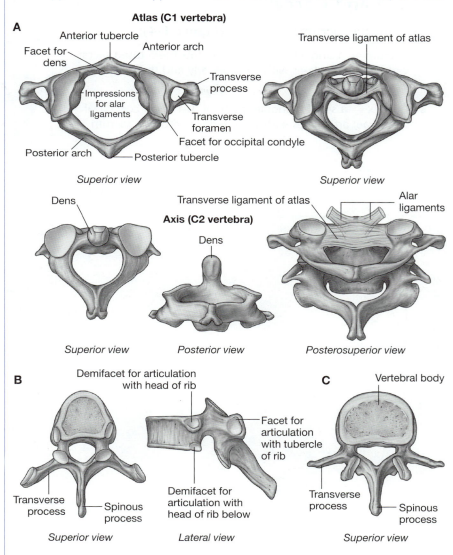

Figure 1-3 Regional vertebrae. **A,** Atlas and axis. **B,** Typical thoracic vertebra. **C,** Typical lumbar vertebra. (From Drake R, Vogl W, Mitchell A: Gray's Anatomy for Students. Philadelphia: Elsevier, 2005, Fig. 2.21B–D)

Sacrum and Coccyx

- Examine the sacrum and coccyx **(Figure 1-4)**:
  - **Sacrum** — a single bone that represents the 5 fused sacral vertebrae; articulates with L5 superiorly and the pelvic bones laterally
  - **Coccyx** — a small triangular bone of 3–4 fused coccygeal vertebrae; articulates with the inferior end of the sacrum

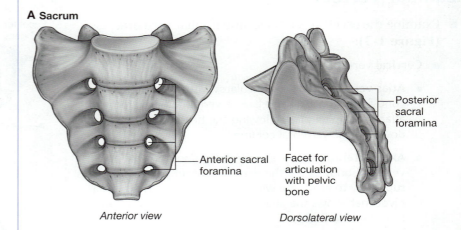

Figure 1-4 Sacrum **(A)** and coccyx **(B)**. (From Drake R, Vogl W, Mitchell A: Gray's Anatomy for Students. Philadelphia: Elsevier, 2005, Fig. 2.21E–F)

Skull and Scapula

■ On an articulated skeleton, identify the following posteriorly (**Figure 1-5**):

- **Skull**
- **Occipital bone**
  - External occipital protuberance
  - Superior nuchal line
  - Inferior nuchal line
- **Temporal bone**
  - Mastoid process
- **Clavicle**
- **Scapula** — a large, flat triangular bone (also known as the shoulder blade)
  - Superior angle
  - Spine
  - Acromion
  - Medial margin
  - Lateral margin
  - Inferior angle

GAFS p 624   ACGA pp 15, 17, 193   NAHA Plates 8, 421

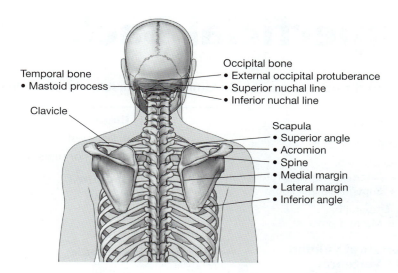

Figure 1-5 Posterior view of the skull and scapula. (Redrawn from Drake R, Vogl W, Mitchell A: Gray's Anatomy for Students. Philadelphia: Elsevier, 2005, Fig. 2.15)

Superficial Back

Lab 2

Prior to dissection, you should familiarize yourself with the following structures:

OSTEOLOGY

Skull
- Occipital b.
  - External occipital protuberance
  - Superior nuchal line
- Temporal b.
  - Mastoid process

Vertebral Column (33 Vertebrae)
- Cervical vertebrae (7)
- Thoracic vertebrae (12)
- Lumbar vertebrae (5)
- Sacrum (5 fused vertebrae)
- Coccyx (4 fused vertebrae)

Vertebral Features
- Spinous process
- Transverse processes
- Transverse foramina (cervical only)
- Laminae
- Pedicles
- Body
- Articular processes (superior and inferior)
- Vertebral foramen
- Intervertebral foramina (notches)
- Intervertebral disc

Ilium
- Iliac crest
- Posterior superior iliac spine

Sacrum

Coccyx

Ribs
- Head
- Tubercle
- Angle

Scapula
- Spine
- Acromion
- Lateral margin
- Medial margin
- Superior angle
- Inferior angle

Miscellaneous
- Triangle of auscultation
- Lumbar triangle
- Midaxillary line

MUSCLES

Superficial (Extrinsic) Back Muscles
- Trapezius m.
- Latissimus dorsi m. (thoracolumbar fascia)
- Rhomboid major m.
- Rhomboid minor m.
- Levator scapulae m.

Intermediate Back Muscles
- Serratus posterior superior m.
- Serratus posterior inferior m.

Deep (Intrinsic) Back Muscles
- Splenius capitis and cervicis mm.

VESSELS AND NERVES

Thyrocervical Trunk
- Transverse cervical a.
  - Superficial branch of transverse cervical a.
- Dorsal scapular (deep branch) a. and n.

Posterior Cutaneous Neurovascular Bundles
- Posterior rami of the spinal nn.
  - Posterior cutaneous nn. (medial and lateral branches)
- Posterior intercostal aa.
  - Posterior cutaneous aa. (medial and lateral branches)

Spinal Accessory N. (CN XI)

Lab 2 Dissection Overview

The purpose of this laboratory session is to learn the anatomy of the superficial back through dissection. You will do so through the following suggested sequence:

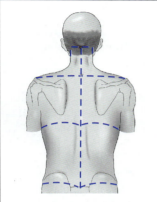

1. Identify surface anatomy and make skin incisions.

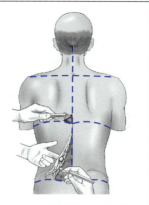

2. Reflect the skin covering the back.

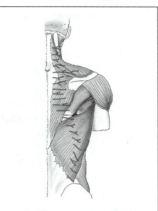

3. Observe cutaneous neurovascular bundles.

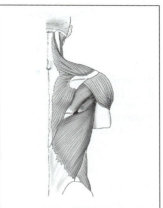

4. Identify the trapezius and latissimus dorsi muscles.

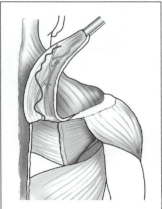

5. Cut and reflect the trapezius muscle. Identify the spinal accessory nerve and transverse cervical artery.

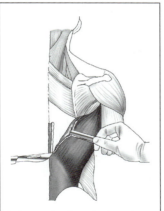

6. Cut and reflect the latissimus dorsi muscle.

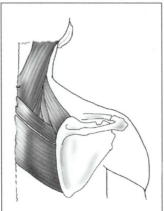

7. Identify the levator scapulae and rhomboid muscles.

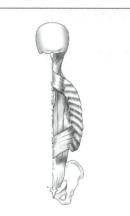

8. Identify the serratus posterior superior, serratus posterior inferior, splenius capitis, and splenius cervicis muscles.

Copyright © 2007, 2004 by Churchill Livingstone, an imprint of Elsevier Inc. All rights reserved.

Table 2-1 Superficial Back Muscles

Muscle	Proximal Attachment	Distal Attachment	Action	Innervation
Trapezius m.	Occipital bone, nuchal ligament, spinous processes of C7–T12 vertebrae	Lateral one third of the clavicle, acromion, spine of the scapula	Elevates, retracts, depresses, and rotates the scapula	Spinal accessory n. (CN IX) and cervical nn. (C3–C4)
Latissimus dorsi m.	Spinous processes of T7 vertebra to sacrum, thoracolumbar fascia, iliac crest, ribs 10–12	Intertubercular groove of the humerus	Extends, adducts, and medially rotates the humerus	Thoracodorsal n. (C6–C8)
Levator scapulae m.	Transverse processes of C1–C4 vertebrae	Upper portion of the medial border of the scapula	Elevates and downward rotates the scapula	Cervical nn. (C3–C4) and dorsal scapular n. (C5)
Rhomboid major m.	Spinous processes of T2–T5 vertebrae	Medial margin of the scapula	Retract and elevate the scapula	Dorsal scapular n. (C4–C5)
Rhomboid minor m.	Nuchal ligament, spinous processes of C7–T1 vertebrae			
Serratus posterior superior m.	C7–T3 vertebrae	Ribs 2–5	Elevates the ribs	Anterior rami of T2–T5 thoracic nn.
Serratus posterior inferior m.	T11–L3 vertebrae	Ribs 9–12	Depresses the ribs	Anterior rami of T9–T12 thoracic nn.

Orientation and Surface Anatomy

■ Place the cadaver prone (face down)

■ Locate the following structures **(Figure 2-1)**. On thin bodies, these structures will appear as projections; on heavier bodies, the structures will need to be palpated:

- **External occipital protuberance**
- **Spinous process of C7 (vertebra prominens)**
- **Acromion of the scapula**
- **Spine of the scapula**
- **Medial margin of the scapula**
- **Superior angle of the scapula**
- **Inferior angle of the scapula**
- **Midaxillary line** — imaginary line coursing vertically from the apex of the axilla along the lateral surface of the trunk
- **Iliac crests**
- **Sacrum**

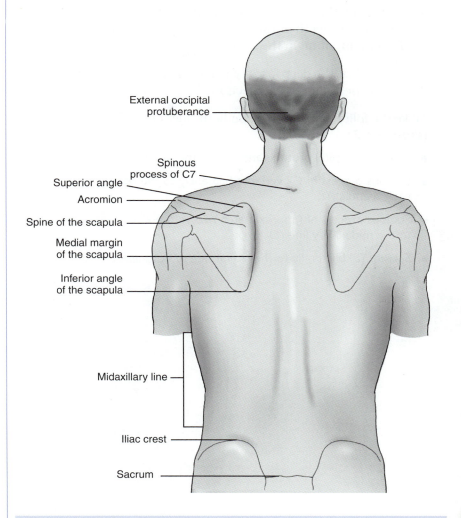

GAFS pp 89–92   ACGA pp 187, 299, 324   NAHA Plate 152

Figure 2-1   Surface anatomy of the back

Skin — Incisions

- The incisions should pass through the skin and superficial fascia, leaving the deep fascia and underlying muscle untouched; the depth of the incision will vary depending on the amount of fat in the superficial fascia

- The "plane" of the deep fascia will most likely be discovered during the next step, skin reflection

- Make the following incisions, on both sides of the back **(Figure 2-2)**:
  - External occipital protuberance *(A)* to the sacrum *(B)*
  - Spinous process of C7 vertebra bilaterally to the acromion of each scapula *(D)*
  - Spinous process of (approximately) T6 vertebra *(C)* bilaterally to the midaxillary line *(E)*
  - Sacrum *(B)* bilaterally to the lateral side of both iliac crests *(F)*

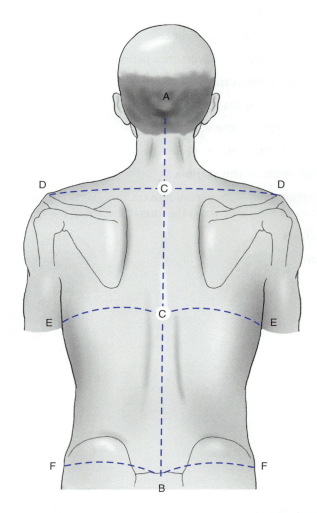

Figure 2-2 Skin incisions of the back

Skin — Reflection

- To reflect the skin of the back **(Figure 2-3)**:
    - Grasp a corner of skin, using a hemostat or forceps (as shown in *I*)
    - Keep pulling up while using a scalpel to cut (reflect) the skin and superficial fascia from the underlying deep fascia and muscles
    - Once enough skin is reflected, use a scalpel to cut a "button-hole" through the skin; place a finger in the "button-hole" and pull up (as shown in *II*); this technique may be more effective than retracting with forceps
    - Reflect the skin and superficial fascia laterally from both sides of the back
        - Do not remove the skin; leave the flaps attached laterally to the body and replace them over the dissected areas when you are finished dissecting to prevent drying
    - Look for neurovascular bundles that course between the deep fascia of the musculature and the superficial fascia being reflected

- As you reflect the superior flap, look for muscle fibers of the trapezius m., *cut no deeper*

- As you reflect the lower flap, look for the change to thoracodorsal fascia (broad, flat, shiny tendon) of the latissimus dorsi m., *cut no deeper*

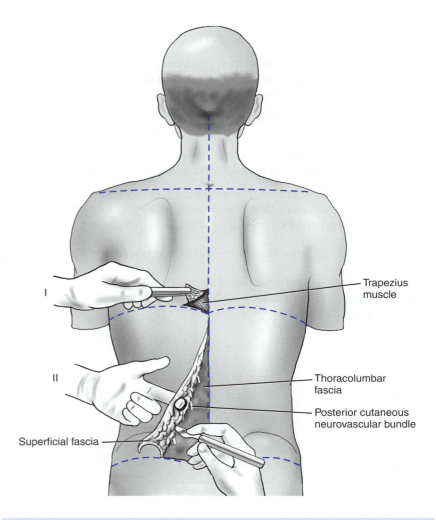

Figure 2-3 Skin reflection of the back

Nerves and Vessels of the Superficial Back

- Identify the following **(Figure 2-4)**:

  - **Posterior cutaneous neurovascular bundles** — pass segmentally through fovea (small holes) in the deep fascia to enter the superficial fascia and skin

    - Located near **spinous processes** of the **cervical** and upper **thoracic** vertebrae

    - In the lower **thoracic** and **lumbar** regions, the bundles are located about three finger widths lateral to the midline

    - *Note:* While attempting to locate these bundles, choose only a small area of the back; you do not need to locate every segmental cutaneous neurovascular bundle

- The posterior cutaneous nn. originate from **posterior rami**

- The posterior cutaneous aa. and vv. originate from **intercostal** and **lumbar vessels** (veins will often have a dark color)

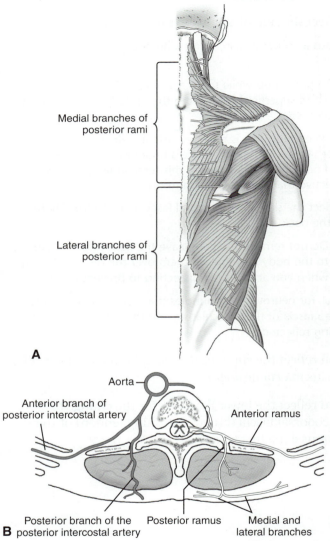

Figure 2-4 Posterior cutaneous neurovascular bundles. **A,** Superficial view of the back, illustrating posterior cutaneous neurovascular bundles. **B,** Cross-sectional view of the posterior cutaneous neurovascular bundles

Superficial (Extrinsic) Back Muscles

- Remove the remaining superficial fascia by grasping the fascia with hemostats and using a scalpel to cut the fascia away from the deeper, underlying muscle to identify the following **(Figure 2-5)**:

  - **Trapezius m.** — identify its attachments to the base of the skull, nuchal ligament, spines of C7–T12 vertebrae, spines of both scapulae, and both acromial processes
    - Observe superior, medial, and inferior divisions of the trapezius m. (respective striations course in different directions)
  - **Latissimus dorsi m.** — identify its attachments from T7 vertebra to the sacrum via the thoracolumbar fascia (the muscle inserts laterally in the intertubercular groove of the humerus; seen later)
  - **Thoracolumbar fascia** — a thick layer of the deep fascia that is made thick by the fused aponeuroses of several muscles; attaches along the spinous processes from T7 vertebra to the sacrum
  - **Triangle of auscultation** — bounded by the medial margin of the scapula and by the trapezius and latissimus dorsi mm.
  - **Lumbar triangle** — bounded by the external oblique m., latissimus dorsi m., and iliac crest

- *Note:* Superficial back muscles are located on the back but act on the upper limbs and will therefore be studied further in the upper limb laboratory sessions

GAFS pp 47–51   ACGA pp 188, 325   NAHA Plates 174, 424

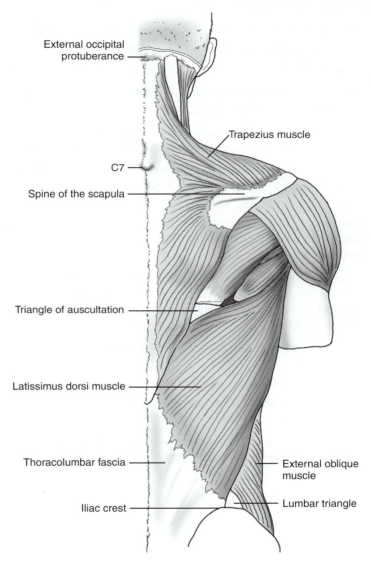

Figure 2-5 Superficial muscles of the back

Trapezius Muscle

- Reflect the trapezius m. in the following manner to allow access to the deeper structures and to preserve its nerve and blood supply:

- To dissect the trapezius m., follow these procedures for both sides of the back **(Figure 2-6)**:
  - Grasp the most inferior attachment of the trapezius m. (spinous process of T12 vertebra) with a hemostat or forceps
  - Free the deep surface of the trapezius m. from the underlying muscles, using a scalpel and your fingers
  - Insert your fingers deep to the free lateral and inferior border of the trapezius m.; you may feel the fat and loose connective tissue separating the trapezius m. from other, deeper musculature
  - Using a scalpel, cut the medial attachment of the trapezius m. from its origin (T12) in a superior direction from all vertebral spines as close to the spinous processes as possible (T12 toward C1)
  - You may need to loosen the muscle with your fingers as you proceed
  - As you approach T1 vertebra, cut the trapezius mm. from the spine of each scapula. (*Note:* Do *not* cut the rhomboid mm. deep to the trapezius mm)
  - With the muscle attached only to the clavicle, reflect the trapezius m. laterally toward the shoulder

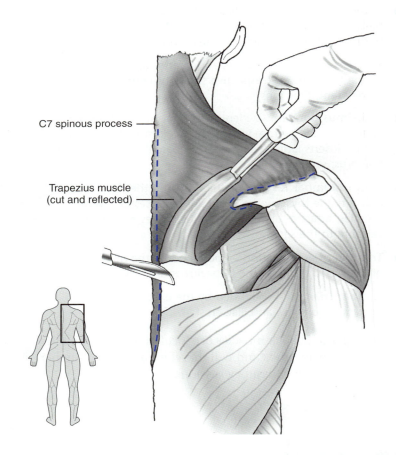

Figure 2-6 Reflection of the trapezius muscle

Trapezius Muscle—cont'd

■ Study the deep surface of the reflected trapezius m. to identify the following nerve and vessels running in parallel within the connective tissue **(Figure 2-7)**:

- **Spinal accessory nerve (cranial nerve XI, CN XI)** — follow the nerve inferiorly to observe the numerous branches into the musculature of the trapezius m.; the nerve exits the skull via the jugular foramen, but do not attempt to follow the nerve back into this region. This area will be dissected in a further laboratory session

- **Superficial branch of the transverse cervical a.** — enters the deep superior surface of the trapezius m.

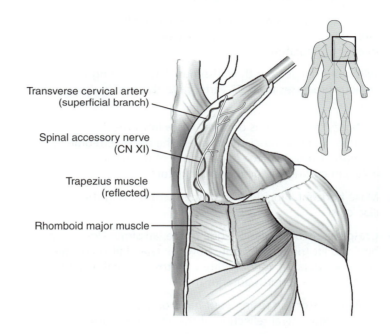

Figure 2-7   Spinal accessory nerve and transverse cervical artery

Latissimus Dorsi Muscle

- To dissect the latissimus dorsi m., follow these procedures for both sides of the body **(Figure 2-8)**:
  - Insert your fingers deep to the superior border of the latissimus dorsi m. and gently lift away from the deeper musculature
  - With your scalpel, cut the latissimus dorsi m. along the spinous processes from T7 vertebra to the sacrum (top of the iliac crest)
    - *Note:* The latissimus dorsi m. arises from the thoracolumbar fascia that covers the deep vertebral musculature (erector spinae mm.) of the back, so try to avoid cutting the deeper musculature
  - Make horizontal incisions from the sacrum along the iliac crest
  - Grasp the medial, inferior edge of the latissimus dorsi m. and begin to lift the muscle; note how the lateral fibers of the latissimus dorsi m. interdigitate with the external oblique m. inferior to the serratus anterior m.
    - Blunt dissection (using your hand or a blunt instrument) will allow lateral reflection of the latissimus dorsi m.
- The thoracodorsal n., a., and v. supplying the latissimus dorsi m. are located on the deep superior surface of the latissimus dorsi m. and will be studied in a further laboratory session

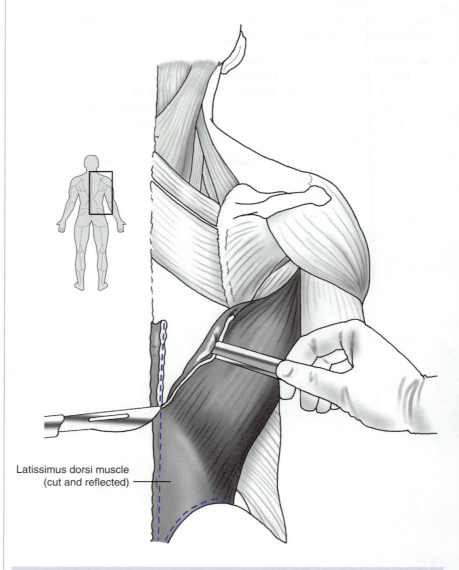

Figure 2-8 Reflection of the latissimus dorsi muscle

Rhomboid and Levator Scapulae Muscles

- Follow these procedures on both sides of the back to dissect the remaining superficial back muscles (**Figures 2-9** and **2-10**):

  - **Rhomboid major and minor mm.** — observe muscle attachments along the spines of C7–T5 vertebrae and the medial margin of the scapula; the two muscles may be fused and appear as one

    - Place your fingers deep to the rhomboid major and minor mm.

    - Dissect, using your scalpel, the muscles' medial attachments from the spinous processes of C7–T5 and reflect the rhomboid mm. laterally (leave them attached to the scapula)

- Identify the following by bluntly dissecting the fat on the deep surface of the rhomboid mm.:

  - **Dorsal scapular n. (C5)** — branches from the C5 root of the brachial plexus

  - **Dorsal scapular (deep branch of the transverse cervical) a.** — exits the posterior triangle of the neck deep to the levator scapulae m. and enters the deep surface of the rhomboid musculature

  - **Levator scapulae m.** — do not dissect the levator scapulae m. at this time; however, observe its attachments on the superior angle of the scapula and transverse processes of C1–C4 vertebrae

GAFS pp 51–53   ACGA pp 189, 191–192   NAHA Plates 174, 424

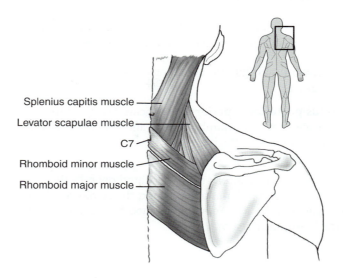

Figure 2-9   Levator scapulae and rhomboid muscles

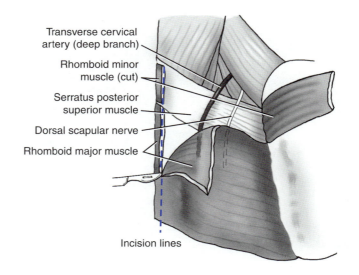

Figure 2-10   Reflection of the rhomboid muscles

Intermediate Back Muscles

- After the superficial back muscles are dissected and reflected, the intermediate back muscles are readily accessible

- Identify the following thin, accessory respiratory muscles **(Figure 2-11)**:

  - **Serratus posterior superior m.** — located deep to the levator scapulae and rhomboid mm. and superficial to the splenius capitis m.; attaches along the spines of C7–T3 vertebrae and the ribs

  - **Serratus posterior inferior m.** — located deep to the latissimus dorsi m. and attached along the spines of T11–L3 vertebrae and the ribs; may be attached to the deep surface of the latissimus dorsi m.

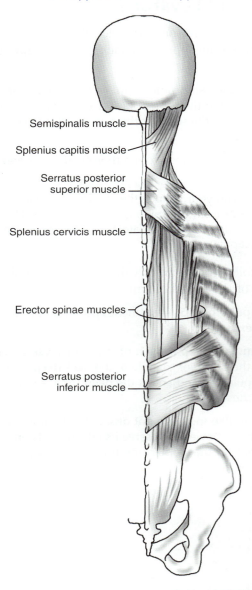

Figure 2-11 Serratus posterior muscles. (*Note:* The picture illustrates continuity of muscles into the neck; at this time your cadaver is not dissected above the C7 vertebra)

Lab 3

Deep Back, Vertebral Column, and Suboccipital Region

Prior to dissection, you should familiarize yourself with the following structures:

DEEP (INTRINSIC) BACK MUSCLES
- Splenius capitis m.
- Splenius cervicis m.
- Erector spinae group
  - Iliocostalis m.
  - Longissimus m.
  - Spinalis m.
- Transversospinalis group
  - Semispinalis m.
  - Multifidus m.
  - Rotatores mm.
- Intertransversarii mm.
- Interspinales mm.
- Levatores costarum mm.

SUBOCCIPITAL REGION
- Superior and inferior nuchal lines
- Nuchal ligament and fascia

Muscles
- Splenius capitis m.
- Splenius cervicis m.
- Longissimus capitis m.
- Semispinalis capitis m.
- Suboccipital mm.
  - Rectus capitis posterior major m.
  - Rectus capitis posterior minor m.
  - Obliquus capitis superior m.
  - Obliquus capitis inferior m.

Vessels and Nerves
- Occipital a.
- Vertebral a.
- Suboccipital n. (posterior ramus of C1)
- Greater occipital n. (posterior ramus of C2)
- Posterior ramus of C3

SUBOCCIPITAL TRIANGLE

Borders
- Rectus capitis posterior major m.
- Obliquus capitis superior m.
- Obliquus capitis inferior m.

Contents
- Vertebral a.
- Suboccipital n. (posterior ramus of C1)

Lab 3 Dissection Overview

The purpose of this laboratory session is to learn the anatomy of the deep aspect of the back through dissection. You will do so through the following suggested sequence:

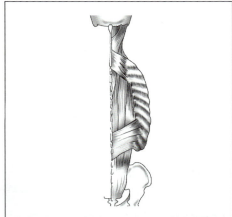

1. Identify the erector spinae musculature.

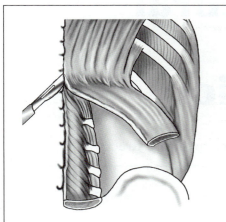

2. Cut the inferior attachments of the erector spinae muscles and reflect.

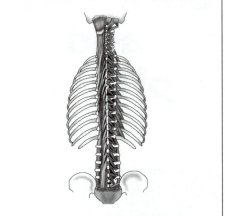

3. Identify the transversospinalis musculature, deep to the erector spinae muscles.

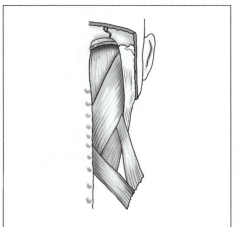

4. Make incisions in the splenius capitis and semispinalis muscles to reveal the suboccipital muscles.

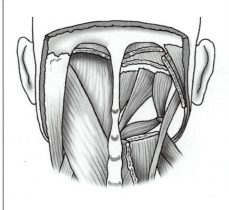

5. Identify the suboccipital musculature.

Table 3-1 Deep Back Muscles

Muscle	Proximal Attachment	Distal Attachment	Action	Innervation
Splenius capitis m.	Nuchal ligament, spinous processes of C7–T4 vertebrae	Mastoid process of the temporal bone and occipital bone	Unilateral: rotate head and neck to one side Bilateral: extend the head and neck	Posterior rami of the middle and lower cervical spinal nn.
Splenius cervicis m.	Spinous processes of T3–T6 vertebrae	Transverse processes of C2–C3 vertebrae		
Erector spinae group — series of muscles that extends from the sacrum to the skull				
• Iliocostalis m.			Unilateral: laterally flex vertebral column Bilateral: extend vertebral column	Segmentally innervated by posterior rami of spinal nn.
• Iliocostalis lumborum	Sacrum, spinous processes of lumbar and T11–T12 vertebrae, and iliac crest	Thoracolumbar fascia and ribs 7–12		
• Iliocostalis thoracis	Angles of ribs 7–12	Ribs 1–6 and transverse process of C7 vertebra		
• Iliocostalis cervicis	Angles of ribs 3–6	Transverse processes of C4–C6 vertebrae		
• Longissimus m.				
• Longissimus thoracis	Thoracodorsal fascia, transverse processes of lumbar vertebrae	Transverse processes of thoracic vertebrae and lower 9 or 10 ribs		
• Longissimus cervicis	Transverse processes of T1–T5 vertebrae	Transverse processes of C2–C6 vertebrae		
• Longissimus capitis	Transverse processes of T1–T5 vertebrae and articular processes of C3–C7 vertebrae	Mastoid process of the temporal bone		
• Spinalis m.				
• Spinalis thoracis	Spinous processes of T11–L2 vertebrae	Spinous processes of T1–T8 vertebrae (varies)		
• Spinalis cervicis	Nuchal ligament and spinous process of C7 vertebra	Spinous process of C2 vertebra (axis)		

Continued

Table 3-1 Deep Back Muscles—cont'd

Muscle	Proximal Attachment	Distal Attachment	Action	Innervation
Transversospinalis group				
Semispinalis m.				
• Semispinalis thoracis	Transverse processes of T6–T10 vertebrae	Spinous processes of C6–T4 vertebrae	Extend the cervical and thoracic regions of the vertebral column and rotate the vertebral column contralaterally	Segmentally innervated by posterior rami of spinal nn.
• Semispinalis cervicis	Transverse processes of T1–T6 vertebrae	Spinous processes of C2–C5 vertebrae		
• Semispinalis capitis	Transverse processes of C7–T6 vertebrae	Between the superior and inferior nuchal lines of the occipital bone	Extends the head, and turns the face toward the opposite side	
Multifidus m.	Sacrum, origin of erector spinae m., posterior superior iliac spine, lumbar vertebrae, thoracic vertebrae, and C4–C7 vertebrae	Spinous processes of lumbar, thoracic, and cervical vertebrae to C2	Extend the vertebral column and rotate the vertebral column contralaterally	
Rotatores mm.	Transverse processes of C2 vertebra to the sacrum	Lamina immediately above vertebra of origin		
Interspinalis mm.	Short paired muscles attached to the spinous processes of continuous vertebrae, one on each side of the interspinous ligament		Aid in extension and rotation of the vertebral column	
Intertransversarii mm.	Small muscles between the transverse processes of contiguous vertebrae		Aid in lateral flexion of the vertebral column; acting bilaterally, stabilize the vertebral column	Posterior rami of spinal nn.
Levatores costarum mm.	Tips of transverse processes of C7–T11 vertebrae	The rib inferior to the vertebral origin, near the tubercle	Elevate the ribs	Posterior rami of C8–T11 spinal nn.

Table 3-1 Deep Back Muscles—cont'd

Muscle	Proximal Attachment	Distal Attachment	Action	Innervation
Suboccipital group of back muscle				
Rectus capitis posterior major m.	Spinous process of C2 (axis) vertebra	Lateral portion of the occipital bone, below the inferior nuchal line	Extends and rotates the head	Posterior ramus of C1 (suboccipital n.)
Rectus capitis posterior minor m.	Posterior tubercle of C1 (atlas) vertebra	Occipital bone below the medial portion of the inferior nuchal line	Extends the head	
Obliquus capitis superior m.	Transverse process of C1 (atlas) vertebra	Occipital bone between the superior and inferior nuchal lines	Extends the head	
Obliquus capitis inferior m.	Spine of C2 (axis) vertebra	Transverse process of C1 (atlas) vertebra	Rotates the head	

Deep (Intrinsic) Back Muscles

- If not already done, cut the thin aponeuroses of both the serratus posterior superior and inferior mm. along their vertebral attachments; reflect both muscles laterally to better reveal the deep back muscles

- The deep muscles of the back include the splenius capitis, splenius cervicis, erector spinae, and transversospinalis musculature; deep to the semispinalis capitis m. are the suboccipital mm.

- Identify the following deep back muscles on both sides of the cadaver **(Figure 3-1)**:

  - **Splenius capitis m.** — superficial to the splenius cervicis m.; attaches along the vertebral column and inserts superiorly into the occipital bone and mastoid process

  - **Splenius cervicis m.** — deep to the splenius capitis m.; attaches along the vertebral column and inserts superiorly into the transverse processes of the upper cervical vertebrae

  - **Erector spinae musculature** — bilateral muscle group formed by long, vertical running muscle bundles along each side of the vertebral column; identify three columns of muscle within the erector spinae group from lateral to medial:

    - **Iliocostalis m.** — most lateral of the erector spinae group; arises from the iliac crest and inserts superiorly into the ribs, hence the name; consists of three parts:

      - **Iliocostalis lumborum** — attaches to the iliac crest and lower six ribs
      - **Iliocostalis thoracis** — attaches to all of the ribs
      - **Iliocostalis cervicis** — attaches to the upper six ribs and transverse processes of lower cervical vertebrae

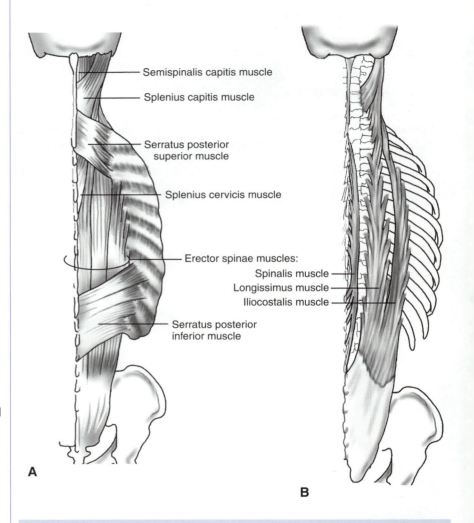

Figure 3-1 Deep back muscles. **A,** Superficial view. **B,** Deep view. (*Note:* The picture illustrates continuity of muscles into the neck; at this time your cadaver is not dissected above the C7 vertebra)

Deep (Intrinsic) Back Muscles—cont'd

- **Longissimus m.** — forms the middle column of the erector spinae group; attaches to the transverse processes along the thoracic and cervical vertebrae. Identify the thoracic (longissimus thoracis) and cervical (longissimus cervicis) portions; the most superior portion (longissimus capitis m.) inserts into the mastoid process of the skull

- **Spinalis m.** — forms the medial column of the erector spinae group; this thin muscle attaches to the spinous processes of the lumbar, thoracic, and cervical vertebrae, hence the name

■ To dissect the erector spinae mm., follow these procedures for both sides of the back **(Figure 3-2)**:

- Use a scalpel to cut the inferior attachment of the erector spinae group along the sacrum and iliac crest
- Continue using a scalpel to cut the erector spinae muscles from the lateral side of the spinous processes, starting at the sacrum and ending at the C7 vertebra

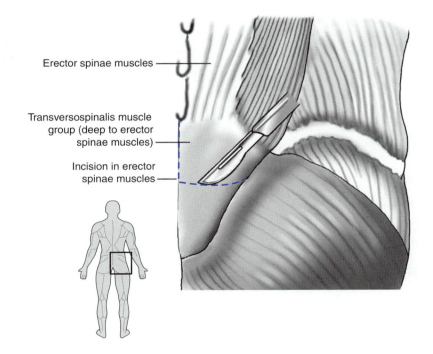

Figure 3-2 Dissection of the erector spinae muscles

Deep (Intrinsic) Back Muscles Continued

Deep (Intrinsic) Back Muscles—cont'd

- Reflect the erector spinae group laterally from the midline of the back; use your fingers to free the erector spinae group from the deeper transversospinalis group, from the sacrum to the C7 vertebra **(Figure 3-3)**

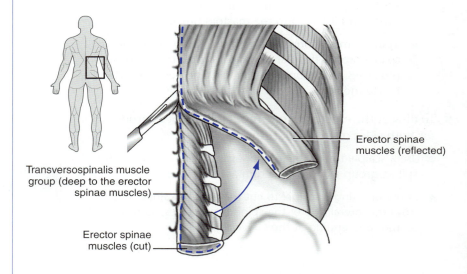

Figure 3-3 Reflection of the erector spinae muscles

Deep (Intrinsic) Back Muscles—cont'd

■ Identify the following **(Figure 3-4A** and **3-4B)**:

- **Transversospinalis group** — with the erector spinae mm. reflected, the space between the spinous and transverse processes will be exposed; observe the muscle fibers that arise from the transverse processes and ascend superiorly and medially to the spinous processes of superior vertebrae; use forceps to separate the following three muscles comprising the transversospinalis group:

  - **Semispinalis mm.** — muscle fibers span 4–6 vertebrae (most superficial)

  - **Multifidus mm.** — muscle fibers span 2–4 vertebrae (intermediate)

  - **Rotatores mm.** — muscle fibers span 1–2 vertebrae (deepest of the transversospinalis group)

  - *Note:* Observe that the muscle striations of the transversospinalis group course from a transverse process *below* to spinous processes *above* (hence the name)

- **Levatores costarum mm.** — between the transverse processes and ribs; observe that the muscle striations descend inferiorly and laterally

- **Intertransversarii mm.** — span adjacent transverse processes

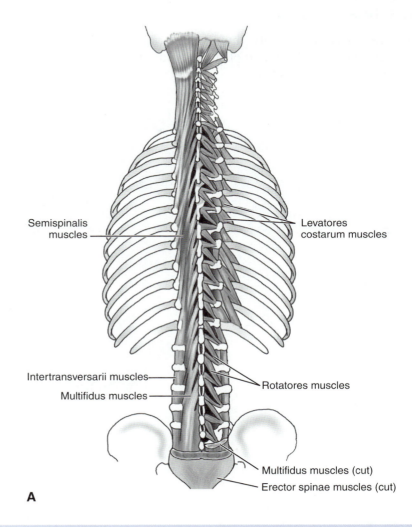

Figure 3-4 Transversospinalis muscles. **A,** Deep view of the back illustrating the transversospinalis muscles   *Continued*

Deep (Intrinsic) Back Muscles Continued

Deep (Intrinsic) Back Muscles—cont'd

- Figure 3-4B is a schematic that demonstrates the vertebral muscle fiber span of the individual transversospinalis mm.

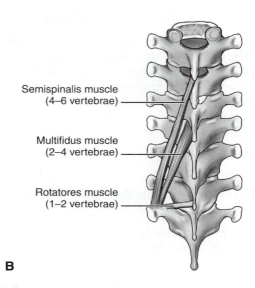

Figure 3-4, cont'd B, Schematic of the transversospinalis muscles. (*Note:* Picture illustrates continuity of muscles into the neck; at this time your cadaver is not dissected above the C7 vertebra)

Suboccipital Triangle Dissection (Right Side Only)

- Inclusion of this dissection will be indicated by your instructor
  - *Note:* Limit this dissection to the right side of the neck to avoid damage to the left posterior triangle of the neck (dissected later)

- Identify the following **(Figure 3-5)**:
  - **Trapezius m.** — attaches to the external occipital protuberance and along the nuchal ligament

- Dissect the following (see Figures 3-5 and 3-6):
  - **Greater occipital n.** — posterior ramus of C2 spinal n.; spend a few moments to find branches of the greater occipital n. and occipital a. in the nuchal fascia overlying the trapezius m.; sharp dissection will be necessary because the fascia in the neck is thick and tough
  - **Trapezius m.** — reflect the trapezius m. inferiorly and laterally by cutting the superior portion of the trapezius from the external occipital protuberance and along the spinous processes (nuchal ligament)
    - Leave the spinal accessory n. (CN IX) and the superficial branch of the transverse cervical a. attached to the deep surface of the trapezius m.

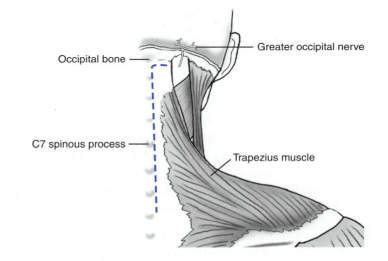

Figure 3-5 Trapezius muscle dissection

Suboccipital Triangle Dissection (Right Side Only) Continued

Suboccipital Triangle Dissection (Right Side Only)—cont'd

- Place a wood block under the superior part of the thorax to allow the neck to flex anteriorly and open the dissection field

- Identify the following **(Figure 3-6)**:
  - **Splenius capitis m.** — observe that the striations course superiorly and laterally at an angle between the vertebrae and mastoid process of the temporal bone
  - **Splenius cervicis m.** — deep to the splenius capitis m.
  - **Semispinalis capitis m.** — part of the transversospinalis group; deep to the splenius capitis m. and attached to the inferior nuchal line of the occipital bone

- To reveal the suboccipital region, use a scalpel to cut the splenius capitis and semispinalis mm. away from the occipital bone; because the muscles are bound tightly, try not to cut deeper than the splenius and semispinalis mm. to preserve deeper muscles; leave the splenius and semispinalis mm. attached to the cervical spinous processes

- Cut the following muscles from their superior attachments (stay close to the skull to spare the greater occipital n. and occipital a.):
  - **Splenius capitis m.** — cut from the mastoid process and superior nuchal line of the occipital bone
  - **Semispinalis capitis m.** — cut from the inferior nuchal line of the occipital bone

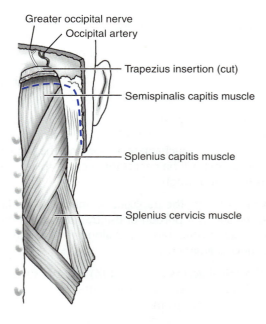

Figure 3-6 Intermediate dissection of the posterior region of the neck

Suboccipital Triangle Dissection (Right Side Only)—cont'd

- With the splenius capitis and semispinalis mm. reflected, the suboccipital region is revealed

- Identify the following muscles deep to the reflected semispinalis and splenius capitis mm. by carefully removing the adipose tissue obscuring the dissection field; watch for and preserve vessels and nerves coursing through the adipose tissue **(Figure 3-7)**:

  - **Rectus capitis posterior major m.** — courses from the spinous process of C2 vertebra to insert on the occipital bone, just below the inferior nuchal ligament

  - **Obliquus capitis superior m.** — courses between the transverse process of C1 vertebra and the occipital bone

  - **Obliquus capitis inferior m.** — larger of the two oblique muscles; courses from the spinous process of C2 vertebra to the transverse process of C1 vertebra

  - **Longissimus capitis m.** — look for its attachment to the mastoid process, lateral to the splenius capitis m.

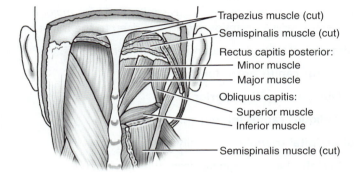

Figure 3-7 Suboccipital triangle muscles

Suboccipital Triangle Dissection (Right Side Only) Continued

Suboccipital Triangle Dissection (Right Side Only)—cont'd

■ Identify the following **(Figure 3-8)**:

- **Greater occipital n.** — posterior ramus of C2 spinal n.; exits the spinal cord between C1 and C2 vertebrae and emerges below the obliquus capitis inferior m. and crosses superficial to the suboccipital triangle in a superior direction (try not to cut this nerve)
- **Rectus capitis posterior minor m.** — cut and reflect the superior attachment of the rectus capitis posterior *major* m.; the rectus capitis posterior *minor* m. is deep to the major m.
- **Suboccipital triangle** — identify the borders:
  - **Rectus capitis posterior major m.**
  - **Obliquus capitis superior m.**
  - **Obliquus capitis inferior m.**
- **Suboccipital triangle** — identify the contents:
  - **Vertebral a.** — originates from the subclavian a. (seen later) and courses through the transverse foramina of the cervical vertebrae
    ◆ Courses horizontally in the groove on the superior surface of the lamina of C1 vertebra (atlas) in the suboccipital triangle
  - **Suboccipital n.** — posterior ramus of C1 spinal n.; courses superior to the C1 vertebra (atlas) to reach the muscles of the suboccipital triangle

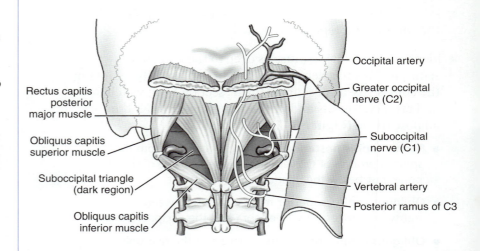

Figure 3-8 Suboccipital triangle borders and contents

Lab 4

Spinal Cord

Prior to dissection, you should familiarize yourself with the following structures:

MENINGES
- Dura mater
  - Epidural space
  - Subdural space
  - Dural sac
- Arachnoid mater
  - Subarachnoid space
- Pia mater
  - Denticulate ligaments
  - Filum terminale

SPINAL CORD
- Posterior median sulcus
- Cervical spinal enlargement
- Lumbar spinal enlargement
- Conus medullaris

SPINAL NERVES
- Anterior roots (rootlets)
- Posterior roots (rootlets)
  - Spinal (dorsal root) ganglion
- Anterior rami
- Posterior rami
- Cauda equina

VERTEBRAL LIGAMENTS
- Nuchal ligament
- Supraspinous ligament
- Interspinous ligament
- Ligamentum flavum
- Intertransverse ligament
- Posterior longitudinal ligament

Lab 4 Dissection Overview

The purpose of this laboratory session is to perform a laminectomy and learn the anatomy of the spinal cord through dissection. You will do so through the following suggested sequence:

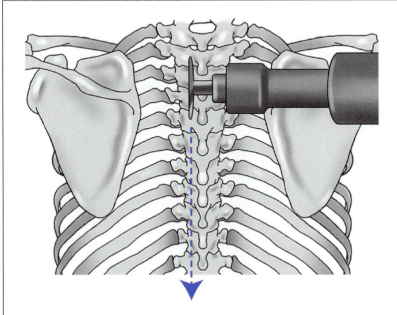

1. Study the vertebral ligaments and then bilaterally cut through the lamina of the vertebral column.

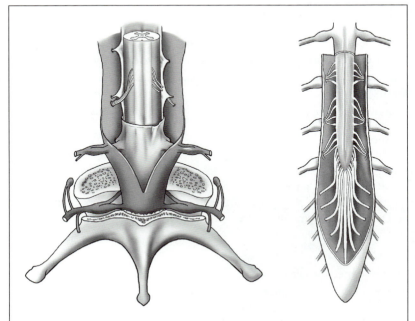

2. Remove the lamina to identify the anatomic parts of the spinal cord.

Ligaments of the Vertebrae

- To prepare for the laminectomy, you should have the vertebral lamina (area between the transverse and spinous processes) devoid of muscle tissue, from the C7 to L5 vertebrae

- Use a scalpel to *cut* and *scrape* the vertebral laminae clean of muscle tissue because the bone saw works well on bones, not on muscles

- This process will destroy the bulk of the transversospinalis group of muscles

- Identify the following ligaments **(Figure 4-1)**:

  - **Supraspinous ligaments** — span the superficial tips of the vertebral spines

  - **Interspinous ligaments** — span the spines of adjacent vertebrae

  - **Intertransverse ligaments** — span the transverse processes of adjacent vertebrae

GAFS pp 43–45   ACGA pp 296, 307   NAHA Plates 158–159

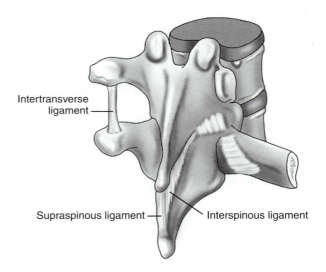

Figure 4-1   Vertebral ligaments

Laminectomy

- Check that the bone-saw switch is in the "off" position before the saw is plugged in; use care with the bone saw; keep your hands and fingers away from the blade

- Refer to **Figures 4-2** and **4-3** for demonstration of the angle of the saw blade

- Turn on the saw and cut into the lamina of C7 vertebra

- As the saw blade cuts through the lamina, you will feel the blade drop; stop cutting when you feel the "drop" to avoid cutting the underlying dura mater; continue this from C7 to the sacrum

  - Repeat for the other side of the vertebral column; it may be necessary to remove some vertebral spines to maintain a straight saw line

  - Use a scalpel to cut and/or a chisel to pry C7 away from C6 and L5 from the sacrum

  - Remove the cut portion of the vertebral column from the cadaver, freeing any remaining attachments with a mallet and chisel

    - Be careful around sharp edges of the remaining parts of the vertebrae

    - Use a mallet to hit (blunt) sharp bony edges

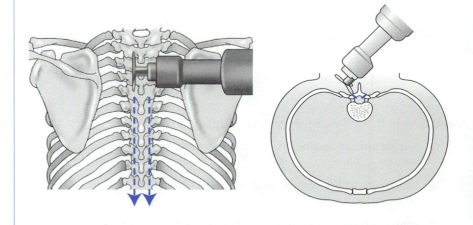

Figure 4-2 Laminectomy

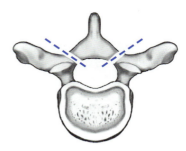

Figure 4-3 Angle of the saw blade (the *dotted lines* indicate the plane of the saw blade)

Inspection of the Removed Laminae

- Review the vertebral ligaments mentioned during this lab

- On the internal aspect of the removed laminae, observe the ligamentum flavum **(Figure 4-4)**; it is yellow because of elastic fibers

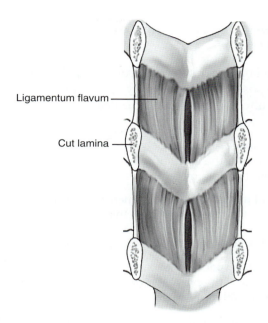

Figure 4-4 Internal view of the removed laminae

Spinal Canal Contents

- Identify the following (**Figures 4-5** and **4-6**):

  - **Epidural fat** — you may notice the vertebral venous plexus in the epidural fat
  - **Dura mater** — a sleeve of dense connective tissue inside the vertebral canal

- Use a scalpel or scissors to cut through the dura mater along its exposed length; carefully reflect and pin the dura mater laterally, trying to retain the deeply positioned arachnoid mater

  - **Subdural space** — region between the dura mater (externally) and the arachnoid mater (internally); use a probe to separate the dura mater from the arachnoid mater
  - **Arachnoid mater** — located immediately deep and loosely attached to the dura mater; very thin

- Cut through a region of the arachnoid mater

  - **Subarachnoid space** — space deep to the arachnoid mater (externally) and the pia mater (internally); cerebrospinal fluid is contained within this space
  - **Pia mater** — intimately covers the spinal cord and cannot be grossly distinguished, with the exception of the denticulate ligaments and filum terminale
  - **Denticulate ligaments** — small bilateral projections of the pia mater that are attached laterally to the surrounding dura mater; seen above the level of L1
  - **Anterior and posterior roots** — observe that the denticulate ligaments separate them
    - Spinal (dorsal root) ganglia — a swelling along each posterior root, in or lateral to the intervertebral foramina

GAFS pp 20–21, 62–71   ACGA pp 297–298   NAHA Plates 170, 172–173

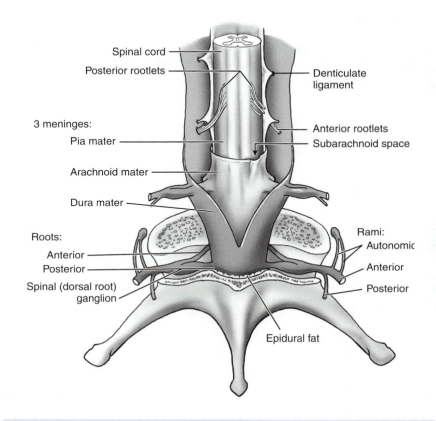

Figure 4-5   Spinal canal contents (posterior view)

Spinal Canal Contents—cont'd

- Identify the following (see Figures 4-5 and 4-6):

  - **Spinal nerves** — exit the spinal canal laterally to traverse the intervertebral foramina

  - **Spinal (dorsal root) ganglion** — a swelling along each posterior root, in or lateral to the intervertebral foramina

  - **Cervical spinal enlargement** — an enlargement of the spinal cord between vertebrae C3 and T2, housing nerve cell bodies for the upper limbs; only a portion of the cervical enlargement will be visible because the laminectomy stopped at the C7 vertebra

  - **Lumbar spinal enlargement** — an enlargement of the spinal cord between vertebrae T9 and T12, housing nerve cell bodies for the lower limbs

  - **Conus medullaris** — inferior region of the spinal cord where the spinal cord tapers into a cone (region of vertebra L2 in the adult)

  - **Cauda equina (horse's tail)** — the aggregate of nerve roots extending from the conus medullaris

  - **Filum terminale** — the pia mater that continues inferiorly from the conus medullaris to the coccyx (usually silver in color)

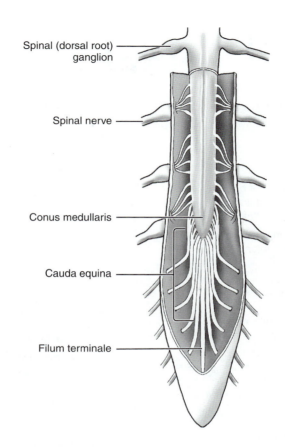

Figure 4-6 Spinal cord

Unit 1 Back Overview

At the end of Unit 1, you should be able to identify the following structures on cadavers, skeletons, and/or radiographs:

Osteology

- Occipital bone
  - External occipital protuberance
  - Superior nuchal line
  - Inferior nuchal line
- Vertebral column (33 vertebrae)
  - Cervical vertebrae (7)
    - Atlas (C1)
    - Axis (C2)
  - Thoracic vertebrae (12)
  - Lumbar vertebrae (5)
  - Sacrum (5 fused vertebrae)
  - Coccyx (4 fused vertebrae)
- Vertebral structures
  - Spinous and transverse processes
  - Laminae and pedicles
  - Vertebral bodies and intervertebral discs
  - Articular processes (superior and inferior)
  - Vertebral arch
  - Vertebral foramina
  - Intervertebral foramina (notches)
  - Transverse foramen (cervical vertebrae only)
- Ilium
  - Iliac crest
  - Posterior superior iliac spine
- Ribs
  - Head, neck, tubercle, angle, costal groove
- Scapula
  - Spine and acromion
  - Lateral and medial margins
  - Superior and inferior angles
- Clavicle

Muscles

- Superficial muscles of the back
  - Trapezius m.
  - Latissimus dorsi m.
  - Levator scapulae m.
  - Rhomboid major m.
  - Rhomboid minor m.
- Intermediate muscles of the back
  - Serratus posterior superior m.
  - Serratus posterior inferior m.
- Deep muscles of the back
  - Splenius capitis m.
  - Splenius cervicis m.
  - Erector spinae group
    - Iliocostalis m.
    - Longissimus m.
    - Spinalis m.
  - Transversospinalis group
    - Semispinalis m.
    - Multifidus m.
    - Rotatores m.
  - Intertransversarii mm.
- Interspinales mm.
- Levatores costarum mm.
- Suboccipital mm.
  - Rectus capitis posterior major m.
  - Rectus capitis posterior minor m.
  - Obliquus capitis superior m.
  - Obliquus capitis inferior m.

Vertebral Ligaments

- Nuchal ligament and nuchal fascia
- Supraspinous ligament
- Interspinous ligament
- Ligamentum flavum
- Intertransverse ligament
- Posterior longitudinal ligament

Miscellaneous

- Triangle of auscultation
- Lumbar triangle
- Thoracolumbar fascia
- Midaxillary line

Vessels (Arteries and Veins)

- Superficial and deep branches of the transverse cervical a.
- Intercostal vessels
  - Posterior and lateral cutaneous aa. and vv.

- Subclavian a.
  - Vertebral a.

Nerves

- Spinal accessory n. (CN XI)
- Dorsal ramus of C1
- Greater occipital n. (posterior ramus of C2)
- Dorsal ramus of C3
- Intercostal nerves
  - Posterior and lateral cutaneous nn.
- Dorsal scapular n. (C5)

Spinal Cord

- Meninges
  - Dura mater
    - Epidural and subdural spaces
    - Dural sac
  - Arachnoid mater
    - Subarachnoid space
  - Pia mater
    - Denticulate ligaments
    - Filum terminale

- Spinal cord
  - Posterior median sulcus
  - Cervical and lumbar spinal enlargements
  - Conus medullaris

Spinal Nerves

- Anterior and posterior roots (rootlets)
  - Spinal (dorsal root) ganglion
- Anterior and posterior rami
  - Cauda equina

Unit 2
Thorax

The purpose of this unit is to learn the anatomic structure of the thorax through dissection.

Lab 5 Osteology of the Thorax	49
Lab 6 Anterior Chest Wall and Breast	55
Lab 7 Thoracic Situs and Lungs	73
Lab 8 Heart	84
Lab 9 Mediastina	102
Unit 2 Thorax Overview	113

Osteology of the Thorax

Lab 5

Prior to dissection, you should familiarize yourself with the following structures:

OSTEOLOGY

Sternum
- Manubrium and jugular notch
- Sternal angle
- Body
- Xiphoid process

Clavicle

Sternoclavicular Joint

Acromioclavicular Joint

Scapula
- Acromion
- Coracoid process

Ribs
- Head
- Neck
- Costal groove
- Costal tubercle

Vertebral Structures
- Spinous process
- Transverse processes
- Laminae
- Pedicles
- Body
- Superior articular processes
- Inferior articular processes
- Vertebral foramina
- Intervertebral foramina (notches)
- Intervertebral disc
- Superior costal facets
- Inferior costal facets
- Transverse costal facets

Lab 5 Dissection Overview

The purpose of this laboratory session is to learn the osteology of the thoracic region. You will do so through the following suggested sequence:

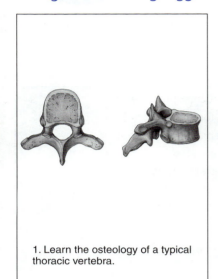

1. Learn the osteology of a typical thoracic vertebra.

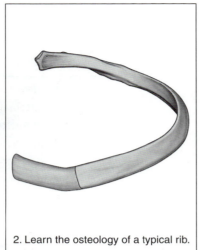

2. Learn the osteology of a typical rib.

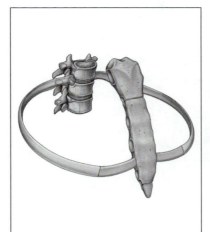

3. Identify the articulations between thoracic vertebrae, ribs, and the sternum.

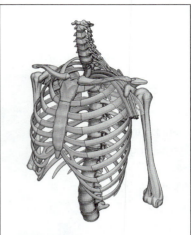

4. Identify the key bony landmarks of the thorax on an articulated skeleton.

Thoracic Vertebrae

- Using a thoracic vertebra, identify the following structures **(Figure 5-1)**:
  - **Vertebral body** — weightbearing part of the vertebra; linked to adjacent vertebral bodies by **intervertebral discs** and ligaments. The size of vertebral bodies increases inferiorly as the amount of weight supported increases
  - **Vertebral arch** — forms the lateral and posterior parts of the vertebral foramen; formed by the right and left pedicles and laminae
  - **Vertebral foramen** — the hole in the center of the vertebra through which the spinal cord courses; combination of all vertebral foramina form the **vertebral canal**
  - **Pedicles** — bony pillars that attach the vertebral arch to the vertebral body
  - **Laminae** — flat sheets of bone that extend from each pedicle to meet in the midline posteriorly
  - **Spinous process** — projects posteriorly and inferiorly from the junction of the two laminae; site for muscle and ligament attachment
  - **Transverse process** — extends posterolaterally from the junction of the pedicle and lamina on each side; a site for articulation with ribs in the thoracic region
  - **Superior and inferior articular processes** — bony projections that articulate with the inferior and superior articular processes, respectively, of adjacent vertebrae
  - **Intervertebral foramina** — formed on each side between adjacent parts of articulating vertebrae invertebral discs; allow structures such as spinal nerves and blood vessels to pass in and out of the vertebral canal
  - **Superior costal facet** — articulates with part of the head of its own rib
  - **Inferior costal facet** — articulates with part of the head of the rib below
  - **Transverse costal facet** — articulates with the tubercle of its own rib

GAFS pp 119–120   ACGA p 306   NAHA Plate 154

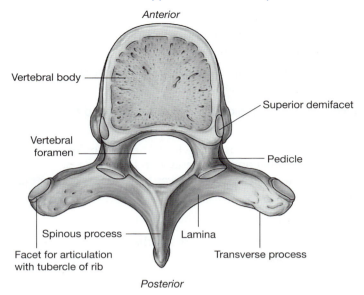

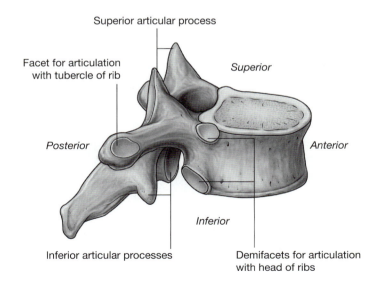

Figure 5-1 Typical thoracic vertebra. (From Drake R, Vogl W, Mitchell A: Gray's Anatomy for Students. Philadelphia: Elsevier, 2005, Fig. 3.18)

Ribs

- There are 12 pairs of ribs; identify the following features of a typical rib **(Figure 5-2)**:

  - **Head** — articulates with the superior and inferior costal facets of the thoracic vertebrae

  - **Neck** — short, flat region that separates the head from the tubercle

  - **Tubercle** — projects posteriorly from the junction of the neck with the shaft and articulates with the transverse process of a thoracic vertebra; serves as a site for ligamentous attachment

  - **Shaft** — long shaft of the rib that is thin and flat

  - **Angle** — region of the rib where the shaft bends forward, lateral to the tubercle

  - **Costal groove** — a longitudinal groove on the inferior margin of the internal surface of a rib; location for the intercostal neurovascular bundle

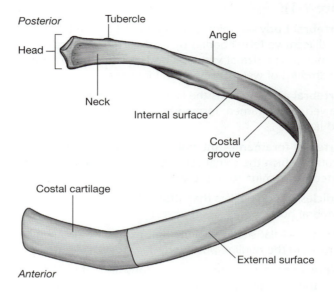

Figure 5-2 Typical rib. (From Drake R, Vogl W, Mitchell A: Gray's Anatomy for Students. Philadelphia: Elsevier, 2005, Fig. 3.21A)

Rib Articulations

- The 12 pairs of ribs articulate with the 12 thoracic vertebrae; observe the following articulations **(Figure 5-3)**:
  - Head of a rib with a superior costal facet
  - Head of a rib with an inferior costal facet
  - Tubercle of a rib with a transverse costal facet
  - Shaft of a rib with the costal cartilage
  - Costal cartilage with the sternum **(Figure 5-4)**
    - True ribs — observe ribs 1–7 articulating directly with the sternum through independent costal cartilages
    - False ribs — observe that ribs 8–10 do not articulate directly with the sternum and that ribs 11 and 12 (floating ribs) do not articulate with the sternum at all

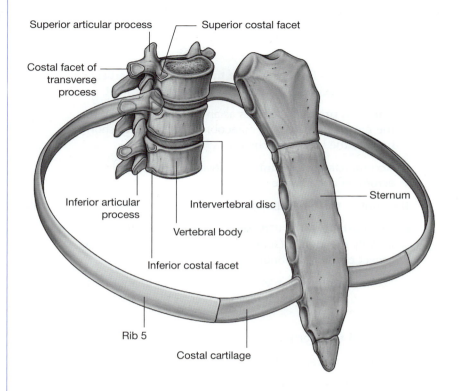

Figure 5-3 Joints between ribs and vertebrae. (From Drake R, Vogl W, Mitchell A: Gray's Anatomy for Students. Philadelphia: Elsevier, 2005, Fig. 3.2)

Thoracic Rib Cage

- Identify the following on an articulated skeleton (see Figure 5-4):

  - **Scapula** — a large, flat triangular bone (also known as the shoulder blade)
    - **Acromion** — forms the tip of the shoulder and articulates with the clavicle to form the acromioclavicular joint
    - **Coracoid process** — serves as an attachment point for the pectoralis minor m., coracobrachialis m., and short head of the biceps brachii m.
    - **Acromioclavicular joint** — synovial joint articulating the acromion and clavicle
  - **Sternum** — the breast bone
    - **Manubrium** — the wide superior segment of the sternum; identify the jugular (suprasternal) notch on the superior aspect of the manubrium
    - **Sternal angle** — marks the junction of the manubrium and the body of the sternum; serves as the marking point for rib 2
    - **Body of the sternum**
    - **Xiphoid process** — pointed, inferior part of the sternum
    - **Sternoclavicular joint** — synovial joint, articulation of the sternum and clavicles

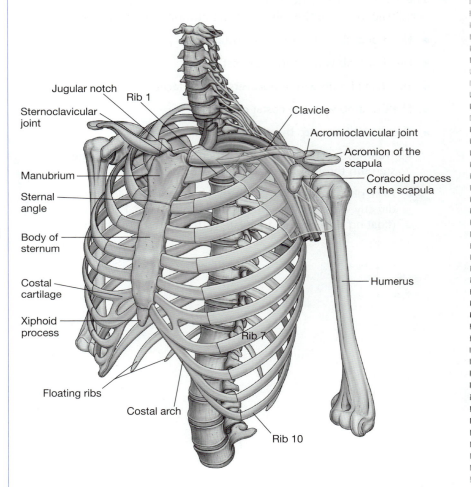

Figure 5-4 Bony landmarks of the thoracic rib cage. (Redrawn from Drake R, Vogl W, Mitchell A: Gray's Anatomy for Students. Philadelphia: Elsevier, 2005, Fig. 7.11)

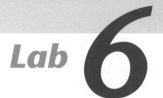

Anterior Chest Wall and Breast

Prior to dissection, you should familiarize yourself with the following structures:

OSTEOLOGY

Sternum
- Manubrium and jugular notch
- Sternal angle
- Body
- Xiphoid process

Clavicle

Sternoclavicular Joint

Scapula
- Acromion
- Coracoid process
- Ribs
  - Head, neck, costal groove, and tubercle

MUSCLES
- Pectoralis major m.
- Pectoralis minor m.
- Serratus anterior m.
- Subclavius m.
- Intercostal mm. (external, internal, innermost)
- Transversus thoracis m.

NERVES

Anterior Rami
- Intercostal nn.
  - Lateral and anterior cutaneous nn.
- Medial pectoral n.
- Lateral pectoral n.

ARTERIES AND VEINS

Thoracic Aorta
- Posterior intercostal vessels
  - Lateral cutaneous aa.

Subclavian Vessels
- Internal thoracic vessels
  - Anterior intercostal vessels
    - Anterior cutaneous aa.

Axillary A.
- Thoracoacromial trunk
  - Deltoid, pectoral, acromial, and clavicular branches
- Lateral thoracic vessels

Superficial Vein
- Cephalic v.

BREAST
- Nipple
- Areola
- Suspensory ligaments
- Lactiferous ducts
- Mammary gland
- Retromammary space

MISCELLANEOUS TERMS AND STRUCTURES
- Deltopectoral triangle
- Clavipectoral fascia
- Midaxillary line
- Parietal pleura
- Sternocostal joints
- Endothoracic fascia

Female cadaver — Turn to page 58 of the dissection guide.

Male cadaver — Turn to page 61 of the dissection guide.

Lab 6 Dissection Overview

The purpose of this laboratory session is to learn the anatomy of the anterior chest wall and the female breast through dissection. You will do so through the following suggested sequence:

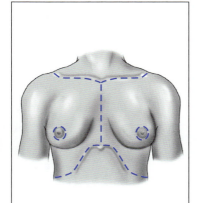

1. Identify surface anatomy, make skin incisions, and study the breast in female cadavers.

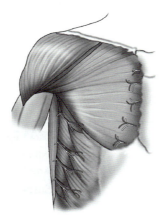

2. Identify cutaneous neurovascular bundles and the pectoralis major muscle.

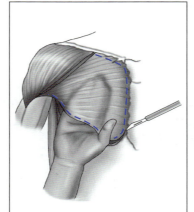

3. Dissect the pectoralis major muscle away from the clavicle, sternum, and rib cage.

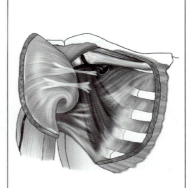

4. Identify the clavipectoral fascia, pectoralis minor, and subclavius muscles as well as the medial and lateral pectoral nerves.

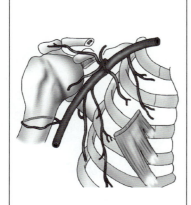

5. Identify branches of the thoracoacromial trunk deep to the pectoralis minor muscle.

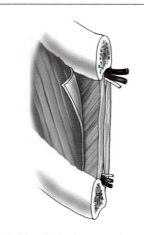

6. Identify the intercostal muscles and associated nerves and vessels.

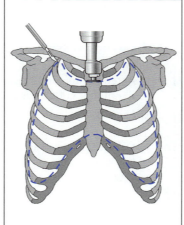

7. Using a scalpel and a bone saw, remove the anterior region of the rib cage.

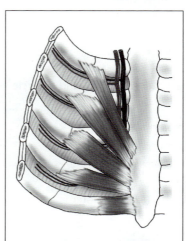

8. Identify the structures on the internal surface of the anterior region of the rib cage.

Table 6-1 Muscles of the Anterior Thoracic Wall

Muscle	Proximal Attachment	Distal Attachment	Action	Innervation
Pectoralis major m.	Medial half of the clavicle, anterior surface of the sternum, and superior six costal cartilages	Lateral lip of the intertubercular groove (humerus)	Adducts, medially rotates, and flexes the humerus at the shoulder joint	Medial (C8–T1) and lateral pectoral (C5–C7) nn.
Pectoralis minor m.	Ribs 3–5 (near their costal cartilages)	Coracoid process (scapula)	Depresses the tip of the shoulder; protracts the scapula	Medial pectoral n. (C8–T1)
Subclavius m.	Rib 1 (near its costal cartilage)	Middle one third of the clavicle (inferior surface)	Depresses and anchors the clavicle	Nerve to the subclavius (C5–C6)
External intercostal mm.	Inferior border of the ribs	Superior border of the ribs below	Move the ribs superiorly	Intercostal nn.
Internal intercostal mm.	Inferior border of the ribs	Superior border of the ribs below	Move the ribs inferiorly	Intercostal nn.
Innermost intercostal mm.	Inferior border of the ribs	Superior border of the ribs below	Act with internal intercostal mm.	Intercostal nn.
Transversus thoracis m.	Lower margins and internal surfaces of ribs 2–6	Inferior aspect of the deep surface of the body of the sternum, xiphoid process, and costal cartilages	Depresses the ribs	Intercostal nn.
Serratus anterior m.	Ribs 8–9	Medial border of the scapula	Protracts and rotates the scapula; keeps the medial border and inferior angle of the scapula opposed to the thoracic wall	Long thoracic n. (C5–C7)

Female Cadaver — Orientation and Incisions

- Turn the cadaver supine (face up)

- Locate the following (on thin bodies, these structures will appear as projections; on heavier bodies, the structures will need to be palpated) **(Figure 6-1)**:

  - **Jugular notch** — superior border of the manubrium; deepened by the medial ends of each clavicle
  - **Sternal body** — main portion, or body, of the sternum
  - **Xiphoid process** — the inferior, pointed tip of the sternum
  - **Sternoclavicular joint** — synovial joint; articulation of the sternum and each clavicle
  - **Acromion of the scapula** — forms the tip of the shoulder; articulates with the clavicle
  - **Acromioclavicular joint** — synovial joint; articulation of the acromion and clavicle
  - **Nipple** — cylindrical prominence centrally located in the areola, where the lactiferous ducts converge; lacks fat, hair, and sweat glands
  - **Areola** — circular pigmented area of skin surrounding the nipple

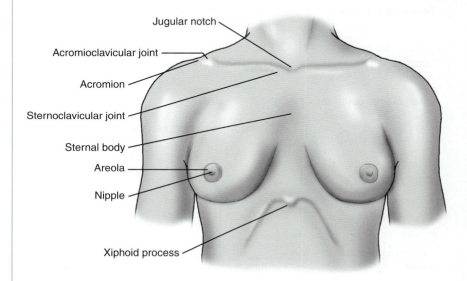

Figure 6-1 Anterior view of the anterior chest wall of the female

Female Cadaver — Orientation and Incisions—cont'd

- Make the following skin incisions bilaterally, using a scalpel **(Figure 6-2)**:
  - Circular incision around each areola
  - Jugular notch *(A)* to the xiphoid process *(B)*
  - Jugular notch *(A)* bilaterally along each clavicle to the lateral tip of the acromion *(C)*
  - Xiphoid process *(B)* bilaterally along the subcostal margin to the midaxillary line *(D)*

- Grasp a corner of skin on one side at point *A* or *B* (with a hemostat) to reflect the skin and superficial fascia laterally, along with the overlying breast; leave the skin flap attached laterally
  - Preserve the underlying pectoralis major mm.

- On the other side of either point *A* or *B*, reflect just the skin, leaving the breast and superficial fascia attached to the cadaver; leave the skin flap attached laterally

- *Note:* Look for neurovascular bundles that course between the deep fascia of the musculature and the superficial fascia

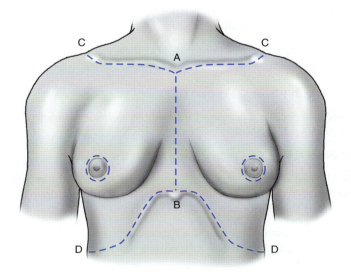

Figure 6-2 Skin incisions on the anterior chest wall of the female

Female Cadaver — Breast Dissection

GAFS pp 115–117   ACGA p 164   NAHA Plate 182

- The **breast** has no capsule and is located in the superficial fascia, superficial to the **pectoralis major m.**

- Make the following incision, with a scalpel, on the breast that is still attached to the thorax:
  - Cut sagittally through the nipple, and then continue the cut through the entire breast

- Identify the following **(Figure 6-3)**:
  - **Areola** — circularly arranged pigmented skin surrounding the nipple
  - **Nipple** — cylindrical prominence within the areola
  - **Lactiferous ducts** — probe the fatty tissue deep to the nipple and areola to locate some of the 15 to 20 ducts that drain milk from the glandular tissue to the nipple
  - **Mammary gland** — probe the subcutaneous fat lobules to look for glandular tissue (oftentimes unidentifiable in the elderly)
  - **Suspensory ligaments of the breast** — fibrous bands that connect the deep fascia to the skin
    - To better observe the suspensory ligaments, you may find it helpful to pull the nipple to put tension on (straighten) the ligaments
  - **Retromammary space** — loose connective tissue region between the deep fascia of the pectoralis major m. and the breast; insert your fingers into this space; the normal breast glides over the retromammary space

- To continue the dissection, please turn to page 63

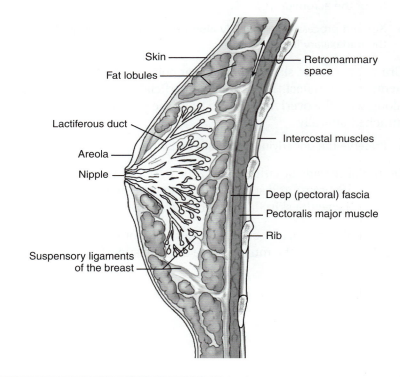

Figure 6-3   Sagittal section of the female breast

Male Cadaver — Orientation and Incisions

- Turn the cadaver supine (face up)

- Locate the following (on thin bodies, these structures will appear as projections; on heavier bodies, the structures will need to be palpated) **(Figure 6-4)**:
  - **Jugular notch** — superior border of the manubrium; deepened by the medial ends of each clavicle
  - **Sternal body** — main portion, or body, of the sternum (breast bone)
  - **Xiphoid process** — the inferior, pointed tip of the sternum
  - **Sternoclavicular joint** — synovial joint; articulation of the sternum and each clavicle
  - **Acromion of the scapula** — forms the tip of the shoulder and articulates with the clavicle
  - **Acromioclavicular joint** — synovial joint; articulation of the acromion and clavicle
  - **Nipple** — cylindrical prominence centrally located in the areola; lacks fat, hair, and sweat glands
  - **Areola** — circular pigmented area of skin surrounding the nipple

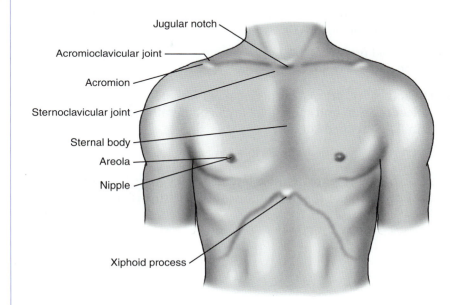

Figure 6-4 Anterior view of the anterior chest wall of the male

Male Cadaver — Orientation and Incisions Continued

Male Cadaver — Orientation and Incisions—cont'd

- Make the following skin incisions, using a scalpel **(Figure 6-5)**:
  - Jugular notch *(A)* to the xiphoid process *(B)*
  - Jugular notch *(A)* bilaterally along each clavicle to the lateral tip of the acromion *(C)*
  - Xiphoid process *(B)* bilaterally along the subcostal margin to the midaxillary line *(D)*

- On both sides, grasp a corner of skin (with a hemostat) and reflect the skin and superficial fascia bilaterally; leave the skin flap attached laterally
  - Preserve the underlying pectoralis major m.

- *Note:* Look for neurovascular bundles that course between the deep fascia of the musculature and the superficial fascia

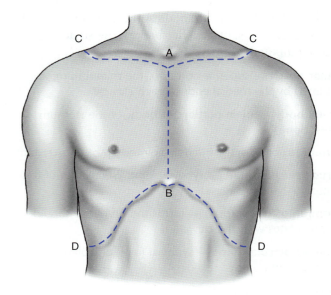

Figure 6-5 Skin incisions on the anterior chest wall of the male

Anterior Wall of the Thorax — Superficial Fascia (Female and Male)

- Use forceps to dissect and identify the following structures **(Figures 6-6** and **6-7)**:

  - **Anterior cutaneous neurovascular bundles** — branches of the **anterior intercostal neurovascular bundles**

    - Upper five anterior cutaneous neurovascular bundles emerge just lateral to the sternum, through slips in the pectoralis major m.

    - Lower six anterior cutaneous neurovascular bundles run inferiorly to the anterior abdominal wall (studied further in another laboratory session)

  - **Lateral cutaneous neurovascular bundles** — branches of the **posterior intercostal neurovascular bundles**

    - Emerge between slips of the serratus anterior m.

- *Note:* Look for cutaneous vv. (which are dark); when you find a cutaneous v., the corresponding a. and n. will accompany it

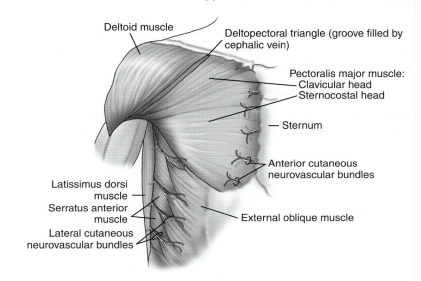

Figure 6-6 Muscles of the pectoral region

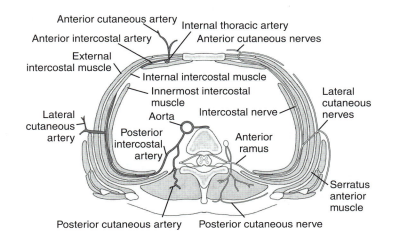

Figure 6-7 Cross-section through the thoracic wall; arteries shown on the cadaver's right side and nerves shown on the cadaver's left

Unit 2 · Lab 6   Anterior Chest Wall and Breast

Anterior Wall of the Thorax

- With a scalpel, remove the remaining superficial fascia and the breast (if you are dissecting a female cadaver) to clarify the borders of the pectoralis major m.

- Identify the following (**Figure 6-8**):
  - **Pectoralis major m.** — observe the clavicular and sternal heads, which are named for their bony attachments, respectively
  - **Deltoid m.** — from the supine perspective, you will see only the anterior half of the deltoid m. attached to the clavicle
  - **Deltopectoral triangle** — triangular space bordered by the clavicle, clavicular head of pectoralis major m., and anterior border of the deltoid m.
    - **Cephalic v.** — using blunt dissection or scissors, find the cephalic v. entering the deltopectoral triangle
      - The cephalic v. may be covered by muscle fibers from the deltoid or pectoralis major m.
      - Do not dissect the cephalic vein into the arm

GAFS pp 116–118, 643–644   ACGA pp 165, 215, 337   NAHA Plates 188, 424

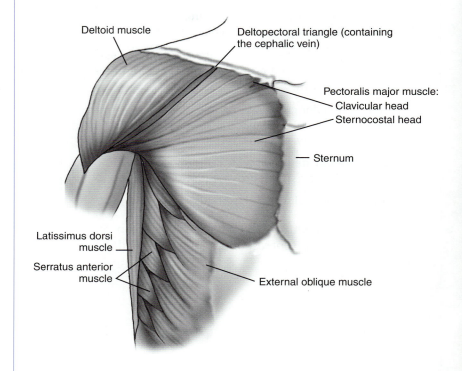

Figure 6-8   Anterior thoracic wall

Anterior Wall of the Thorax—cont'd

- Follow these instructions to dissect the pectoralis major m. from the thoracic wall **(Figure 6-9)**:
  - Gently insert your fingers deep to the inferior border of the pectoralis major m.
  - Slide your fingers back and forth along the inferior border of the pectoralis major m. to break the fascial connections between the muscle and rib cage; if necessary, use scissors or a scalpel to cut an opening in the deep fascia along the inferior border of the muscle
  - Using your scalpel, cut the pectoralis major m. along its sternal attachment *(A)* to its clavicular attachment *(B)*
  - As you detach the pectoralis major m. and reflect it laterally, look for neurovascular bundles entering the deep surface of the muscle
    - The neurovascular bundles contain the lateral pectoral n., medial pectoral n., and branches of the thoracoacromial a.
  - Repeat these dissection steps on the other pectoralis major m.

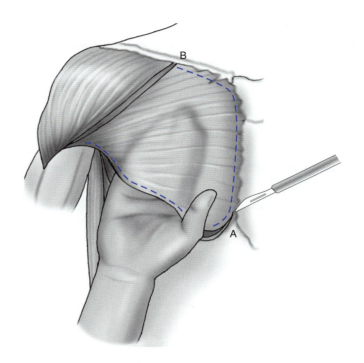

Figure 6-9 Incision to dissect the pectoralis major muscle

Anterior Wall of the Thorax — Deltopectoral Triangle

■ Identify the following (**Figures 6-10** and **6-11**):

- **Clavipectoral fascia** — deep to the pectoralis major m.; originates on the clavicle and envelops the subclavius and pectoralis minor mm.; extends between the two muscles as a single sheet

  - **Suspensory ligament of the axilla** — continuation of the clavipectoral fascia into the axillary region (do not dissect into the axilla)

- **Subclavius m.** — attached to the inferior surface of the clavicle and rib 1

- **Pectoralis minor m.** — attached from the coracoid process to ribs 3–5

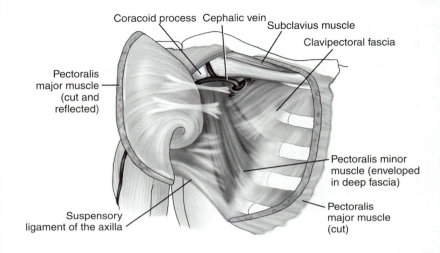

Figure 6-10 Clavipectoral fascia

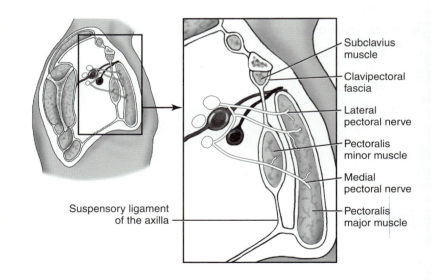

Figure 6-11 Parasagittal section through the axilla to demonstrate the clavipectoral fascia

Anterior Wall of the Thorax—Deltopectoral Triangle Contents

■ Dissect, using forceps, the clavipectoral fascia between the pectoralis minor and subclavius mm.; preserve the structures that pass through it:

- Cephalic v. (not shown in illustration)
- Thoracoacromial trunk
- Branches of the medial and lateral pectoral nn.

■ Identify the following structures by removing the fat between the clavicle and pectoralis minor m. **(Figures 6-12** and **6-13):**

- **Lateral pectoral n.** — originates from the lateral cord of the brachial plexus (not seen at this point); enters the superior deep surface of pectoralis major m., after passing through the clavipectoral fascia

- **Medial pectoral n.** — originates from the medial cord of the brachial plexus (not seen at this point) and passes through the pectoralis minor m. to enter the deep surface of the pectoralis major m.

  - Note: The names *medial* and *lateral* pectoral n. are derived from the cords of the brachial plexus from which each nerve arises, not their anatomic position, which is opposite to their names in the pectoral region

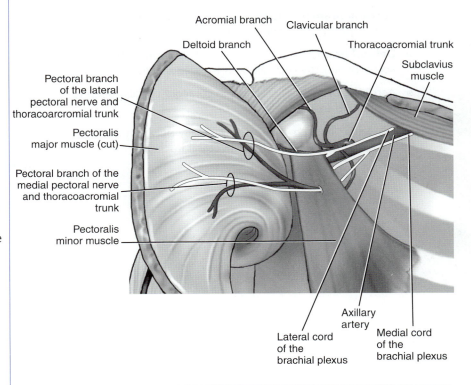

Figure 6-12 Branches of the thoracoacromial trunk

Anterior Wall of the Thorax — Deltopectoral Triangle Contents Continued

Anterior Wall of the Thorax — Deltopectoral Triangle Contents—cont'd

- **Cephalic v.** — follow the cephalic v. to its termination into the **axillary v.** (not shown in illustration)

- **Thoracoacromial trunk/artery** — originates from the axillary a.; courses deep to the pectoralis minor m.; the thoracoacromial trunk is short (2–4 mm) and divides into four branches, according to their respective fields of distribution; find the trunk by following one or two of its branches proximally:

  - **Pectoral branch** — follows the pectoral nn. into the deep surface of the pectoralis major m.

  - **Deltoid branch** — may arise from the acromial branch; accompanies the cephalic v. in the deltopectoral triangle

  - **Acromial branch** — crosses the coracoid process deep to the deltoid m.

  - **Clavicular branch** — ascends medially between the pectoralis major m. and clavipectoral fascia

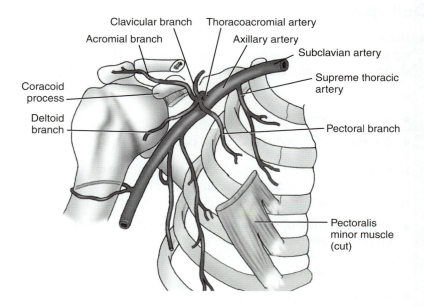

Figure 6-13 Branches of the thoracoacromial trunk artery

Intercostal Structures

- Dissect and identify the following structures in an intercostal space (the upper intercostal spaces are usually best to demonstrate the following details) **(Figure 6-14)**:

  - **External intercostal mm.** — superficial layer of intercostal mm.
    - The muscle fibers course in an oblique fashion (superior and lateral to inferior and medial)
    - The muscle belly fills the intercostal spaces posteriorly and laterally; anteriorly it is a membrane
    - Using a scalpel, carefully cut through the external intercostal mm. and their membrane and reflect them to expose the underlying internal intercostal mm.

  - **Internal intercostal mm.** — intermediate layer of intercostal mm.
    - The fibers course at a right angle and deep to the external intercostal mm.
    - The muscle belly fills the intercostal spaces anteriorly and laterally; posteriorly it is a membrane

  - **Innermost intercostal mm.** — deepest layer of intercostal mm.
    - The fibers follow the same course as the internal intercostal mm.
    - The muscle belly fills the intercostal spaces laterally; anteriorly and posteriorly it is a membrane
    - Oftentimes, the only delineation between the internal and innermost intercostal mm. is the presence of the intercostal v., a., and n.

  - **Intercostal v., a.,** and **n.** — use forceps to separate the internal intercostal mm. from the innermost intercostal mm. along the inferior border of each rib to identify the intercostal v., a., and n. (the v., a., and n. will be in the superior region of the intercostal space, deep to the costal groove)

  - **Collateral intercostal v., a.,** and **n.** — located along the superior border of each rib; you may not see them during this dissection because they are smaller than the intercostal v., a., and n.

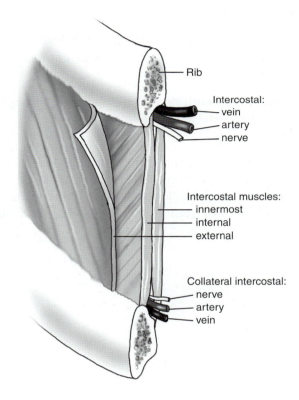

Figure 6-14 Intercostal structures

Removal of the Anterior Thoracic Wall

- Using a scalpel, cut a window through the intercostal mm., immediately lateral to the sternum, in the first intercostal space **(Figure 6-15)**:

- Identify and transect the **internal thoracic vessels**, which course from superior to inferior, about 1 cm lateral to the sternum

- Repeat this process on both sides of the sternum, through the first seven intercostal spaces, bilaterally

- Use forceps or your fingers to separate the internal thoracic vessels from the intercostal mm., in preparation for removing the anterior portion of the rib cage, without removing the internal thoracic vessels (this is not an easy task and most likely will result in breakage of the internal thoracic vessels)

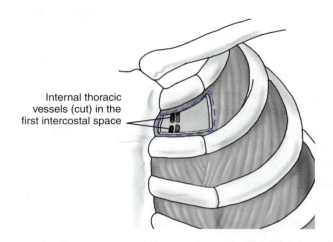

Figure 6-15 Intercostal incision

Removal of the Anterior Thoracic Wall—cont'd

- Use a scalpel to cut all structures down to the ribs along the perimeter of the anterior thoracic wall **(Figure 6-16)**; cut the structures as follows:
  - From the sternal angle
  - From the first intercostal space (inferior to rib 1), bilaterally
  - From the midaxillary line, bilaterally
  - Along the eighth or ninth intercostal space, from the midaxillary line to the sternum, bilaterally
  - From the sternoxiphoid joint

- *With a bone saw or rib cutter:* Cut through the sternum and ribs (remember to only cut through the bone, *not* deeper, to avoid cutting the internal thoracic vessels, parietal pleura, and the lungs); using your fingers, push the underlying parietal pleura away from the ribs as you progress

- *With a scalpel:* Cut through the intercostal muscles and other soft tissues

- Lift the rib cage away from the body
  - Use your fingers to open the space in the **endothoracic fascia** (a thin fascial layer between the internal intercostal mm./membrane and the **parietal pleura**) while separating the rib cage from the parietal pleura
  - *Note:* Many pathologic conditions cause adhesions of the parietal pleura to the visceral pleura; you may not be able to open the pleural space without shredding the pleurae
  - Attempt to leave the internal thoracic vessels intact as the anterior portion of the rib cage is removed

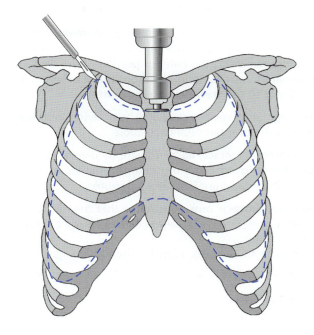

Figure 6-16 Rib cage incisions and saw cuts

Examination of the Removed Anterior Thoracic Wall

- Look at the inside surface of the removed rib cage to identify the following structures **(Figure 6-17)**:
  - **Internal thoracic vessels** — (seen if the internal thoracic vessels were not separated from the inside surface of the rib cage before removing the anterior portion of the rib cage); the internal thoracic aa. originate from the **subclavian a.**, just posterior to the **sternoclavicular joint**
    - The internal thoracic vessels are the anterior contribution to the anterior intercostal circulation
    - Both internal thoracic aa. terminate by dividing into **superior epigastric** and **musculophrenic aa.** at about rib 6 (studied in a future laboratory session)
  - **Transversus thoracis mm.** — observe that the muscle is attached to the sternal body and costal cartilage of ribs 2–6

- On the cut ends of the ribs, identify the following:
  - **External intercostal mm.**
  - **Internal intercostal mm.**
  - **Intercostal vv., aa., and nn.**
  - **Innermost intercostal mm.**

- Return the dissected rib cage to its anatomic position on the cadaver when you are finished with this and subsequent dissections

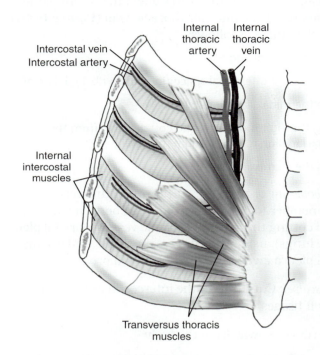

Figure 6-17 Internal surface of the rib cage and sternum

Lab 7

Thoracic Situs and Lungs

Prior to dissection, you should familiarize yourself with the following structures:

PLEURAL SPACE
- Endothoracic fascia
- Parietal pleura
  - Costal pleura
  - Mediastinal pleura
  - Diaphragmatic pleura
  - Cervical pleura
- Pleural space
- Visceral pleura
  - Same regions as the parietal pleura

PLEURAL RECESSES
- Costomediastinal recess
- Costodiaphragmatic recess

ROOT OF THE LUNGS
- Pulmonary aa.
- Pulmonary vv.
- Bronchi
- Pulmonary ligaments
- Bronchial aa.
- Lymph nodes

NERVES AND VESSELS
- Phrenic nn.
- Vagus nn.
  - Recurrent laryngeal nn.
- Pericardiacophrenic vessels

LEFT LUNG
- Apex
- Costal, mediastinal, and diaphragmatic surfaces
- Hilum
  - Pulmonary ligament
  - Bronchi, pulmonary aa. and vv.
- Superior (upper) and inferior (lower) lobes
- Oblique fissure
- Cardiac notch
- Lingula
- Contact impressions after fixation
  - Cardiac impression
  - Aortic groove impression
  - Descending aorta impression
- Bronchi
  - Primary
  - Secondary
  - Tertiary
- Bronchopulmonary (hilar) lymph nodes

RIGHT LUNG
- Apex
- Costal, mediastinal, and diaphragmatic surfaces
- Hilum
  - Pulmonary ligament
  - Bronchi, pulmonary aa. and vv.
- Superior (upper), middle, and inferior (lower) lobes
- Oblique and horizontal fissures
- Contact impressions after fixation
  - Cardiac impression
  - Esophageal impression
- Bronchi
  - Primary
  - Secondary
  - Tertiary
- Bronchopulmonary (hilar) lymph nodes

Lab 7 Dissection Overview

The purpose of this laboratory session is to observe the thoracic organs in situ (thoracic situs). In addition, you will learn the anatomy of the lungs through dissection. You will do so through the following suggested sequence:

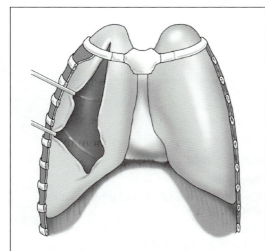

1. Identify pleural membranes, pleural space, lungs, and heart in situ.

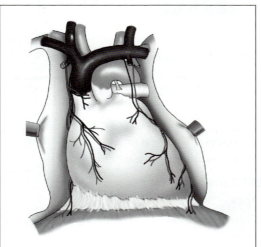

2. Identify the phrenic nerves and pericardiacophrenic vessels.

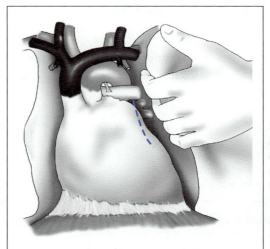

3. Reveal the root of the lungs, and cut the pulmonary vessels and bronchial tree to remove both lungs.

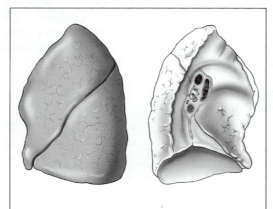

4. Identify the anatomic structures on the left lung.

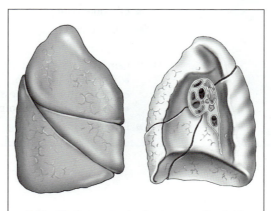

5. Identify the anatomic structures on the right lung.

Pleural Spaces

- Identify the following, but do not cut **(Figure 7-1)**:
  - **Middle mediastinum** — contains the pericardial sac and heart
  - **Parietal pleura** — serous membrane that is subdivided into four regions, identified by structures contacted:
    - **Costal parietal pleura** — lines the internal surface of the ribs and intercostal mm.
    - **Mediastinal parietal pleura** — lines the mediastinum
    - **Diaphragmatic parietal pleura** — lines the superior surface of the diaphragm
    - **Cervical parietal pleura** — extends into the thoracic inlet, superior to rib 1, and is often called the cupola; near its summit, the cervical portion of the parietal pleura is crossed anteriorly by the subclavian artery, which can usually be felt through the parietal pleura
- Make a longitudinal incision, using scissors or a scalpel, through the parietal pleura (if still intact) from the apex of the chest to the diaphragm; then reflect the cut edges of the parietal pleura laterally and medially
  - **Visceral pleura** — attached directly to the lung's surface and as such cannot be distinguished from the lung itself, except at the pulmonary ligaments, where the visceral and parietal pleurae are contiguous
  - **Pleural spaces** — left and right pleural spaces are between the parietal and visceral pleurae
- Using your hands, break adhesions, if present, between the parietal and visceral pleura while exploring the pleural spaces

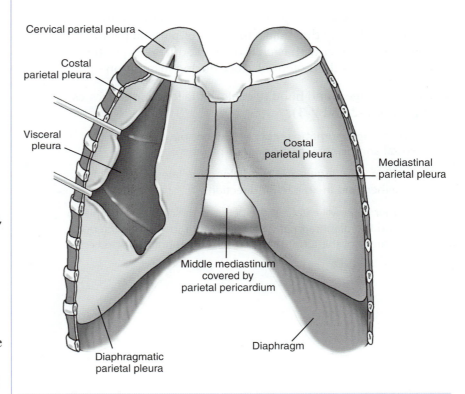

Figure 7-1 Pleural sacs

Pleural Recesses

- **Pleural recesses** — regions where the parietal pleura reflects so sharply that adjacent layers of parietal pleura come into contact with each other (e.g., during expiration); lung tissue fills this potential space during inspiration

- Use your fingers and hand to explore the following recesses **(Figures 7-2** and **7-3)**:
  - **Costodiaphragmatic recess** — pleural space between the costal and diaphragmatic parietal pleurae
    - Slide your fingers and hand along the lateral aspect of either lung in an inferior direction
    - Your hand will enter a space between the costal parietal pleura and the diaphragmatic parietal pleura, below the inferior margin of the lung; this is the costodiaphragmatic recess

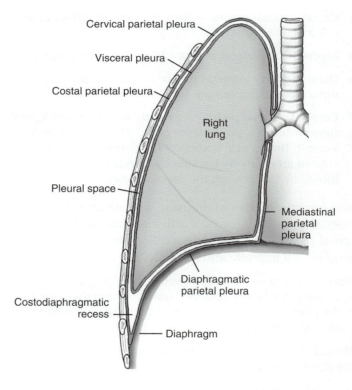

Figure 7-2 Coronal view of the pleural cavity and recesses

Pleural Recesses—cont'd

- **Costomediastinal recess** — pleural space between the costal and mediastinal parietal pleurae

  - Using your fingers, explore the region of the cardiac notch, where the costal parietal pleura reflects from the anterior thoracic wall and continues as the mediastinal parietal pleura

  - The costomediastinal recess occurs on each side but is largest on the left side, in the region anterior to the heart

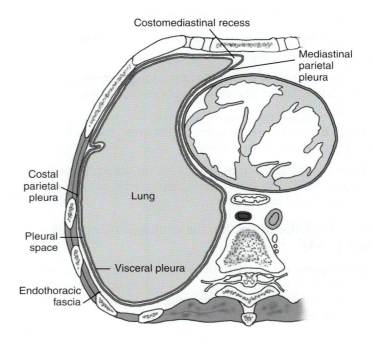

Figure 7-3 Cross-sectional view of the pleural cavity

Phrenic Nerves and Pericardiacophrenic Vessels

- To identify the phrenic nn. and pericardiacophrenic aa. and vv., take the following steps:
  - Gently pull the medial margin of the lungs laterally to reveal the **pericardial sac** (the thick, fibrous sac containing the heart)
  - Look along the anterolateral surface of the pericardial sac to locate the neurovascular bundles containing the phrenic nn. and pericardiacophrenic vessels
  - Dissect, using sharp forceps, through the fibrous tissue to reveal and observe the neurovascular bundle on both sides of the pericardial sac

- Identify the following within the neurovascular bundles **(Figure 7-4)**:
  - **Left phrenic n.** — look between the left subclavian a. and v., deep to the clavicle, to locate the left phrenic n.; courses along the left side of the pericardial sac, anterior to the root of the left lung, to enter the diaphragm
    - Look for a descending band (the neurovascular bundle) about 1.5 cm anterior to the root of the left lung; bluntly dissect and free the phrenic n. and accompanying pericardiacophrenic vessels from the mediastinum (do not cut)
  - **Right phrenic n.** — look lateral to the superior vena cava to locate the right phrenic n.; courses along the right side of the pericardial sac, anterior to the root of the right lung
    - Locate the right phrenic n. in the same manner as the left phrenic n.
  - **Pericardiacophrenic a. and v.** — branch from the internal thoracic a. and v.; accompany the phrenic nn. between the mediastinal parietal pleura and the pericardial sac
  - Avoid cutting the phrenic n. or the pericardiacophrenic a. or v. when making the subsequent incisions through the root of the lungs

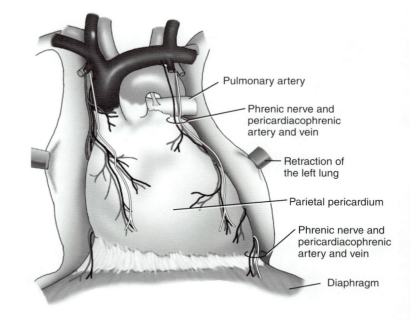

Figure 7-4 Phrenic nerves and pericardiacophrenic vessels

Removal of the Lungs from the Thoracic Cavity

- The phrenic nn. pass anterior, and the vagus nn. pass posterior, to the roots of each lung; try not to damage these nerves during removal of the lungs

- To remove the lungs, follow these instructions **(Figure 7-5)**:
  - Expose and palpate the root of the lung to verify its attachment to the mediastinum by placing your hand between the lung and pericardium and pulling the lung laterally, thereby drawing out and exposing the root of the lung
  - Using a scalpel, *carefully* transect the root of the lung midway between the lung and pericardium; do not cut your fingers or the heart
  - Repeat this procedure for the other lung

- *Note:* Some pathologic conditions cause lung adhesions to surrounding structures; break the adhesions with fingers or cut them with scissors

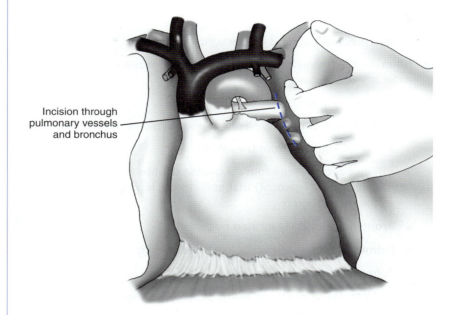

Figure 7-5 Incisions at the root of the lungs

Left Lung

- Examine the excised lungs; if available, use a hand air pump or compressed air hose to inflate bronchopulmonary segments

- Identify the following **(Figures 7-6 and 7-7)**:
  - **Apex**
  - **Base**
  - **Costal, mediastinal, and diaphragmatic surfaces**
  - **Hilum** — the region where air passages and vessels either enter or exit the lung
    - **Pulmonary ligament**
      - Transition of parietal pleura to visceral pleura
      - Hangs inferiorly from the hilum
      - The parietal pleura forms a double membrane (pulmonary ligament) that anchors the lung to the mediastinum
    - **Bronchi** — generally located posteriorly
    - **Pulmonary aa.** — generally located superiorly
    - **Pulmonary vv.** — generally located inferiorly
      - *Note:* These positional terms depend on where the hilum is cut; generally the cut will demonstrate segmental bronchi and branches of the pulmonary a.
    - **Bronchial aa.** and **bronchopulmonary lymph nodes** (usually dark colored)

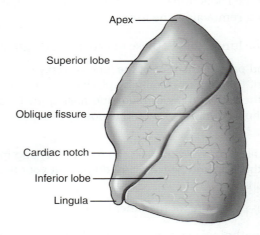

Figure 7-6 Lateral view of the left lung

Left Lung—cont'd

- **Superior and inferior lobes** — separated by the oblique fissure
- **Cardiac notch** — gap in the superior lobe where the heart lies
- **Lingula** — most anterior and inferior portion of superior lobe; wraps around the heart
- **Contact impressions** — cardiac impression, aortic arch groove, and descending aorta impression
- **Bronchi** — generally located posteriorly

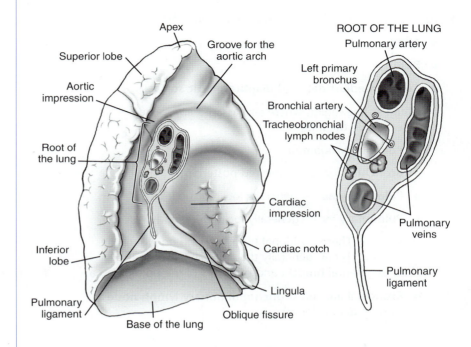

Figure 7-7 Medial view of the left lung

Right Lung

- Identify the following **(Figures 7-8 and 7-9)**:
  - **Apex**
  - **Base**
  - **Costal, mediastinal, and diaphragmatic surfaces**
  - **Hilum** — the region where air passages and vessels either enter or exit the lung
    - **Pulmonary ligament**
    - **Bronchi** — generally located posteriorly
    - **Pulmonary aa.** — generally located superiorly
    - **Pulmonary vv.** — generally located inferiorly
      - *Note:* These positional terms depend on where the hilum is cut; generally the cut will demonstrate segmental bronchi and branches of the pulmonary a.
    - **Bronchial aa.** and **bronchopulmonary lymph nodes** (usually dark colored)

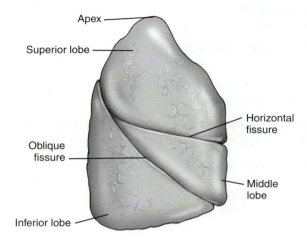

Figure 7-8 Lateral view of the right lung

Right Lung—cont'd

- **Superior lobe** — separated from the middle lobe by the horizontal fissure
- **Inferior lobe** — separated from the superior lobe and middle lobe by the oblique fissure
- **Contact impressions** — cardiac impression and esophageal impression
- **Bronchi** — follow the bronchi into one lung, using blunt dissection; find two or three lobar segments

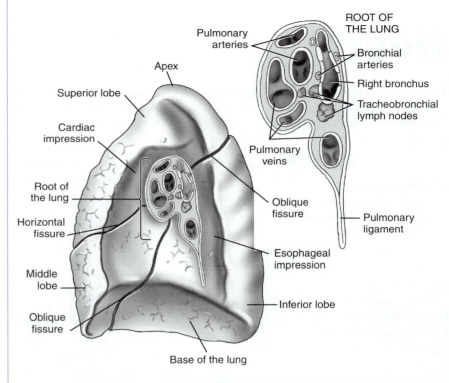

Figure 7-9 Medial view of the right lung

Lab 8

Heart

Prior to dissection, you should familiarize yourself with the following structures:

ANTERIOR MEDIASTINUM
- Thymus

MIDDLE MEDIASTINUM

Pericardial Sac
- Parietal pericardium
  - Fibrous and serous layers
- Pericardial cavity
- Visceral pericardium (epicardium)
- Transverse pericardial sinus
- Oblique pericardial sinus
- Left vagus n.
  - Recurrent laryngeal n.
- Ligamentum arteriosum
- Phrenic n.

Heart
- Right and left atria
- Right and left ventricles
- AV* sulcus
- Interventricular groove
- Apex
- Base

CORONARY VESSELS

Coronary Arteries
- Left coronary a.
  - Anterior interventricular branch
  - Circumflex branch
    - Left (obtuse) marginal branch
- Right coronary a.
  - Atrial a.
    - SA* branch
  - Right (acute) marginal branch
  - Posterior interventricular branch

Coronary Veins
- Coronary sinus
  - Great cardiac v.
  - Middle cardiac v.
  - Small cardiac v.
  - Anterior cardiac vv.

RIGHT HEART

Right Atrium (Auricle)
- Pectinate mm.
- Sulcus terminalis
- Crista terminalis
- Sinus venarum
- Superior and inferior venae cavae
- Coronary sinus
- Fossa ovalis
- Tricuspid valve
- SA* and AV* nodes

Right Ventricle
- Tricuspid valve (right AV* valve)
- Anterior, posterior, and septal cusps
- Chordae tendineae
- Papillary mm.
- Trabeculae carneae
- Supraventricular crest
- Septomarginal trabecula (moderator band)
- Conus arteriosus
- Orifice for the pulmonary trunk

Pulmonary Trunk
- Pulmonary valve (right, left, and anterior cusps)

LEFT HEART

Left Atrium (Auricle)
- Pulmonary vv. (4)
- Bicuspid orifice
- Foramen ovale and its valve
- Bicuspid valve (mitral or left AV* valve)

Left Ventricle
- Bicuspid valve
- Anterior and posterior cusps
- Chordae tendineae
- Papillary mm.
- Trabeculae carneae
- Orifice for the aorta
- Interventricular septum

Aorta
- Aortic valve (right, left, and posterior cusps)

*AV, atrioventricular; SA, sinuatrial

Lab 8 Dissection Overview

The purpose of this laboratory session is to learn the anatomy of the heart through dissection. You will do so through the following suggested sequence:

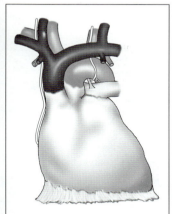

1. Identify the pericardial sac and the heart in situ.

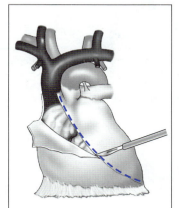

2. Make an incision through the parietal pericardium to observe the heart within the pericardial sac.

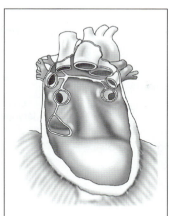

3. Remove the heart from the pericardial sac and observe the cut elements of the vasculature associated with the heart.

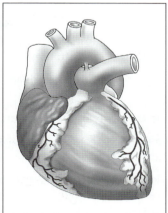

4. Study the external surface of the heart.

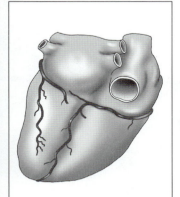

5. Identify coronary arteries and cardiac veins.

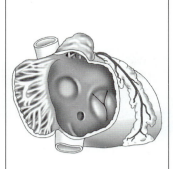

6. Dissect the right atrium of the heart.

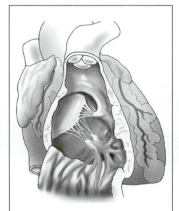

7. Dissect the right ventricle of the heart.

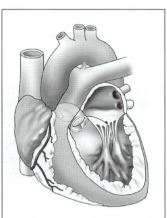

8. Dissect the left atrium and left ventricle of the heart.

Orientation

■ Identify the following **(Figure 8-1)**:

- **Thymus gland** — directly posterior to the manubrium (in the anterior mediastinum); overlies the aortic arch, left brachiocephalic v., trachea, and the pericardium
  - The thymus gland may be absent (involuted) or present as organized fat (not shown in illustration)
- **Aorta** — arches superiorly over the pulmonary trunk
- **Pulmonary trunk (a.)** — bifurcates into the right and left pulmonary aa. in the concavity of the aortic arch
- **Superior vena cava (SVC)** — courses along the right side of the ascending portion of the aortic arch
- **Ligamentum arteriosum** — fibrosed arterial connection (ductus arteriosus) between the pulmonary trunk and aortic arch; bluntly dissect the area between the bifurcation of the pulmonary trunk and the aorta to find the ligamentum arteriosum
- **Left vagus n.** — courses across the aortic arch, immediately lateral to the ligamentum arteriosum
  - After crossing anterior to the aortic arch, the left vagus n. courses posterior to the left pulmonary a. and hilum of the left lung
  - **Left recurrent laryngeal n.** — branches from the left vagus n. at the level of the ligamentum arteriosum; loops around the aortic arch to ascend to the larynx
- **Right vagus n.** — to locate the right vagus n., probe the area where it passes between the right brachiocephalic a. and v. and posterior to the hilum of the right lung

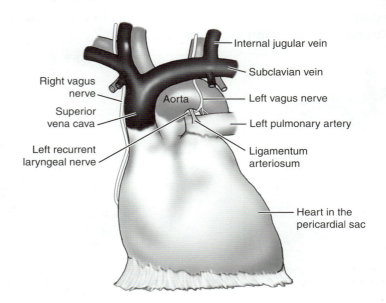

Figure 8-1 Heart in situ

Opening the Pericardial Sac

- Identify the following **(Figure 8-2)**:

  - **Pericardial sac** — fibroserous membrane surrounding the heart; must be opened before the heart can be studied and removed from the middle mediastinum

    - The pericardial sac may be obscured if the body donor had open-heart surgery (e.g., valve replacement or coronary artery bypass graft)

- To open the pericardial sac, take the following steps:

  - Pinch a fold of the pericardial sac with forceps
  - Cut the fold with a scalpel or scissors; make a longitudinal incision from the SVC to the apex of the heart to completely open the sac

- Fold back the parietal pericardium to identify the following:

  - **Fibrous layer** — the external surface of the parietal pericardium
  - **Serous layer** — the internal surface of the parietal pericardium
  - **Pericardial cavity (space)** — the space between the parietal pericardium and the visceral pericardium
  - **Visceral pericardium** — covers the surface of the heart, including the adipose (fat) tissue that may envelop the heart

- Dissect the entire anterior portion of the pericardial sac to better investigate the heart; do not dissect the posterior portion of pericardial sac at this time

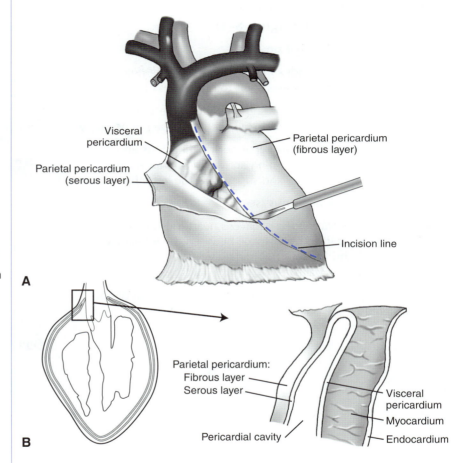

Figure 8-2 Pericardium. **A,** Incision line in the pericardium. **B,** Coronal section through the heart to demonstrate the pericardial sac

Pericardial Sinuses

■ Identify the following, which will be useful for the subsequent dissection **(Figure 8-3)**:

- **Transverse pericardial sinus**
  - Push your right index finger posterior to the pulmonary trunk, from the cadaver's left to right sides of the heart
  - Continue to push your finger between the ascending aorta and SVC, immediately superior to the pulmonary vv.
  - This space is the **transverse pericardial sinus** and lies posterior to the ascending aorta and pulmonary trunk, anterior to the SVC, and superior to the left atrium
- **Oblique pericardial sinus** (see Figure 8-5)
- On the left border of the cadaver's heart, push your fingers behind the heart into the space between the **inferior vena cava** (IVC) and the four pulmonary vv. (the heart will be cupped by your palm)
- The **oblique pericardial sinus** is a serous-lined cul-de-sac bordered by the pulmonary veins and the IVC

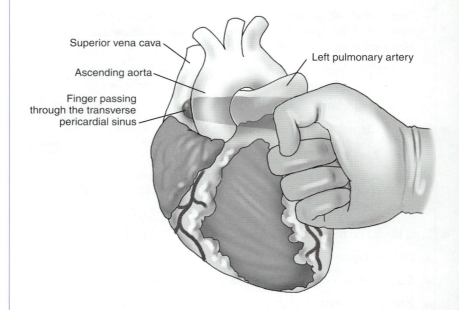

Figure 8-3 Transverse pericardial sinus

Removal of the Heart from the Middle Mediastinum

- Using a scalpel, completely transect the following structures; avoid cutting the vagus nn. if possible **(Figure 8-4)**:

  - **Pulmonary trunk** — cut across the pulmonary trunk before the bifurcation of the pulmonary aa.
  - **Ascending aorta** — cut across the ascending aorta at the site of the transverse pericardial sinus
  - **SVC** — cut across the SVC, about 2 cm superior to its union with the right atrium (inferior to the **azygos v.**)
  - **IVC** — transect the IVC as inferiorly as possible prior to the site where it passes through the diaphragm; avoid cutting the diaphragm
  - **Pulmonary vv.** — lift the apex of the heart anteriorly and superiorly to stretch the four pulmonary vv. from the remaining pericardial sac to expose the oblique pericardial sinus; transect each pulmonary v.

- The only thing holding the heart in place at this point is the connective tissue between the transverse and oblique pericardial sinuses

- Use blunt dissection or scissors to break the connections to remove the heart from the pericardial sac

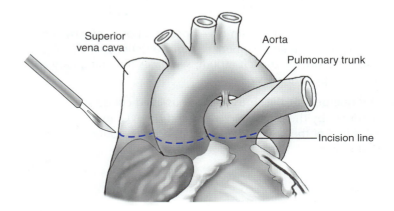

Figure 8-4 Incisions for removal of the heart

Removal of the Heart from the Middle Mediastinum Continued

Removal of the Heart from the Middle Mediastinum—cont'd

- Identify the following **(Figure 8-5)**:

  - **Pericardial sac** — examine the posterior aspect of the pericardial sac after the heart has been removed

  - **Transverse pericardial sinus** — bordered posteriorly by the ascending aorta and pulmonary trunk, anteriorly by the SVC, and superiorly by the left atrium; separates the pulmonary aa. from the pulmonary vv.

  - **Oblique pericardial sinus** — a serous-lined cul-de-sac bordered by the pulmonary veins and the IVC; formed by reflection of the parietal pericardium onto the pulmonary vv. of the heart

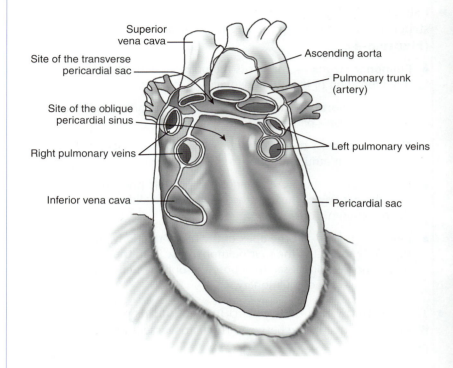

Figure 8-5 Pericardial sac (empty)

Inspection of the Removed Heart

GAFS pp 158–161   ACGA pp 352–354   NAHA Plate 212

- Identify the following surfaces and structures **(Figure 8-6)**:

  - **Anterior (sternocostal) surface** — formed mostly by the right ventricle

  - **Inferior (diaphragmatic) surface** — formed mostly by the left ventricle

  - **Left (pulmonary) surface** — formed mostly by the left ventricle, which creates the cardiac notch in the left lung

  - **Superior** and **inferior venae cavae** — aligned along the right border of the heart

  - **Pulmonary trunk** — bifurcates inferior to the aortic arch

  - **Ascending aorta** — the right atrium may overlap the ascending aorta

  - **Pulmonary vv.** — four located posterior and inferior to the pulmonary trunk; the two right pulmonary vv. are positioned between the superior and inferior venae cavae

  - **Coronary sulcus** — oblique groove that separates the atria from the ventricles; filled by coronary vessels and adipose tissue

  - **Anterior interventricular groove** — filled by the left anterior interventricular (descending) coronary a., great cardiac v., and adipose tissue

  - **Posterior interventricular groove** — filled by the right posterior interventricular coronary a., middle cardiac v., and adipose tissue

  - **Apex** — the inferolateral portion of left ventricle; lies posterior to the fourth or fifth intercostal space, about one hand width from the midsagittal line

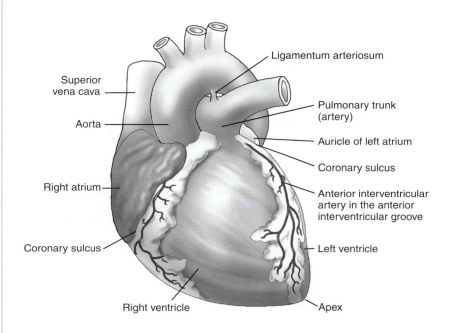

Figure 8-6 Surface features of the heart

Right Coronary Artery

GAFS pp 170–174   ACGA pp 352–353, 358   NAHA Plates 216, 218–219

- Identify the following **(Figure 8-7)**:

  - **Right coronary a.** — arises from the aortic arch, directly superior to the right cusp of the aortic valve; the artery's orifice is inside of the ascending aorta

    - Follow the right coronary a. distally between the right atrium and right ventricle (coronary sulcus), using blunt dissection and the scraping technique to remove the pericardial fat; locate the following branches of the right coronary a.:

      - **Atrial branch** — first branch from the right coronary a.; supplies the right atrium
      - **Sinuatrial (SA) (nodal) branch** — division of the atrial branch; supplies the SA node
      - **Right (acute) marginal a.** — supplies the right surface of the right ventricle; courses toward the apex along the inferior border of the heart
      - **Posterior interventricular a.** (posterior descending a.) — descends in the posterior interventricular groove toward the apex

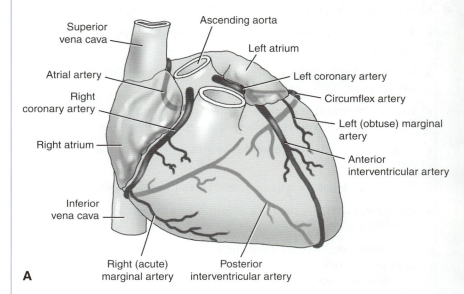

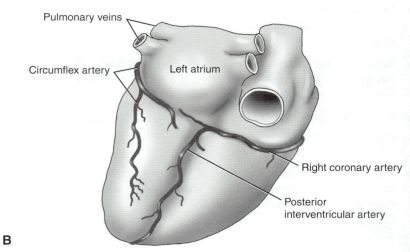

Figure 8-7 Coronary arteries. **A,** Anterior view of the heart. **B,** Posterior view of the heart

Left Coronary Artery

- Identify the following **(Figure 8-8)**:
  - **Left coronary artery** — arises from the aortic arch, directly superior to the left cusp of the aortic valve; the artery's orifice is inside of the ascending aorta
    - Follow the left coronary a. distally to its first division at the left atrium using blunt dissection and the scraping technique to remove the pericardial fat; locate the following branches of the left coronary a.:
      - **Anterior interventricular branch** (left anterior descending a.; LAD branch) — courses in the anterior interventricular groove to the apex; may anastomose with the posterior interventricular branch of the right coronary a. at the apex
      - **Circumflex branch** — follows the coronary sulcus around the left border of the heart and gives off marginal aa., including the left (obtuse) marginal a.; may anastomose with the posterior interventricular branch of the right coronary a. in the coronary sulcus

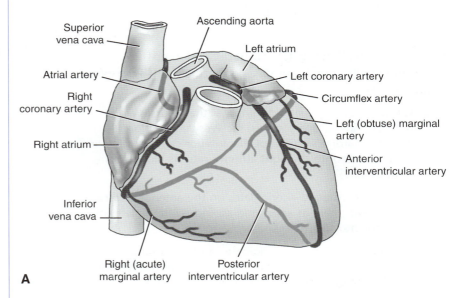

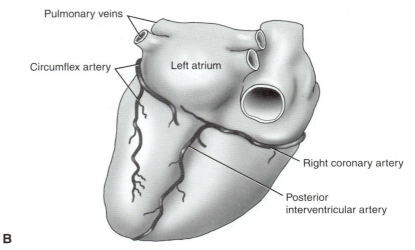

Figure 8-8 Coronary arteries. **A,** Anterior view of the heart. **B,** Posterior view of the heart

Cardiac Veins

- The cardiac veins are named differently than the coronary arteries

- Identify the following; use blunt dissection or the scraping technique to remove pericardial fat **(Figures 8-9 and 8-10)**:

  - **Coronary sinus** — large tributary v. that courses along the posterior coronary sulcus; receives venous blood from all of the cardiac vv. (except the anterior cardiac vv., which drain directly into the right atrium); returns blood to the right atrium

    - **Great cardiac v.** — originates on the anterior surface of the heart, near its apex, and ascends with the left anterior interventricular (descending) coronary a.

    - **Middle cardiac v.** — originates on the posterior surface of the heart, in the posterior interventricular groove; ascends with the posterior interventricular coronary a.

    - **Small cardiac v.** — originates on the anterior surface of the heart, along the inferior margin of the right ventricle; ascends with the right (acute) marginal coronary a.

    - **Anterior cardiac vv.** — drain the wall of the right atrium and empty directly into the right atrium

- *Note:* Often, two each of the previously identified veins flank the corresponding coronary artery

GAFS pp 175–176 ACGA pp 352–354 NAHA Plate 216

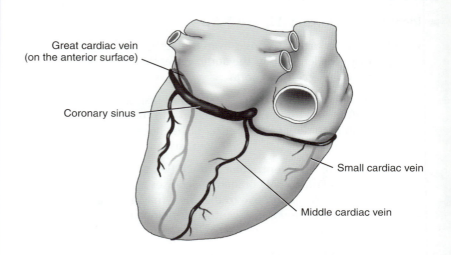

Figure 8-9 Posterior view of the heart to demonstrate the cardiac veins

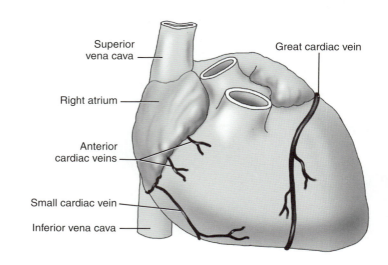

Figure 8-10 Anterior view of the heart to demonstrate the cardiac veins

Right Atrial Incisions

- Make the following incisions through the wall of the right atrium to expose its lumen **(Figure 8-11)**:
  - Horizontally from *A* to the anterior border *(B)*
  - Longitudinally from *B* to the inferior border *(C)*
  - Horizontally from *C* to the posterior–inferior border (not shown)

- Open the cut flap posteriorly, exposing the internal contents; use forceps to remove blood clots; wash the atrium with water

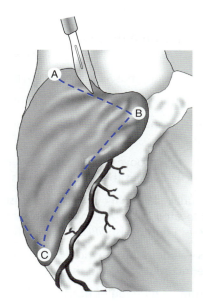

Figure 8-11   Right atrial incisions

Right Atrial Internal Structures

- This chamber receives venous blood from the superior and inferior venae cavae and from the coronary sinus

- Identify the following within the right atrium **(Figure 8-12)**:

  - **Pectinate mm.** — rough, muscular anterior wall region
  - **Sinus venarum** — smooth, thin-walled posterior region
  - **Crista terminalis** — separates the smooth and rough parts of the atrial wall *internally*
  - **Sulcus terminalis** — a groove on the external surface of the right atrium; directly overlies the crista terminalis
  - **SA node** — its surface landmark is where the crista terminalis meets the SVC; located in the atrial wall, between the sulcus terminalis and crista terminalis; *difficult to identify*
  - **Coronary sinus** — opens into the right atrium, between the apertures of the tricuspid valve and the IVC
  - **Interatrial septum** — partition of heart muscle that separates the two atria
  - **Fossa ovalis** — a depression in the interatrial septum, superior to the IVC (was the foramen ovale in the fetus)
  - **Tricuspid valve** — observe the superior border of the three cusps
  - **Atrioventricular (AV) node** — located in the AV septum, above the opening of the coronary sinus; *also difficult to identify*

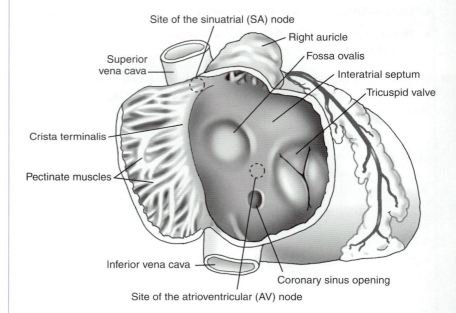

Figure 8-12 Right atrial structures

Right Ventricular Incisions

- Push a blunt instrument through the lumen of the pulmonary trunk into the right ventricle to serve as an internal guide while opening the right ventricle

- Make the following incisions through the wall of the right ventricle to expose its lumen **(Figure 8-13)**:
  - Horizontally from *A* to *B*, inferior to the pulmonary valve (use the blunt instrument that you placed in the right ventricle as a guide)
  - Make another incision about 1 cm inferior and parallel to the coronary groove toward the inferior border *(C)*
  - Make an additional incision about 2 cm to the left of and parallel to the anterior interventricular groove toward the inferior border *(D)* of the right ventricle
  - Open the cut ventricular flap inferiorly; use forceps to remove blood clots; wash the ventricle with water

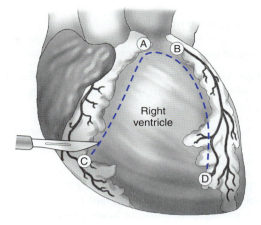

Figure 8-13 Right ventricular incisions

Right Ventricular Internal Structures

- Identify the following **(Figure 8-14)**:

    - **Trabeculae carneae** — irregular muscular elevations

    - **Papillary mm.** — myocardial pillars attached to the tricuspid valve via chordae tendineae (attach the cusps of the tricuspid valve to the papillary mm.)

        - **Anterior papillary m.** (largest) — arises from the anterior, inner surface of the right atrial wall; attaches to the anterior and posterior cusps of the tricuspid valve

        - **Posterior papillary m.** — arises from the inferior surface of the right atrial wall; attaches to the posterior and septal cusps of the tricuspid valve

        - **Septal papillary m.** — arises from the interventricular septum; attaches to the anterior and septal cusps of the tricuspid valve

    - **Septomarginal trabecula** (moderator band) — muscular bundle that runs between the interventricular septum and the anterior papillary m. (present in about 60% of hearts)

    - **Conus arteriosus** — smooth surface of the right ventricle, immediately inferior to the pulmonary trunk

    - **Supraventricular crest** — separates the smooth conus arteriosus from the rough muscular portion of the right ventricle

    - **Pulmonary valve** — observe the anterior, left, and right cusps; they are named for their anatomic position

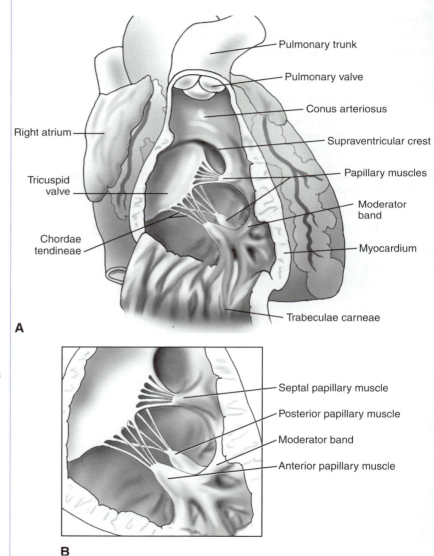

Figure 8-14 Right ventricular structures. **A,** Right ventricle open. **B,** Papillary muscles of the right ventricle

Left Atrial Incisions and Structures

- Make an inverted U-shaped incision through the wall of the left atrium, between the pulmonary vv., to expose the lumen of the left atrium **(Figure 8-15)**

- Fold the flap of the left atrium inferiorly; remove blood clots; wash the atrium with water

- Identify the following:
  - **Four pulmonary vv.** (two on each side) — enter the lateral aspects of the left atrium
  - **Bicuspid (mitral) valve** — observe the superior border of the two cusps
  - **Pectinate mm.** — rough, muscular region of the auricular appendage of the left atrium

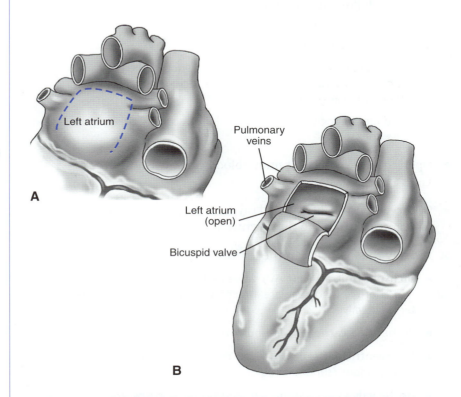

Figure 8-15 Left atrium. **A,** Left atrial incisions. **B,** Left atrium open.

Left Ventricular Incisions and Internal Structures

- Make the following incision through the wall of the left ventricle **(Figure 8-16)**:
  - *Note:* Some coronary vessels will be cut
  - Start inferior to the ascending aorta (inferior to the right and left coronary cusps) and continue the incision parallel to the interventricular groove to the apex
  - Continue the incision through the length of the left ventricle to its apex

- Open the left ventricle; remove blood clots; wash the ventricle with water

- Observe that the lateral wall myocardium is thicker for the left ventricle than the right ventricle

- Identify the following in the left ventricle (see Figure 8-16):
  - **Bicuspid (mitral) (left AV) valve** — two papillary mm. and chordae tendineae are attached to the two cusps of the bicuspid valve
  - **Trabeculae carneae** — irregular muscular elevations
  - **Interventricular septum** — has muscular (inferior) and membranous (superior) regions
  - **Aortic valve** — has right, left, and posterior cusps; the fibrous thickenings at the midpoint of the edge of each cusp are called **nodules**

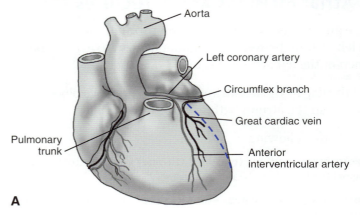

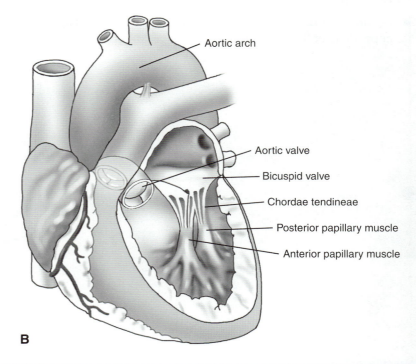

Figure 8-16 Left ventricular structures. **A,** Left ventricular incision. **B,** Left ventricle open

Valves of the Heart

- Identify the following cusps of the valves from a superior view of the heart **(Figure 8-17)**:
  - **Tricuspid (right AV) valve**
    - Anterior cusp
    - Septal (medial) cusp
    - Posterior cusp
  - **Pulmonary semilunar valve**
    - Anterior cusp
    - Right cusp
    - Left cusp
  - **Bicuspid (left AV) (mitral) valve**
    - Anterior cusp
    - Posterior cusp
  - **Aortic semilunar valve**
    - Right cusp — associated with the opening (os) of the right coronary a.
    - Left cusp — associated with the opening (os) of the left coronary a.
    - Posterior cusp

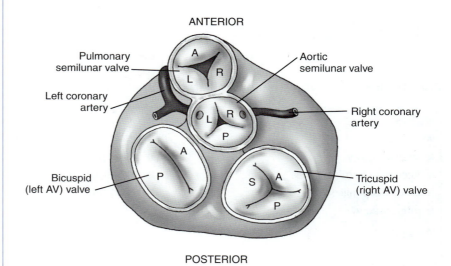

Figure 8-17 Valves of the heart

Lab 9

Mediastina

Prior to dissection, you should familiarize yourself with the following structures:

VEINS
- Azygos v.
- Hemiazygos v.
- Accessory hemiazygos v.
- Brachiocephalic vv.
- Intercostal vv.

ARTERIES
- Aortic arch
  - Brachiocephalic a.
  - Left common carotid a.
  - Left subclavian a.
- Descending aorta
  - Intercostal aa.
  - Bronchial aa.
  - Esophageal aa.

NERVES
- Thoracic spinal nerves
- Sympathetic ganglia
- Sympathetic trunks
- Gray and white rami communicantes
- Greater splanchnic nn. (T5–T9)
- Lesser splanchnic nn. (T10–T11)
- Least splanchnic nn. (T12)
- Intercostal nn.
- Vagus nn.
  - Recurrent laryngeal nn.
  - Cardiac plexus
  - Pulmonary plexus
  - Esophageal plexus
    - Anterior vagal trunk
    - Posterior vagal trunk

MUSCLES
- Innermost intercostal mm.
- Subcostal mm.

MISCELLANEOUS
- Trachea
  - Carina
- Esophagus
- Thoracic duct
- Anterior longitudinal ligament

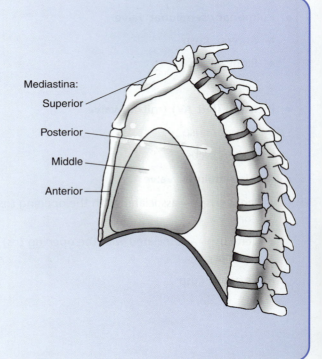

Mediastina:
- Superior
- Posterior
- Middle
- Anterior

Lab 9 Dissection Overview

The purpose of this laboratory session is to learn the anatomy of the mediastina through dissection. You will do so through the following suggested sequence:

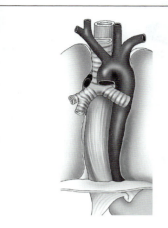

1. Study the esophagus, bronchial tree, aorta, and associated structures.

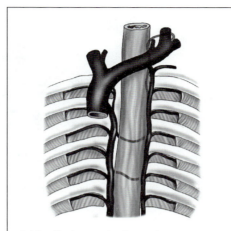

2. Identify the caval veins and azygos system of veins.

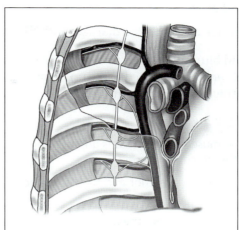

3. Dissect the posterior intercostal nerves and sympathetic trunk.

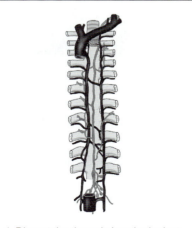

4. Dissect the thoracic lymphatic duct.

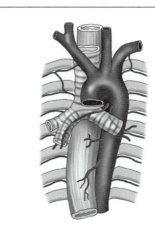

5. Dissect the branches of the aorta to the esophagus, bronchi, and intercostals.

Posterior Mediastinum

- Identify the borders of the posterior mediastinum **(Figure 9-1)**:
  - **Vertebral bodies T5–T12** (posterior border)
  - **Posterior surface of the pericardial sac** (anterior border)
- Use scissors and blunt dissection to carefully remove the pericardial sac from the mediastinum (leave the pericardium attached to the diaphragm)
- Identify the following:
  - **Esophagus** — muscular tube that is anterior and slightly to the right of the descending aorta
  - **Descending aorta** — posterior and slightly to the left of the esophagus
  - **Vagus nn.** — bluntly dissect the already exposed right and left vagus nn. superiorly and inferiorly to follow their continuity
    - **Right vagus n.** — posterior to the root of the right lung; medial to the azygos v.
    - **Left vagus n.** — posterior to the root of the left lung; anterior to the aortic arch
      - **Left recurrent laryngeal n.** — branch from the left vagus n.; immediately left to the ligamentum arteriosum; hooks (recurs) back up the neck
  - **Esophageal plexus** — the vagus nn. branch and become a plexus on the esophagus (you may need to clean the esophagus to identify parts of the plexus)
    - **Anterior vagal trunk** — at the distal end of the esophagus, the esophageal plexus converges on the *left* side to form the anterior vagal trunk
    - **Posterior vagal trunk** — at the distal end of the esophagus, the esophageal plexus converges on the *right* side to form the posterior vagal trunk

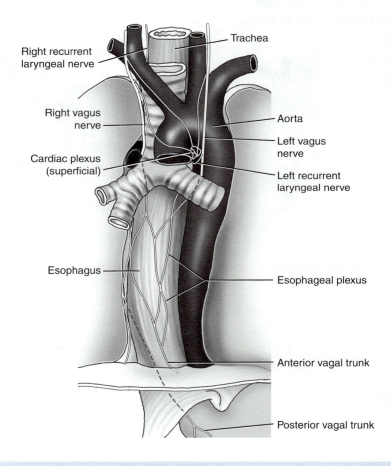

Figure 9-1 Esophageal plexus and vagus nerves

The Trachea and Related Structures

- Identify the following **(Figure 9-2)**:

  - **Trachea** — the windpipe; located anterior to the esophagus and posterior to the aortic arch

    - **Tracheal rings** — palpate the trachea to identify the tracheal C-shaped rings (they are not complete rings)

  - **Carina** — the distal point of the trachea, where it bifurcates into the right and left primary bronchi; used as a landmark during bronchoscopy

  - **Primary bronchi** — the trachea bifurcates into two primary bronchi (right and left)

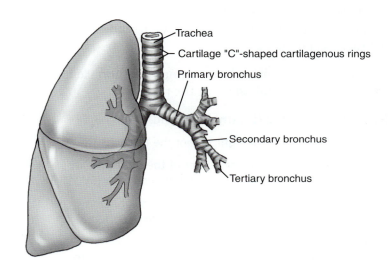

Figure 9-2   Trachea

Azygos System of Veins

- *Note:* Expect variation with the azygos system of veins; the superior and supreme intercostal vv. usually drain into the brachiocephalic vv.

- Peel the remaining parietal pleura and endothoracic fascia away from the internal aspect of the rib cage

- Identify the following (**Figures 9-3** and **9-4**):

  - **Azygos v.** — drains the right side of the thoracic wall
    - Arches over the superior border of the right primary bronchus to drain into the superior vena cava (SVC)
    - Courses along the posterior thoracic wall inferiorly to the diaphragm, along the right side of vertebral bodies T4–T12
    - **Right intercostal vv.** — drain into the azygos v.; to identify intercostal structures on obese bodies, it may be necessary to use the scraping technique to minimize fat in the intercostal spaces

  - **Hemiazygos v.** — drains part of the left side of the thoracic wall, in combination with the accessory hemiazygos v.
    - Courses along the posterior thoracic wall, from the diaphragm along the left side of vertebral bodies T9–T12
    - At about T9 vertebra, crosses to the right side, posterior to the aorta, thoracic duct, and esophagus, to join the azygos v.

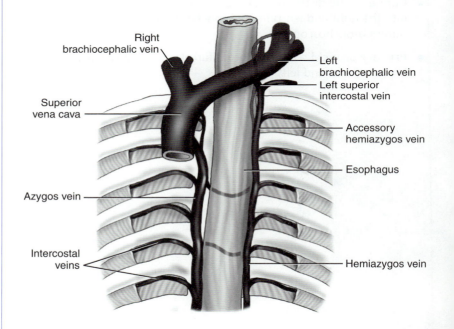

Figure 9-3 Azygos system of veins

Azygos System of Veins—cont'd

- **Accessory hemiazygos v.** — also drains the left side of the thoracic wall
  - Originates at the fourth or fifth intercostal space and descends on the left side of the thoracic vertebrae to about T8
  - At about T8 vertebra, crosses to the right side, posterior to the aorta, thoracic duct, and esophagus, to join the azygos v.
  - **Left intercostal vv.** — drain into the hemiazygos system of veins

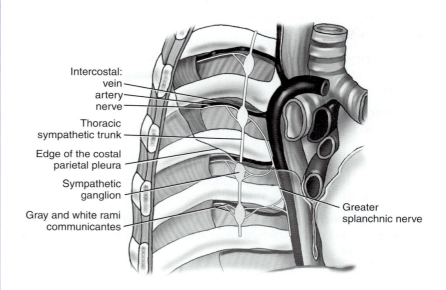

Figure 9-4 Lateral view of the azygos vein

Lymphatic System in the Thorax

■ Identify the following, using the blunt dissection technique (**Figure 9-5**):

- **Thoracic duct** — very fragile yet the largest lymphatic vessel in the body; to identify it, pull the esophagus to the right side
  - Located deep and parallel to the esophagus and descending aorta; 3–4 mm in diameter and may look dull white
  - Terminates superiorly in the neck by emptying into the junction of the left internal jugular v. and left subclavian v. (studied further in another laboratory session)
- **Tracheobronchial lymph nodes** — located below and on either side of the tracheal bifurcation; large; should be identifiable

GAFS pp 132, 149–150, 196–197   ACGA p 340   NAHA Plates 206, 239

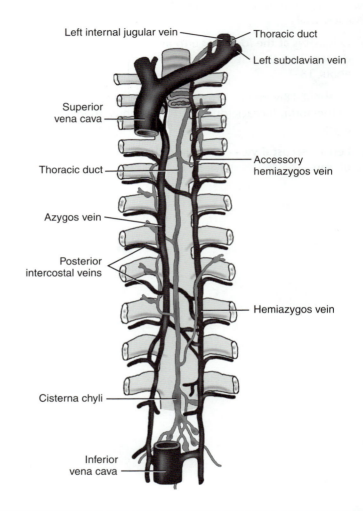

Figure 9-5   Thoracic duct

Nerves in the Posterior Mediastinum

■ Identify the following by probing the intercostal spaces near the vertebral bodies on one side of the thorax **(Figure 9-6)**:

- **Thoracic sympathetic (nerve) trunk** — located bilaterally on the following:
  - The heads of the ribs in the superior part of the thorax
  - The costovertebral joints in the midthorax
  - The vertebral bodies in the inferior part of the thorax
- **Rami communicantes** — thread-sized communications located between the sympathetic trunks and intercostal nn.
- **Greater splanchnic nn.** (spinal levels T5–T9) — located on the lateral surface of the vertebral bodies T6–T12
- **Lesser splanchnic nn.** (spinal levels T10–T11) — located on the lateral surface of the vertebral bodies T10–T11
- **Least splanchnic nn.** (spinal level T12) — located on the lateral surface of T12 vertebral body
- **Intercostal neurovascular bundles (v., a., and n.)** — review them

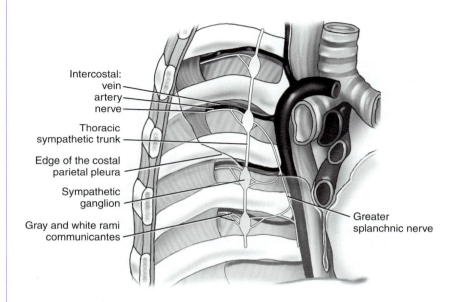

Figure 9-6 Thoracic sympathetic nerves

Superior Mediastinum

- Identify the inferior border of the superior mediastinum:
  - Located superior to a horizontal plane from the sternal angle anteriorly to the T4–T5 intervertebral disc posteriorly

- To gain wider access to this region, remove the inferior portion of the manubrium with a bone saw or rib cutter (leave the sternoclavicular and sternocostal joints for rib 1 intact)

- Cut the SVC transversely, immediately superior to the azygos v., and reflect the cut end superiorly

- To identify the following you may need to remove additional pleura, pericardium, and fascia to clarify these structures **(Figure 9-7)**:
  - **Brachiocephalic vv.** — unite to form the SVC
  - **Aortic arch** — located deep to the left brachiocephalic v.; arches over the left bronchus and becomes the descending thoracic aorta (the thread-sized nerves in this area are part of the **cardiac plexus**)
    - *Note:* Do not take the time to completely display the autonomic nervous system plexuses and their branches of origin and distribution at this time; however, they are of great physiologic importance, and it is wise to have a general knowledge of their location so that they can be observed as the dissection proceeds

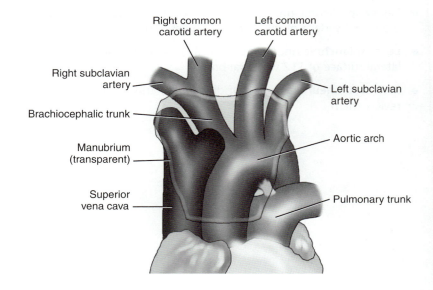

Figure 9-7 Aortic arch branches

Superior Mediastinum—cont'd

- Three branches of the aortic arch:
  - **Brachiocephalic trunk** — first branch; 4–5 cm long; bifurcates to form the right common carotid and right subclavian aa.
  - **Left common carotid a.** — second branch
  - **Left subclavian a.** — third branch
- Branches of the descending thoracic aorta (**Figures 9-8 and 9-9**):
  - **Esophageal aa.** — very small and hard to identify
  - **Bronchial aa.** — small; look at the hilum of either lung to identify these vessels
  - **Posterior intercostal aa.** — originate from the descending thoracic aorta; easiest to find

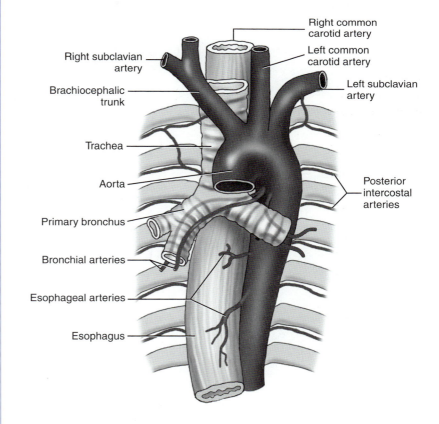

Figure 9-8 Descending aorta branches of the thorax

Superior Mediastinum Continued

Superior Mediastinum—cont'd

- Branches of the descending thoracic aorta (**Figures 9-8** and **9-9**):
  - **Esophageal aa.** — very small and hard to identify
  - **Bronchial aa.** — small; look at the hilum of either lung to identify these vessels
  - **Posterior intercostal aa.** — originate from the descending thoracic aorta; easiest to find

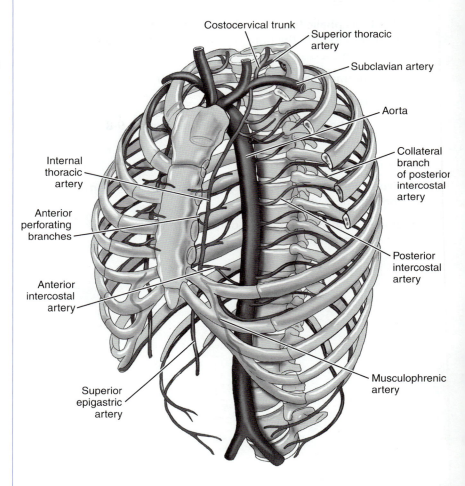

Figure 9-9 Distribution of arterial branches arising from the descending aorta. (Redrawn from Drake R, Vogl W, Mitchell A: Gray's Anatomy for Students. Philadelphia: Elsevier, 2005, Fig. 3.29)

Unit 2 Thorax Overview

At the end of Unit 2, you should be able to identify the following structures on cadavers, skeletons, and/or radiographs:

Osteology
- Vertebral column (33 vertebrae)
  - Cervical vertebrae (7)
  - Thoracic vertebrae (12)
- Vertebral structures
  - Transverse processes
  - Pedicles
  - Bodies and intervertebral discs
  - Articular processes (superior and inferior)
  - Vertebral foramina
  - Intervertebral foramina (notches)
  - Superior and inferior costal facets
  - Transverse costal facet
- Ribs
  - Head, neck, tubercle, angle, costal groove
- Scapula
  - Spine and acromion
  - Coracoid process
  - Lateral and medial margins
  - Superior and inferior angles
- Sternum
  - Manubrium and jugular notch
  - Sternal angle
  - Body and xiphoid process
- Clavicle
- Sternoclavicular joint
- Acromioclavicular joint

Muscles
- Pectoralis major m.
- Pectoralis minor m.
- Subclavius m.
- Intercostal mm. (external, internal, innermost)
- Transversus thoracis m.
- Subcostal m.
- Serratus anterior m.

Miscellaneous
- Deltopectoral triangle
- Clavipectoral fascia
- Midaxillary line
- Parietal pleura
- Sternocostal joints
- Trachea
- Carina
- Esophagus
- Thoracic duct
- Thymus
- Anterior longitudinal ligament

Breast
- Nipple, lactiferous ducts, and areola
- Mammary gland
- Suspensory ligaments
- Retromammary space

Vessels (Arteries and Veins)
- Intercostal vessels
  - Lateral and anterior cutaneous aa. and vv.
- Cephalic v.
- Subclavian a. and v.
  - Vertebral a.
  - Internal thoracic a. and v.
- Axillary a.
  - Thoracoacromial trunk
  - Deltoid, pectoral, acromial, and clavicular branches
- Superior vena cava
  - Brachiocephalic vv.
  - Azygos v.
  - Hemiazygos v.
  - Accessory hemiazygos v.
- Aortic arch
  - Brachiocephalic a.
  - Left common carotid a.
  - Left subclavian a.
- Descending thoracic aorta
  - Intercostal aa.
  - Bronchial aa.
  - Esophageal aa.

Nerves
- Thoracic spinal nerves
- Sympathetic ganglion
- Sympathetic trunk
- Gray and white rami communicantes

Nerves—cont'd

- Greater splanchnic n. (T5-T9)
- Lesser splanchnic n. (T10-T11)
- Least splanchnic n. (T12)
- Intercostal nerves
  - Lateral and anterior cutaneous nn.
- Lateral and medial pectoral nn.
- Phrenic nn.
- Vagus nn.
  - Recurrent laryngeal nn.
  - Cardiac plexus
  - Pulmonary plexus
  - Esophageal plexus
    - Anterior vagal trunk
    - Posterior vagal trunk

Lung

- Endothoracic fascia
- Pleural cavity
  - Parietal pleura
    - Costal, mediastinal, diaphragmatic, and cervical pleurae
  - Pleural space
  - Visceral pleura (same regions as the parietal pleura)
- Pleural recesses
  - Costomediastinal recess
  - Costodiaphragmatic recess
- Left lung
  - Apex
  - Costal, mediastinal, and diaphragmatic surfaces
  - Hilum
    - Pulmonary ligament
    - Bronchi, bronchial aa., lymph nodes, pulmonary aa. and vv.
  - Superior/inferior lobes and oblique fissure
  - Cardiac notch and lingula
  - Contact impressions
    - Cardiac impression
- Aortic groove impression
- Descending aorta impression
- Bronchi
  - Primary, secondary, and tertiary
- Hilar lymph nodes
- Right lung
  - Apex
  - Costal, mediastinal, and diaphragmatic surfaces
  - Hilum
    - Pulmonary ligament
    - Bronchi, bronchial aa., pulmonary aa. and vv.
  - Superior, middle, and inferior lobes
  - Oblique and horizontal fissures
  - Contact impressions
    - Cardiac impression
    - Esophageal impression
  - Bronchi
    - Primary, secondary, and tertiary
  - Hilar lymph nodes

Heart

- Pericardial sac
  - Parietal pericardium
    - Fibrous and serous layers
  - Pericardial space
  - Visceral pericardium (epicardium)
  - Transverse and oblique pericardial sinuses
  - Ligamentum arteriosum
- Heart
  - Right and left atria and ventricles
  - Atrioventricular sulcus
  - Interventricular groove
  - Apex and base
- Coronary arteries
  - Left coronary a.
    - Anterior interventricular branch
    - Circumflex branch
      - Obtuse marginal branch
  - Right coronary a.
    - Atrial a.
    - Sinuatrial branch
    - Acute marginal branch
    - Posterior interventricular branch
- Coronary veins
  - Coronary sinus
    - Great, middle, and small cardiac vv.
  - Anterior cardiac vv.
- Right atrium (auricle)
  - Pectinate muscles
  - Sulcus and crista terminalis
  - Sinus venarum
  - Superior and inferior venae cavae
  - Coronary sinus
  - Fossa ovalis and tricuspid valve
  - SA and AV nodes
- Right ventricle
  - Tricuspid valve (right AV valve)
  - Anterior, posterior, and septal cusps
  - Chordae tendineae and papillary mm.
  - Trabeculae carneae
  - Septomarginal trabecula (moderator band)
  - Conus arteriosus
  - Supraventricular crest
- Pulmonary trunk
  - Pulmonary valve (right, left, and anterior cusps)
- Left atrium (auricle)
  - Pulmonary vv. (4)
  - Bicuspid orifice
  - Foramen ovale/fossa ovalis
- Left ventricle
  - Bicuspid valve (mitral or left AV valve)
  - Anterior and posterior cusps
  - Chordae tendineae
  - Papillary mm.
  - Trabeculae carneae
  - Orifice for aorta
  - Interventricular septum
- Aorta
  - Aortic valve (right, left, and posterior cusps)

Unit 3
Abdomen, Pelvis, and Perineum

The purpose of this unit is to learn the anatomic structures of the abdomen, pelvis, and perineum through dissection.

Lab 10 Osteology of the Abdomen, Pelvis, and Perineum   117

Lab 11 Anterior Abdominal Wall and Inguinal Canal   129

Lab 12 Peritoneum and Foregut   147

Lab 13 Midgut and Hindgut   170

Lab 14 Posterior Abdominal Wall   183

Lab 15 Gluteal Region and Ischioanal Fossa   196

Lab 16 Urogenital Triangle   203

Lab 17 Pelvis and Reproductive Systems   226

Unit 3 Abdomen, Pelvis, and Perineum Overview   245

Osteology of the Abdomen, Pelvis, and Perineum

Lab 10

Prior to dissection, you should familiarize yourself with the following structures:

Sternum
- Xiphoid process

Ribs (12 Pairs)
- Costal margin
- Costal cartilage

Sacrum
- Promontory
- Anterior and posterior sacral foramina
- Ala
- Sacral canal
- Sacral hiatus

Os Coxae (Ilium, Ischium, Pubis)
- Acetabulum
- Ischiopubic (conjoint) ramus
- Obturator foramen
- Greater sciatic notch/foramen
- Pelvic brim, inlet, and outlet
- False and true pelvis
- Linea terminalis (arcuate line, pecten pubis, and pubic crest)
- Ilium
  - Iliac crest and fossa
  - Arcuate line
  - Anterior superior iliac spine
  - Posterior superior/inferior iliac spine
- Ischium
  - Ischial ramus (ischiopubic ramus)
  - Ischial tuberosity and spine
  - Lesser sciatic notch/foramen
- Pubis
  - Pubic tubercle
  - Pubic crest
  - Superior pubic ramus
    - Pecten pubis/pectineal line
  - Pubic symphysis and arch
  - Inferior pubic ramus (ischiopubic ramus)

Lab 10 Dissection Overview

The purpose of this laboratory session is to learn the osteology of the abdomen, pelvis, and perineum through dissection. You will do so through the following suggested sequence:

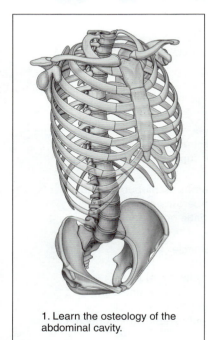

1. Learn the osteology of the abdominal cavity.

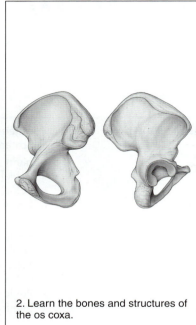

2. Learn the bones and structures of the os coxa.

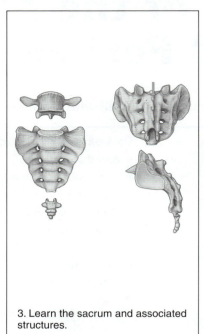

3. Learn the sacrum and associated structures.

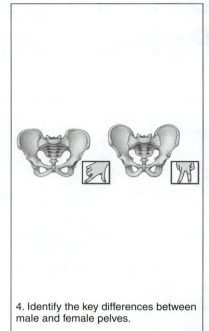

4. Identify the key differences between male and female pelves.

Abdominal Wall Osteology

- Locate the following structures on an articulated skeleton **(Figure 10-1)**:
  - Sternum
  - Xiphoid process
  - Costal margin
  - Costal cartilage
  - Rib 12
  - Lumbar vertebra 1 (L1)
  - Lumbar vertebra 5 (L5)
  - Sacrum
  - Iliac crest
  - Iliac fossa
  - Anterior superior iliac spine
  - Pubic tubercle
  - Pectineal line
  - Pubic symphysis

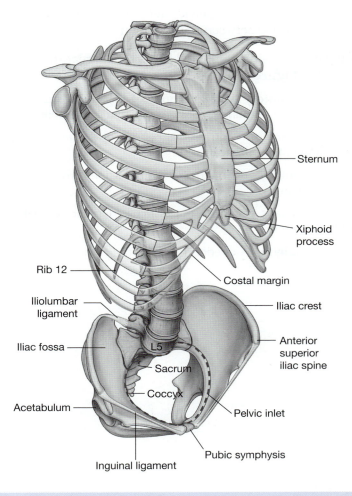

Figure 10-1 Abdominal osteology overview. (From Drake R, Vogl W, Mitchell A: Gray's Anatomy for Students. Philadelphia: Elsevier, 2005, Fig. 4.1)

Pelvic Inlet (Superior Pelvic Aperture)

- The pelvic inlet is the circular opening between the abdominal cavity and the pelvic cavity through which structures traverse between the abdomen and pelvis

- Identify the following bones and joints that border the pelvic inlet **(Figure 10-2)**:
  - **Sacral promontory (vertebral body of S1)** — protrudes into the pelvic inlet, forming its posterior margin in the midline
  - **Ala of the sacrum** — forms on either side of the promontory the margin of the pelvic inlet
  - **Sacroiliac joint** — the margin of the pelvic inlet crosses the sacroiliac joint
  - **Linea terminalis** — consists of the arcuate line, pecten pubis, and pubic crest
  - **Pubic symphysis** — anterior margin of the pelvic inlet; in the midline

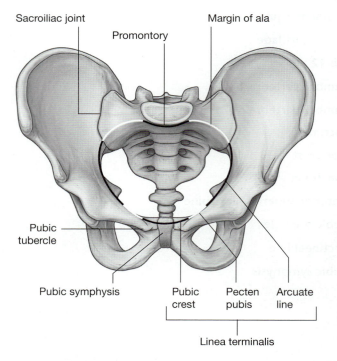

Figure 10-2 Pelvic inlet. (From Drake R, Vogl W, Mitchell A: Gray's Anatomy for Students. Philadelphia: Elsevier, 2005, Fig. 5.28)

Pelvic Walls

- Walls of the true pelvis consist of the sacrum, coccyx, the pelvic bones inferior to the linea terminalis, two ligaments, and two muscles

  - The two ligaments are important architectural elements because they link each pelvic bone to the sacrum and coccyx and help define the apertures between the pelvic cavity and adjacent regions through which structures pass **(Figure 10-3)**

    - **Sacrotuberous ligament** — triangular shaped; superficial to the sacrospinous ligament; its base has a broad attachment that extends from the posterior superior iliac spine of the pelvic bone, along the posterior aspect and lateral margin of the sacrum and coccyx; laterally the apex of the ligament is attached to the medial margin of the ischial tuberosity

    - **Sacrospinous ligament** — triangular shaped, with its apex attached to the ischial spine and its base attached to the related margins of the sacrum and coccyx

    - **Greater sciatic notch** — between the ischial spine and posterior superior iliac spine; sacrotuberous and sacrospinous ligaments convert it into the greater sciatic foramen (lies superior to the sacrospinous ligament and the ischial spine)

    - **Lesser sciatic notch** — between the ischial spine and ischial tuberosity; sacrotuberous and sacrospinous ligaments convert it into the lesser sciatic foramen (lies inferior to the ischial spine and sacrospinous ligament between the sacrospinous and sacrotuberous ligaments)

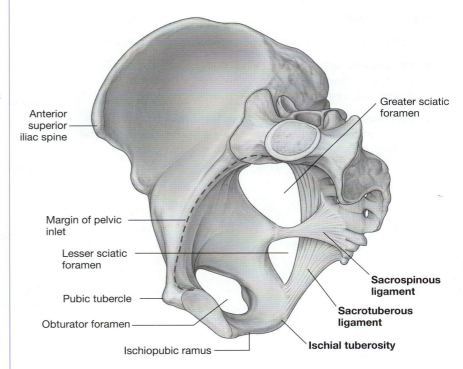

Figure 10-3 Pelvic walls. (From Drake R, Vogl W, Mitchell A: Gray's Anatomy for Students. Philadelphia: Elsevier, 2005, Fig. 5.5)

Pelvic Outlet (Inferior Pelvic Aperture)

- Diamond shaped, the pelvic outlet is formed anteriorly by bone and posteriorly by ligaments; terminal parts of the urinary and gastrointestinal tracts and the vagina pass through; the area enclosed by the boundaries of the pelvic outlet and below the pelvic floor is the perineum

- Identify the following borders of the pelvic outlet **(Figure 10-4)**:

  - **Pubic symphysis** — forms the anterior margin in the midline
  - **Ischiopubic ramus** — the pelvic outlet extends laterally and posteriorly along each side of the inferior border of the ischiopubic ramus to the ischial tuberosity
  - **Sacrotuberous ligament** — from the ischial tuberosities, the boundaries continue posteriorly and medially along the sacrotuberous ligament on both sides of the coccyx

GAFS p 390   ACGA pp 446, 481   NAHA Plates 357, 359

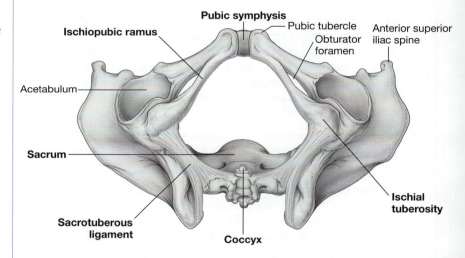

Figure 10-4 Pelvic outlet. (From Drake R, Vogl W, Mitchell A: Gray's Anatomy for Students. Philadelphia: Elsevier, 2005, Fig. 5.32)

Pelvic Bone

- The pelvic bone consists of the right and left os coxae, which articulate with the sacrum posteriorly and the pubic symphysis anteriorly

- Identify the following on an os coxa **(Figure 10-5)**:

  - **Acetabulum** — articular socket on the lateral surface, which, together with the head of the femur, forms the hip joint

  - **Obturator foramen** — located inferior to the acetabulum; most of the foramen is closed by a flat connective tissue membrane, the **obturator membrane**; a small obturator canal remains open superiorly between the membrane and the adjacent bone, providing communication between the lower limb and the pelvic cavity

  - **Greater sciatic notch** — posterior margin of the os coxa, superior to the ischial spine

  - **Lesser sciatic notch** — posterior margin of the os coxa, inferior to the ischial spine

  - **Pubic symphysis** — fibrocartilaginous joint that articulates the two pubic bones

- Each os coxa is formed by three bones (see Figure 10-5):

  - **Ilium** — most superior part

  - **Ischium** — most posterior part

  - **Pubis** — anterior and inferior parts of the os coxa

  - At birth, these three bones are connected by cartilage in the area of the acetabulum; in adulthood, they fuse into a single bone

GAFS pp 379–381   ACGA p 436   NAHA Plate 486

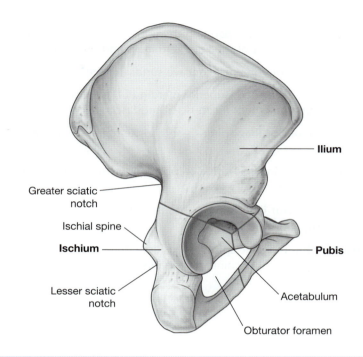

Figure 10-5 The os coxa: ilium, ischium, and pubis. (From Drake R, Vogl W, Mitchell A: Gray's Anatomy for Students. Philadelphia: Elsevier, 2005, Fig. 5.20)

Pelvic Bone Components — Ilium

■ The most superior of the three bones that form the os coxa; identify the following parts **(Figure 10-6)**:

- **Articular surface** — large L-shaped surface that articulates with the sacrum
- **Arcuate line** — ridge separating the upper and lower parts of the ilium; forms part of the linea terminalis and pelvic brim
- **Iliac fossa** — anteromedial concave surface of the ilium
- **Iliac crest** — thickened, superior margin of the ilium that serves as an attachment for muscles and fascia
- **Anterior superior iliac spine** — anterior termination of the iliac crest
- **Posterior superior iliac spine** — posterior termination of the iliac crest
- **Anterior inferior iliac spine** — positioned inferior to the anterior superior iliac spine
- **Posterior inferior iliac spine** — positioned inferior to the posterior superior iliac spine, on the posterior border of the sacral surface of the ilium

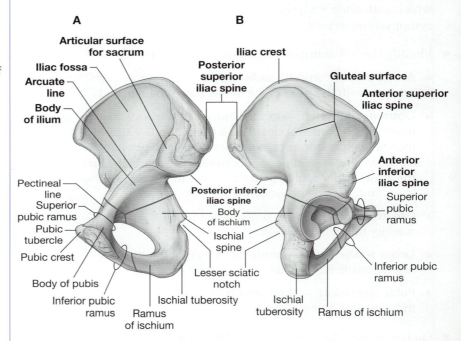

Figure 10-6 Ilium: components of the pelvic bone. **A,** Medial surface. **B,** Lateral surface. (From Drake R, Vogl W, Mitchell A: Gray's Anatomy for Students. Philadelphia: Elsevier, 2005, Fig. 5.21)

Pelvic Bone Components — Pubis

- The anterior and inferior bone of the os coxa is the **pubis**; has a body and two branches (rami); identify the following parts **(Figure 10-7)**:

  - **Pubic tubercle** — a rounded projection on the superior surface of the pubis

  - **Superior pubic ramus** — projects posterolaterally from the body of the pubis and joins the ilium and ischium; the superior pubic ramus is positioned toward the acetabulum

  - **Pectineal line (pecten pubis)** — sharp, superior margin on the superior pubic ramus; forms part of the linea terminalis and the pelvic inlet

  - **Pubic crest** — anteriorly, continuation of the pectineal line; also part of the linea terminalis and pelvic inlet

  - **Inferior pubic ramus** — projects laterally and inferiorly to join with the ramus of the ischium; the inferior pubic ramus and ischial ramus are termed the **ischiopubic (conjoint) ramus**

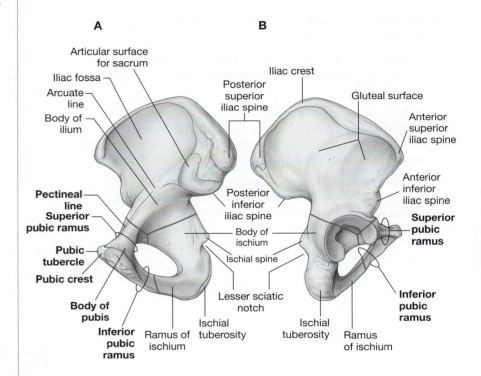

Figure 10-7 Ischium: components of the pelvic bone. **A,** Medial surface. **B,** Lateral surface. (From Drake R, Vogl W, Mitchell A: Gray's Anatomy for Students. Philadelphia: Elsevier, 2005, Fig. 5.21)

Pelvic Bone Components — Ischium

- The posterior and inferior bone of the os coxa; identify the following parts **(Figure 10-8)**:

  - **Ischial body** — projects superiorly to join with the ilium and the superior pubic ramus
  - **Ischial spine** — a pointed projection on the posterior margin of the ischium that separates the lesser and greater sciatic notches
  - **Ischial tuberosity** — the most prominent feature of the ischium; large bone protuberance on the posteroinferior aspect of the ischium; an important site for lower limb muscle attachments and for supporting the body when sitting
  - **Ischial ramus** — projects anteriorly to join with the inferior ramus of the pubis; the ischial ramus and inferior pubic ramus are oftentimes called the **ischiopubic ramus** or **conjoint ramus**

GAFS pp 382–383 ACGA pp 445–447 NAHA Plate 486

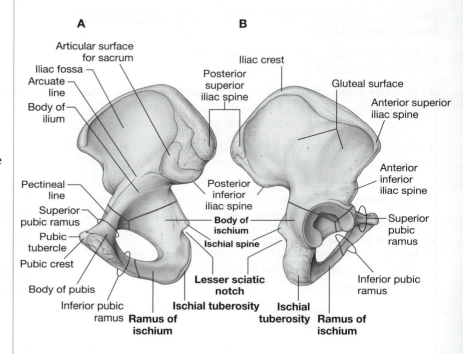

Figure 10-8 Pubis: components of the pelvic bone. **A,** Medial surface. **B,** Lateral surface. (From Drake R, Vogl W, Mitchell A: Gray's Anatomy for Students. Philadelphia: Elsevier, 2005, Fig. 5.21)

Sacrum and Coccyx

- Identify the following **(Figure 10-9)**:

  - **Sacrum** — formed by the fusion of the five sacral vertebrae; articulates with L5; its apex articulates with the coccyx

    - **Articular facet** — large L-shaped facet on the lateral surface of the sacrum for articulation with the ilium of the pelvis

    - **Promontory** — the anterior edge of the first sacral vertebra (S1)

    - **Ala** — broad, winglike transverse processes that flank the superior surface of the sacrum (superior aspect of S1)

    - **Anterior sacral foramina** (four pairs) — for the anterior rami of spinal nerves

    - **Posterior sacral foramina** (four pairs) — for the posterior rami of spinal nerves

    - **Sacral canal** — continuation of the vertebral canal that terminates in the sacral hiatus

  - **Coccyx** — the small terminal part of the vertebral column, consisting of four fused coccygeal vertebrae; articulates with the sacrum

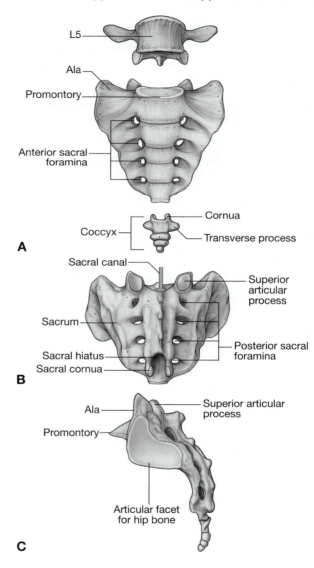

Figure 10-9 Sacrum and coccyx. **A,** Anterior view. **B,** Posterior view. **C,** Lateral view. (From Drake R, Vogl W, Mitchell A: Gray's Anatomy for Students. Philadelphia: Elsevier, 2005, Fig. 5.22)

Gender Differences

- The pelves of women and men differ in a number of ways, many having to do with a passageway for a fetus during parturition through a woman's pelvic cavity; note the following **(Figure 10-10)**:

  - **Pelvic inlet** — the typical female pelvic inlet is more circular in shape compared to the typically heart-shaped male pelvic inlet

  - **Pubic arch** — the angle formed by the two arms of the pubic bone is typically larger in women (80–85 degrees) than it is in men (50–60 degrees); the angle formed by the pubic arch can be approximated by the angle between the thumb and index finger for females and that between the index finger and middle finger for males, as shown in the insets

  - **Ischial spines** — generally do not project as far medially into the pelvic cavity in women as they do in men

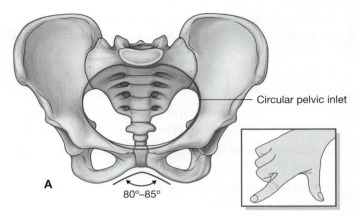

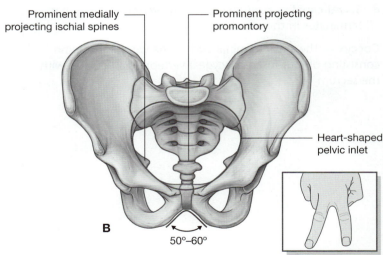

Figure 10-10 Gender differences of the bony pelvis. **A**, Female. **B**, Male. (From Drake R, Vogl W, Mitchell A: Gray's Anatomy for Students. Philadelphia: Elsevier, 2005, Fig. 5.27)

Anterior Abdominal Wall and Inguinal Canal

Lab 11

Prior to dissection, you should familiarize yourself with the following structures:

OSTEOLOGY
- Ribs (costal margin)
- Xiphoid process
- Pubis
  - Pubic symphysis
  - Pubic crest and tubercle
  - Pecten pubis
- Ilium
  - Iliac crest
  - Anterior superior iliac spine

MUSCLES
- Rectus abdominis m.
  - Tendinous intersections
  - Rectus sheath
    - Anterior and posterior layers
    - Arcuate line
- Pyramidalis m.
- External oblique m.
  - Inguinal ligament
    - Lacunar ligament
    - Superficial inguinal ring
- Internal oblique m.
- Transversus abdominis m.
  - Conjoint tendon (inguinal falx)
  - Deep inguinal ring

NERVES AND VESSELS
- Internal thoracic a. and v.
  - Superior epigastric aa. and vv.
  - Musculophrenic aa. and vv.
- Subcostal n. (T12)
- Iliohypogastric n. (L1)
- Ilioinguinal n. (L1)
- Genital branch of the genitofemoral n. (L1–L2)
- Lower intercostal and lumbar v., a., and n.
  - Lateral cutaneous v., a., and n.
  - Anterior cutaneous v., a., and n.
- External iliac a.
  - Inferior epigastric a. and v.
  - Deep circumflex iliac a. and v.
- Femoral a.
  - Superficial circumflex iliac a. and v.
  - Superficial epigastric a. and v.
- Lateral thoracic v.
  - Thoracoepigastric v.
- Paraumbilical vv.

SUPERFICIAL INGUINAL RING
- Medial and lateral crura
- Intercrural fibers
- Spermatic cord/round ligament of the uterus

ANTERIOR ABDOMINAL WALL (INTERNAL)
- Median umbilical fold (obliterated urachus)
- Medial umbilical folds (obliterated umbilical aa.)
- Lateral umbilical folds (inferior epigastric aa. and vv.)
- Superior epigastric aa. and vv.
- Falciform ligament (liver)
  - Ligamentum teres hepatis (obliterated umbilical v.)

Layers of the Anterolateral Abdominal Wall
- Skin
- Superficial fascia
  - Superficial (fatty) layer (Camper's fascia)
  - Deep (membranous) layer (Scarpa's fascia)
- External oblique m./aponeurosis
- Internal oblique m./aponeurosis
- Transversus abdominis m./aponeurosis
- Transversalis fascia
- Extraperitoneal fat
- Parietal peritoneum

OTHER STRUCTURES
- Umbilicus
- Linea alba
- Linea semilunaris
- Inguinal triangle
- Inguinal canal

Lab 11 Dissection Overview

The purpose of this laboratory session is to learn the anatomy of the anterior abdominal wall through dissection. You will do so through the following suggested sequence:

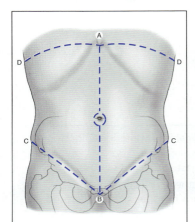

1. Identify surface anatomy landmarks, and make skin incisions.

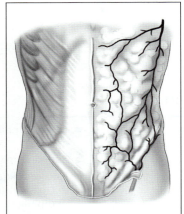

2. Identify cutaneous veins, superficial and deep fascia, and superficial abdominal muscles.

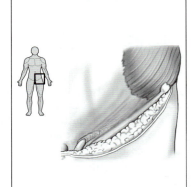

3. Identify the inguinal ligament, superficial inguinal ring, and associated structures.

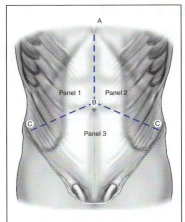

4. Make incisions in the anterior abdominal wall to study the muscle and fascial layers.

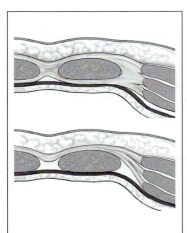

5. Identify the contributing layers to the rectus sheath above and below the arcuate line.

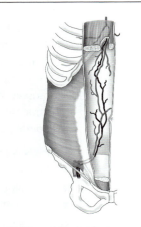

6. Dissect the lumbar vessels and nerves and the superior and inferior epigastric vessels.

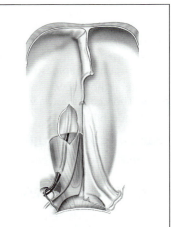

7. Study the internal surface of the anterior abdominal wall.

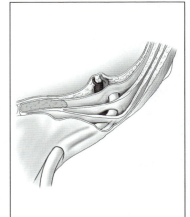

8. Study the inguinal canal and associated structures.

Table 11-1 Muscles of the Anterior Abdominal Wall

Muscle	Proximal Attachment	Distal Attachment	Action	Innervation
External oblique m.	Outer surfaces of ribs 5–12	Iliac crest; aponeurosis ending in the midline raphe (linea alba)	Compresses the abdominal contents; both muscles flex the trunk; each muscle bends the trunk to the same side, turning the anterior part of the abdomen to the opposite side	Anterior rami of spinal nerves T7–T12
Internal oblique m.	Thoracolumbar fascia; iliac crest and lateral two thirds of the inguinal ligament	Inferior border of ribs 9–12; aponeurosis ending in the linea alba; pubic crest and pectineal line	Compresses the abdominal contents; both muscles flex the trunk; each muscle bends the trunk and turns the anterior part of the abdomen to the same side	Anterior rami of spinal nerves T7–T12 and L1
Transversus abdominis m.	Thoracolumbar fascia; iliac crest; lateral one third of the inguinal ligament; costal cartilages of ribs 7–12	Aponeurosis ending in the linea alba; pubic crest and pectineal line	Compresses the abdominal contents	
Rectus abdominis m.	Pubic crest, pubic tubercle, and pubic symphysis	Costal cartilages of ribs 5–7; xiphoid process	Compresses the abdominal contents; flexes the vertebral column; tenses the abdominal wall	Anterior rami of spinal nerves T7–T12
Pyramidalis m.	Pubis and pubic symphysis	Linea alba	Tenses the linea alba	Anterior ramus of spinal nerve T12

Table 11-2 Layers of the Abdominal Wall and Scrotum (Male)

Layers of the Abdominal Wall	Corresponding Layers in the Scrotum
1. Skin	1. Skin
Superficial fascia	
2. Fatty (Camper's)	2. Disappears because the scrotum contains no fat
3. Membranous (Scarpa's)	3. Dartos muscle and fascia
4. External oblique m.	4. External spermatic fascia
5. Internal oblique m.	5. Cremaster muscle and fascia
6. Transversus abdominis m.	6. No contribution
7. Transversalis fascia	7. Internal spermatic fascia
8. Extraperitoneal fatty tissue	8. Areolar connective tissue
9. Peritoneum	9. Tunica vaginalis

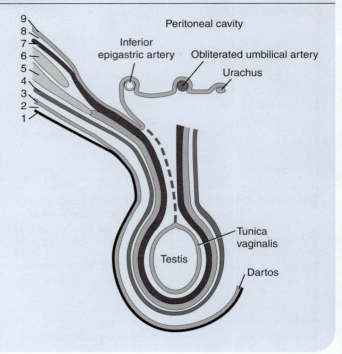

Orientation

- Locate the following surface structures. On thin bodies, these structures will appear as projections; on heavier bodies, the structures will need to be palpated **(Figure 11-1)**:
  - **Xiphoid process**
  - **Costal margin**
  - **Iliac crest**
  - **Anterior superior iliac spine**
  - **Location of the inguinal ligament**
  - **Pubic crest and tubercle**
  - **Umbilicus**

- During this dissection, you will explore nine layers of tissue that make up the anterolateral abdominal wall:
  1. Skin
  2. Camper's fascia (fatty layer of the superficial fascia) — variable in its thickness, depending on whether the cadaver is thin or fat
  3. Scarpa's fascia (membranous layer of the superficial fascia)
  4. External oblique m. — enveloped by deep fascia
  5. Internal oblique m. — enveloped by deep fascia
  6. Transversus abdominis m. — enveloped by deep fascia
  7. Transversalis fascia
  8. Extraperitoneal fat
  9. Parietal peritoneum

- Refer to **Figure 11-2** throughout this dissection as reference

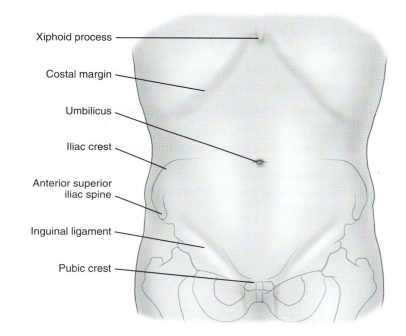

Figure 11-1 Abdominal surface anatomy

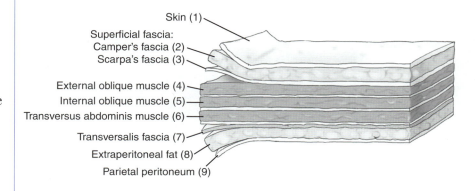

Figure 11-2 Layers of the anterolateral abdominal wall

Unit 3 • **Lab 11** Anterior Abdominal Wall and Inguinal Canal

Abdominal Skin Incisions

- With a scalpel, make the following incisions bilaterally to reflect the skin, but leave the superficial fascia (fat) intact **(Figure 11-3)**:

  - Xiphoid process *(A)* to the pubic symphysis *(B)* (cut circumferentially around the umbilicus)

  - Pubic symphysis *(B)* bilaterally to each iliac crest *(C)* along a straight line

  - Xiphoid process *(A)* bilaterally to each midaxillary line *(D)*

- After the incisions are made, reflect the skin flaps laterally to expose the superficial fascia; do not remove the skin from its lateral attachment

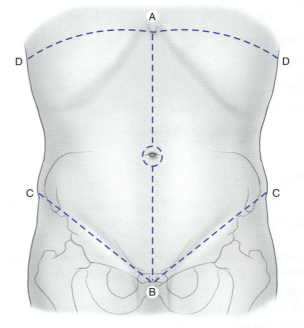

Figure 11-3 Abdominal skin incisions

Superficial Fascia

- On just one side, identify the two layers of the subcutaneous (superficial) fascia of the anterolateral abdominal wall **(Figure 11-4)**:

  - **Fatty (superficial) layer (Camper's fascia)** — the most external layer, composed mainly of fat that may be several centimeters thick or may be absent in emaciated bodies

  - **Membranous (deep) layer (Scarpa's fascia)** — inferior to the umbilicus; use a scalpel to make a midline incision through the superficial fascia, as shown in Figure 11-4

    - With forceps, reflect the margins of the cut fascia laterally to identify Camper's fascia externally (the fat) and Scarpa's fascia internally (the shiny, tougher membrane, much like plastic wrap, covering the deep surface of Camper's fascia)

- While reflecting the superficial fascia, explore the space between Scarpa's fascia and the deep fascia

  - Insert a finger into the space between Scarpa's fascia and the rectus sheath (very thick fascia that is immediately deep to Scarpa's fascia)

  - Push your finger in all directions (especially inferiorly into the upper region of the scrotal sac or labia majora)

  - Note the **fundiform ligament** superior to the penis or clitoris; a midline elevation/fold of fascia that helps to support the penis or clitoris (see Figure 11-5); to be dissected in a future laboratory session

  - *Note:* You cannot push your finger into the thigh because Scarpa's fascia is fused to the fascia lata (deep fascia of the thigh), 2.5 cm inferior to the inguinal ligament

- Reflect both flaps of the superficial fascia laterally to the midaxillary line; leave the umbilicus attached to the muscular abdominal wall; leave the flaps attached laterally

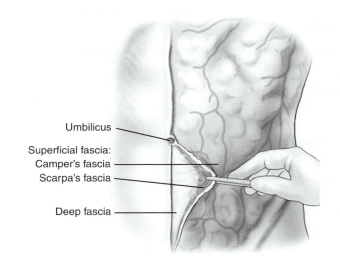

Figure 11-4 Superficial fascia inferior to the umbilicus

Cutaneous Nerves

- Use forceps to dissect and identify the following superficial veins and nerves on either side of the abdomen; use blunt dissection and the scraping technique to remove the fat **(Figure 11-5)**:

  - **Thoracoepigastric v.** — tributary of the lateral thoracic v., which is a tributary of the axillary v.

  - **Superficial epigastric v.** — probe through the fat between the umbilicus and inguinal region; tributary to the femoral v. (femoral v. will be dissected in a future laboratory session)

  - **Superficial circumflex iliac v.** — inferior and parallel to the inguinal ligament; tributary to the femoral v.

  - **Paraumbilical vv.** — tributaries to the lateral thoracic v.; also anastomose with deep veins, such as the portal v.; paraumbilical vv. contribute to the portal–caval anastomoses

  - **Anterior cutaneous nn.** — immediately lateral to the linea alba; pierce the anterior wall of the rectus sheath

    - **T7, T8, and T9 nn.** supply the skin region superior to the umbilicus

    - **T10 n.** supplies skin around the umbilicus

    - **T11, T12 (subcostal n.), and L1 (iliohypogastric and ilioinguinal nn.)** supply the skin region inferior to the umbilicus; the iliohypogastric n. is about 4 cm superior to the pubic symphysis, just superior to the superficial inguinal ring

  - **Lateral cutaneous nn.** — emerge through the serratus anterior and external oblique mm.

    - **T12 (subcostal) nn.** — emerge superior to the iliac crest and descend to supply that region of the skin

    - **L1 (iliohypogastric and ilioinguinal) nn.** — also emerge superior to the iliac crest (inferior and parallel to the subcostal n.) and descend to supply that region of the skin

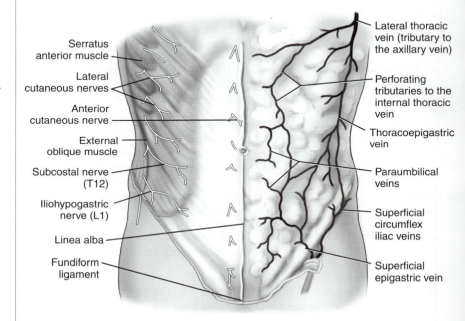

Figure 11-5 Cutaneous nerves and veins

Anterior Abdominal Wall Musculature

- Reflect or remove all superficial fascia on the anterior abdominal wall to identify the following **(Figure 11-6)**:

  - **External oblique m.** — observe the direction of its striations, which is from superolateral to inferomedial

  - **External oblique aponeurosis** — the anterior tendinous membrane of the external oblique m.; forms part of the anterior lamina of the **rectus sheath**

  - **Rectus sheath** — a tendinous sheath formed by the aponeuroses of the external and internal oblique and transversus abdominis mm.; surrounds the rectus abdominis m.

  - **Linea semilunaris** — superficial crease formed by the lateral border of the rectus sheath

  - **Tendinous intersections** — superior, middle, and inferior tendinous slips that anchor the anterior layer of the rectus sheath to the rectus abdominis m.

  - **Linea alba** — strong tendinous seam between the two rectus sheaths

  - **Pyramidalis m.** (often absent) — located deep to the anterior layer of the rectus sheath and anterior to the inferiormost portion of the rectus abdominis m.

    - To see the pyramidalis m., use a scalpel to make a short, vertical incision through the linea alba, immediately superior to the pubic symphysis; reflect the fascia to reveal the pyramidalis m. deep to the rectus sheath

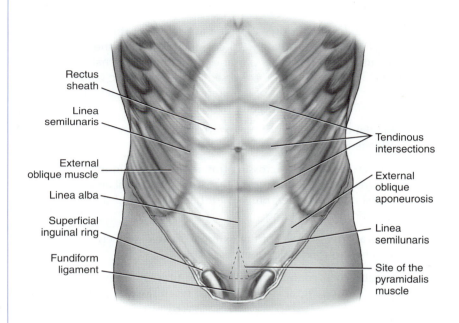

Figure 11-6 Anterior abdominal wall musculature

Superficial Inguinal Ring

- Dissect, using forceps, to identify the following **(Figure 11-7)**:
  - **Superficial inguinal ring** — located at the end of the inguinal canal approximately 2.5 cm superolateral to the pubic tubercle; a triangular passage through the external oblique aponeurosis that is traversed by the spermatic cord (male) or round ligament of the uterus (female); borders of the superficial inguinal ring are the following:
    - **Medial crus** — fibers of the external oblique aponeurosis attached to the pubic symphysis
    - **Intercrural fibers** — crossing (intercrural) fibers in the external oblique aponeurosis that hold the medial and lateral crura together; prevent further widening of the superficial inguinal ring
    - **Lateral crus** — fibers of the external oblique aponeurosis attached to the pubic tubercle
  - **Spermatic cord/round ligament of the uterus** — passes through the superficial inguinal ring to reach the perineum
  - **Inguinal ligament** — the inferior border of the external oblique aponeurosis between the anterior superior iliac spine laterally and the pubic tubercle medially (a better view of the inguinal ligament will be provided once the anterior abdominal wall is opened in a future laboratory session)
- *Note:* A thin layer of connective tissue overlies the superficial inguinal ring; you will need to dissect through it with forceps to get a clear view of the ring

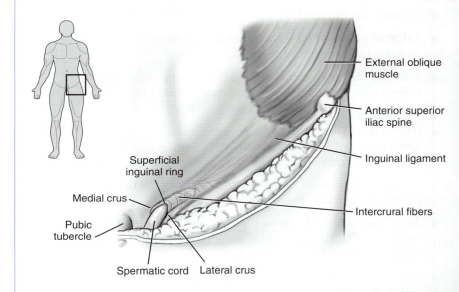

Figure 11-7 Superficial inguinal ring

Abdominal Wall Incisions

- With a scalpel, make the following abdominal incisions through the anterolateral abdominal wall **(Figure 11-8)**:
  - To avoid cutting the underlying viscera, make a 1-cm sagittal incision at *B*
  - Push a blunt probe through the hole and lift up the linea alba to extend the incision to the following points:
    - The xiphoid process *(A)*
    - About 2 cm above the anterior superior iliac spine *(C)* on both sides
- Fold the flaps laterally (see panels 1 and 2 in Figure 11-8) or inferiorly (see panel 3 in Figure 11-8) to expose the abdominal contents
- Panels 1, 2, and 3 from Figure 11-8 will be referred to in subsequent dissections of the anterior abdominal wall

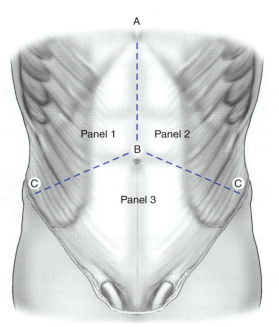

Figure 11-8 Abdominal wall incisions

Layers of the Anterior Abdominal Wall

- Use a probe to separate the layers in the cut edges of panels 1 and 2 of the abdominal wall

- Identify the following **(Figure 11-9)**:

  - **External oblique m.** — the most superficial of the three flat anterolateral abdominal wall muscles; muscle fibers course in an inferomedial direction; its large aponeurosis covers the anterior part of the abdominal wall to the midline
    - Approaching the midline, the aponeuroses are entwined, forming the **linea alba**, which extends from the xiphoid process to the pubic symphysis
  - **Internal oblique m.** — intermediate muscle layer deep to the external oblique m.; the striations course at right angles to the external oblique m. in a superomedial direction
    - Anteriorly the internal oblique aponeuroses blend into the linea alba at the midline
  - **Transversus abdominis m.** — deep muscle layer (deep to the internal oblique); the striations course, for the most part, in the transverse plane
    - Anteriorly the aponeuroses blend with the linea alba at the midline
  - **Rectus abdominis m.** — courses longitudinally from the sternum and costal margin to the pubis; the paired muscles are separated by the linea alba
  - **Transversalis fascia** — a thin continuous layer of fascia between the transversus abdominis m. and rectus abdominis m. (superficially) and the extraperitoneal fat (deep)
  - **Extraperitoneal fat** — located between the transversalis fascia and parietal peritoneum
  - **Parietal peritoneum** — serous lining on the internal surface of the abdominal wall

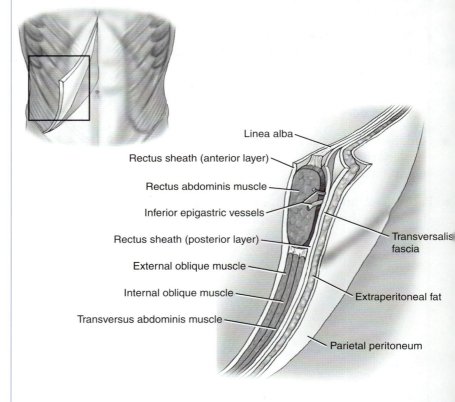

Figure 11-9 Layers of the anterior abdominal wall

Anterior Abdominal Wall — Rectus Sheath

- Using blunt dissection to tease the layers apart, identify the following **(Figures 11-10, 11-11,** and **11-12)**:

  - **Rectus abdominis m.** — long, flat muscle that extends the vertical length of the anterior abdominal wall; a paired muscle, separated in the midline by the linea alba; widens and thins as it ascends from the pubic symphysis to costal cartilages 5–7

    - **Linea alba** — a dense aponeurotic band running from the xiphoid process to the pubic symphysis; intervenes between the two rectus abdominis mm.

  - **Rectus sheath** — tendinous sheath surrounding the rectus abdominis m., formed by the aponeuroses of the external oblique, internal oblique, and transversus abdominis mm.; contains the superior and inferior epigastric vessels and anterior cutaneous neurovascular bundles

    - With scissors or a scalpel, make a vertical incision to open the anterior layer of the rectus sheath to display its contents; observe that, along its course, the rectus abdominis m. is intersected by three or four tendinous insertions; sever these connections with a scalpel and observe the following:

      - In its upper three quarters (above the arcuate line), the rectus sheath consists of an anterior layer (formed by the aponeuroses of the external and internal oblique mm.) and a posterior layer (formed by the aponeuroses of the internal oblique and transversus abdominis mm.)

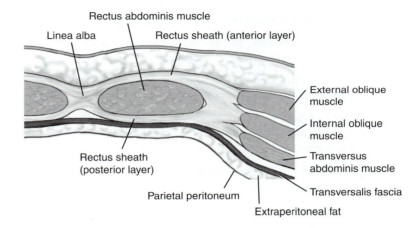

Figure 11-10 Cross-section of the rectus sheath superior to the arcuate line

Anterior Abdominal Wall — Rectus Sheath Continued

Anterior Abdominal Wall — Rectus Sheath—cont'd

- ♦ In its lower one quarter, the rectus sheath consists of an anterior layer only (formed by the aponeuroses of all three anterior abdominal wall muscles)
- ♦ At the **arcuate line**, the inferior edge of the posterior layer of the rectus sheath is distinct
- ♦ Inferior to the arcuate line, the rectus abdominis m. is in direct contact with the transversalis fascia

- **Transversalis fascia** — a thin aponeurotic membrane between the transversus abdominis m., rectus abdominis m., and the extraperitoneal fat
- **Extraperitoneal fat** — located between the transversalis fascia and parietal peritoneum
- **Parietal peritoneum** — serous lining on the internal surface of the abdominal wall

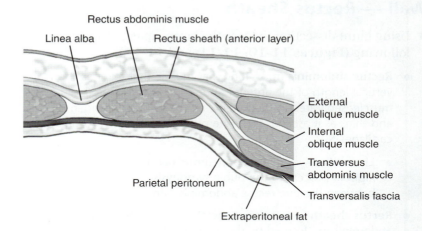

Figure 11-11   Cross-section of the rectus sheath inferior to the arcuate line

Epigastric Vessels Deep to the Rectus Abdominis Muscle

GAFS pp 253–256   ACGA pp 426–428   NAHA Plates 251, 253, 255–256

- Bluntly dissect the rectus abdominis m. from the posterior layer of the rectus sheath

- Identify the following **(Figure 11-12)**:

  - **Superior epigastric vessels** — found on the deep surface of the rectus abdominis m.; terminal branches of the internal thoracic vessels; usually smaller than the inferior epigastric vessels

  - **Inferior epigastric vessels** — arise from the external iliac vessels, superior to the inguinal ligament; course superiorly in the transversalis fascia to reach the posterior surface of the rectus abdominis m. in the vicinity of the arcuate line; course deep to the posterior layer of the rectus sheath above the arcuate line

    - The superior and inferior epigastric vessels anastomose on the deep surface of the rectus abdominis m.

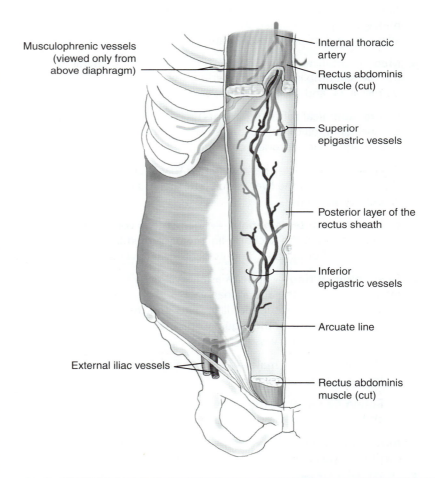

Figure 11-12 Epigastric vessels

Anterior Abdominal Wall — Internal Surface

- Identify the following structures on the internal surface of the abdominal wall **(Figure 11-13)**:

  - **Med*ian* umbilical fold (ligament)** — unpaired fold in the midsagittal plane; formed by the urachus (obliterated allantois) and its peritoneal covering

  - **Med*ial* umbilical folds (ligaments)** — paired folds lateral to the median umbilical fold; formed by the obliterated umbilical aa. and their peritoneal covering

  - **Lateral umbilical folds (ligaments)** — paired folds lateral to the medial umbilical folds; formed by the inferior epigastric vessels and their peritoneal covering

  - **Falciform ligament** — peritoneal fold that spans between the umbilicus and the liver (studied further in another laboratory session)

    - **Ligamentum teres hepatis** — ligamentous cord in the free margin of the falciform ligament; formed by the obliterated umbilical v. and its peritoneal covering

  - **Deep inguinal ring** — appears as an oval defect on the internal surface of the abdominal wall; located midway between the anterior superior iliac spine and the pubic symphysis, superior to the inguinal ligament and lateral to the inferior epigastric vessels

    - **Ductus deferens (male)** — exits the abdominal cavity via the deep inguinal ring

    - **Round ligament of the uterus (female)** — exits the abdominal cavity via the deep inguinal ring

  - **Inguinal triangle** — bounded by the rectus abdominis m. medially, inguinal ligament inferiorly, and inferior epigastric vessels laterally

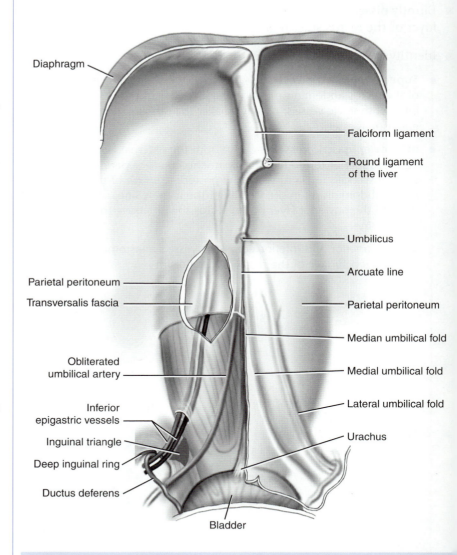

Figure 11-13 Internal view of the anterior abdominal wall; the peritoneum is removed from the left side

Inguinal Canal — Borders

GAFS pp 256–265   NAHA Plates 259–261

- **Inguinal canal** — the passageway (about 2–3 cm long) through the inferior part of the abdominal wall that lies parallel and superior to the inguinal ligament; located between the superficial and deep inguinal rings **(Figure 11-14)**

- With scissors or a scalpel, make a cut through the external abdominal aponeurosis, about 5 cm above the inguinal ligament, from the region of the superficial to deep inguinal ring to the muscular portion of the external abdominal m. (see Figure 11-14A)

- Bluntly dissect the external oblique m. from the internal oblique m.; identify the following borders of the inguinal canal (see Figure 11-14B and 11-14C):
  - **External opening** — superficial inguinal ring
  - **Roof** — fascia of the internal oblique and transversus abdominis mm.
  - **Floor** — formed by the lacunar, pectineal, and inguinal ligaments
    - **Lacunar ligament** — formed by the external oblique aponeurosis; wraps underneath and medial to the contents of the inguinal canal; attaches along the pectineal line
    - **Pectineal ligament** — fibers of the lacunar ligament that continue laterally along the pecten pubis
  - **Anterior wall** — aponeurosis of the external oblique m.
  - **Posterior wall** — transversalis fascia and conjoint tendon
    - **Conjoint tendon** — formed by fusion of the inferior, medial fibers of both the internal oblique and transversus abdominis mm.; attaches to the pubic crest and pecten pubis
  - **Internal opening** — deep inguinal ring

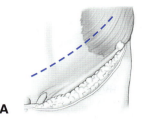
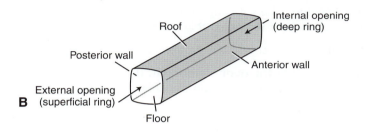
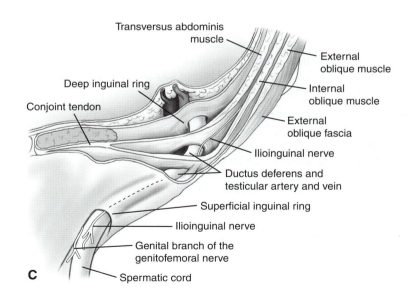

Figure 11-14   Inguinal canal borders. **A,** Incision line. **B,** Schematic of the inguinal canal. **C,** Expanded view of the inguinal region on the left side

BOTH SEXES

Inguinal Canal — Contents

- Identify the following **(Figure 11-15)**:

  - **Ilioinguinal n. (L1)** — descends into the inguinal canal, between the internal and external oblique mm.
    - **Male** — traverses the inguinal canal, coursing along the inferior aspect of the spermatic cord to the superficial inguinal ring, where it contributes to cutaneous innervation from the upper thigh, scrotum, and penis
    - **Female** — same course but supplies the labia majora
  - **Genital branch of the genitofemoral n. (L1–L2)** — also enters the inguinal canal through the deep inguinal ring
    - **Male** — supplies the cremaster m. and the scrotal skin
    - **Female** — supplies the skin of the mons pubis and labia majora
  - **Spermatic cord** (male) — courses from the prostate gland (pelvic cavity), through the deep inguinal ring lateral to the inferior epigastric vessels, inguinal canal, and superficial inguinal ring; extends to the scrotum to reach the posterior border of the testis
  - **Round ligament of the uterus** (female) — courses from the uterus (pelvic cavity), through the deep inguinal ring, inguinal canal, and superficial inguinal ring; spreads into fibrous strands within the labia majora

- The inguinal canal also contains blood and lymphatic vessels

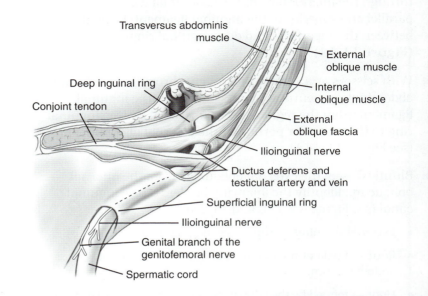

Figure 11-15 Contents of the inguinal canal on the left side

Lab 12

Peritoneum and Foregut

Prior to dissection, you should familiarize yourself with the following structures:

PERITONEUM
- Mesentery
  - Root of the mesentery
- Mesocolon
  - Transverse mesocolon
  - Sigmoid mesocolon
  - Mesoappendix
- Lesser omentum
  - Hepatophrenic ligament
  - Hepatogastric ligament
  - Hepatoduodenal ligament
- Greater omentum
  - Gastrosplenic ligament
  - Splenorenal ligament
- Peritoneal attachments of the liver
  - Coronary ligament
    - Falciform ligament
    - Triangular ligaments
    - Hepatorenal ligament
- Recesses, fossae, and folds
- Peritoneal cavity
  - Greater sac
  - Lesser sac (omental bursa)
    - Omental (epiploic) foramen
- Paravesical fossa
- Rectovesical pouch
- Vesicouterine pouch
- Rectouterine pouch

ARTERIES
- Celiac trunk
  - Left gastric a.
    - Esophageal a.
  - Splenic a.
    - Left gastro-omental a.
    - Short gastric aa.
  - Common hepatic a.
    - Hepatic a. proper
      - Right gastric a.
      - Left and right hepatic aa.
        - Cystic a.
    - Gastroduodenal a.
      - Supraduodenal a.
      - Anterior/posterior superior pancreaticoduodenal a.
      - Right gastro-omental a.

STOMACH
- Greater and lesser curvatures
- Pylorus and pyloric sphincter
- Body, cardia, and fundus
- Gastric rugae

SMALL INTESTINE
- Duodenum
  - Duodenojejunal junction
  - Suspensory ligament of the duodenum
- Jejunum and ileum
- Ileocecal junction

LARGE INTESTINE
- Cecum
  - Vermiform appendix
- Ascending colon
- Transverse colon
- Descending colon
- Sigmoid colon
- Rectum
- Anus

LIVER
- Diaphragmatic and visceral surfaces
- Left and right lobes
- Quadrate and caudate lobes
- Falciform and round ligaments (ventral mesentery)
- Porta hepatis
- Subphrenic recess
- Bare area
- Common hepatic duct
  - Cystic duct
  - Common bile duct

OTHER ABDOMINAL ORGANS
- Gallbladder
- Spleen
- Pancreas

Lab 12 Dissection Overview

The purpose of this laboratory session is to learn the anatomy of the peritoneum and foregut through dissection. You will do so through the following suggested sequence:

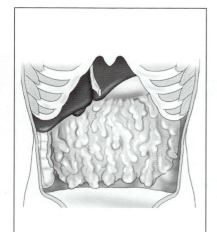

1. Identify the greater omentum, lesser omentum, greater sac, lesser sac, and omental foramen.

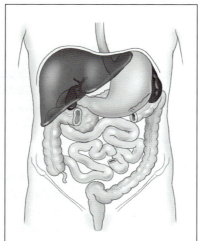

2. Gain an overview of the organs of the abdominal cavity.

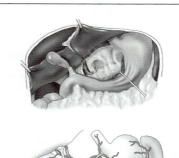
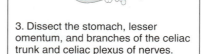

3. Dissect the stomach, lesser omentum, and branches of the celiac trunk and celiac plexus of nerves.

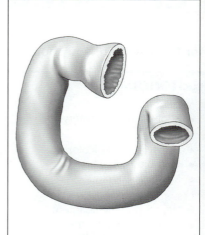

4. Dissect the duodenum.

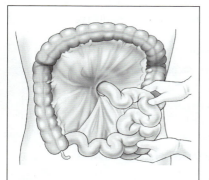

5. Identify the duodenojejunal junction, and observe the intraperitoneal and retroperitoneal regions of the duodenum.

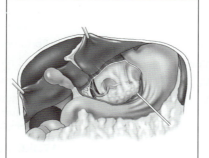

6. Dissect the spleen.

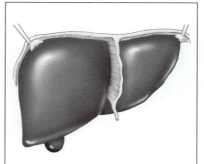

7. Study the surfaces, lobes, ligaments, and internal structure of the liver.

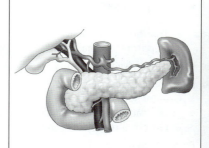

8. Dissect the porta hepatis, which consists of the portal vein, hepatic artery proper, and common bile duct.

Peritoneal Cavity — Greater Omentum

- As a result of incisions already made through the abdominal wall (previous lab), you have cut through the anterior layer of the parietal peritoneum

- Identify the following (do not cut) **(Figures 12-1 and 12-2)**:

  - **Peritoneal cavity** (greater sac) — the potential space between the visceral and parietal layers of peritoneum; divided into two regions—the greater and lesser sacs:

    - **Greater sac** — the space between the parietal and visceral peritoneum, not including the sac deep to the stomach (lesser sac)

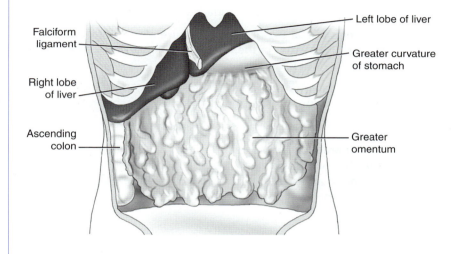

Figure 12-1 Greater omentum in situ

Peritoneal Cavity — Greater Omentum Continued

Peritoneal Cavity — Greater Omentum—cont'd

- **Greater omentum** — apron of adipose and connective tissue covering the abdominal viscera; consists of a double sheet that folds upon itself to create four layers of peritoneum:
  - One sheet descends from the anterior surface of the stomach, the other from the posterior surface of the stomach
  - Both sheets fuse at the **greater curvature** of the stomach and descend, in front of the transverse colon and small intestine, toward the pelvis
  - This membrane turns upon itself and ascends; at the **transverse colon**, it forms the gastrocolic ligament
    - *Note:* In most adults, the four layers are fused
  - The left border of the greater omentum is continuous with the **gastrosplenic ligament**; the right border extends to the **duodenum** (studied further in another laboratory session); expect variations

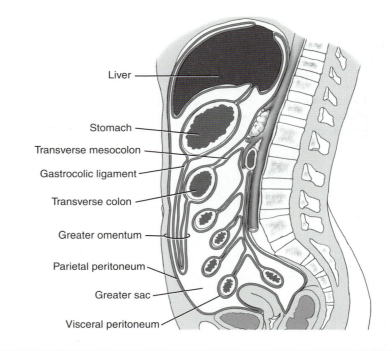

Figure 12-2 Female abdominopelvic cavity (sagittal section)

Peritoneal Cavity — Lesser Omentum

- Lift up the liver to identify the following (do not cut) (**Figures 12-3** and **12-4**):

  - **Lesser omentum** — two layers of peritoneum that course from the anterior and posterior surfaces of the stomach and proximal part of the duodenum, fuse at the **lesser curvature** of the stomach, and ascend to the liver; two ligaments comprise the lesser omentum:

    - **Hepatogastric ligament** — the part of the lesser omentum between the liver and the stomach

    - **Hepatoduodenal ligament** — the part of the lesser omentum between the liver and the duodenum

      - **Porta hepatis** — enclosed in the free border of the hepatoduodenal ligament; contains the common bile duct, hepatic a., and portal v.

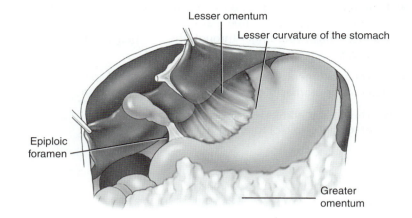

Figure 12-3 Lesser omentum in situ

Peritoneal Cavity — Lesser Omentum Continued

Peritoneal Cavity — Lesser Omentum—cont'd

- **Omental (epiploic) foramen** — located on the right side of the midline, deep to the free margin of the hepatoduodenal ligament; push your finger through the foramen into the lesser sac
- **Lesser sac** (omental bursa) — potential peritoneal space deep to the stomach, duodenum, and lesser omentum
  - The greater and lesser sacs communicate through the omental (epiploic) foramen

GAFS pp 225, 230, 266–271   ACGA pp 390–391   NAHA Plates 272–273, 275

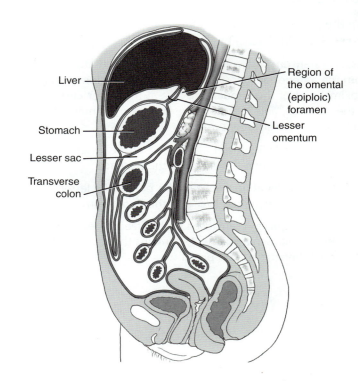

Figure 12-4 Lesser omentum and lesser sac

Overview of the Abdominal Viscera

- Identify the following within the abdominal cavity (do not cut) **(Figure 12-5)**:

  - **Liver** — positioned in the right upper quadrant
  - **Gallbladder** — attached to the inferior surface of the liver (may be absent due to surgical removal)
  - **Stomach** — left upper quadrant, inferior to the left lobe of the liver
  - **Spleen** — left upper quadrant, posterior and lateral to the stomach; touches the diaphragm and the tail of the pancreas; slide your right hand into the peritoneal cavity, lateral to the stomach, to cup the spleen in your hand

- Reflect the greater omentum superiorly to expose the intestine, and identify the following. (*Note:* It may be necessary to bluntly dissect or cut omental adhesions during reflection).

  - Most of the **duodenum** (first segment of the small intestine) and all of the **pancreas** are retroperitoneal and cannot be seen at this time
  - **Jejunum** — second segment of the small intestine
  - **Ileum** — third segment of the small intestine
  - **Ileocecal junction** — right lower quadrant; union of the ileum to the cecum
  - **Cecum** and the **vermiform appendix** — right lower quadrant; the appendix is located on the inferior border of the cecum (appendix may be absent following surgical removal; do not search for the appendix at this time)
  - **Ascending, transverse, descending, and sigmoid colon** — extend from the right lower quadrant to the left lower quadrant
  - **Kidneys** and **adrenal glands** — retroperitoneal; the right kidney is inferior to the liver; the left kidney is slightly superior to the right kidney because of the liver; palpate but do not dissect the kidneys at this time; the kidneys will be studied further in another laboratory session

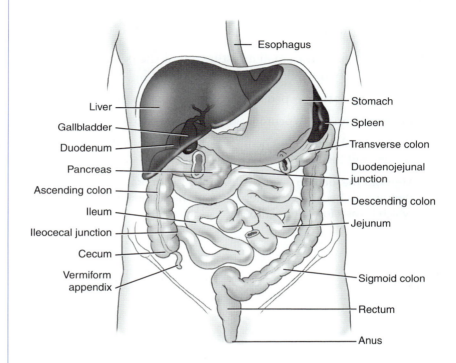

Figure 12-5 Abdominal viscera in situ

Pelvic Peritoneum — Male

- The instructions on this page aim to help you, the student, understand the continuation of the peritoneum into the pelvic cavity (do *not* dissect the pelvic organs at this time)

- Gently lift loops of the small intestine out of the pelvic basin to identify the following **(Figure 12-6)**:

  - **Paravesical fossae** — peritoneal recesses lateral to the bladder
  - **Pararectal fossae** — peritoneal recesses lateral to the rectum
  - **Rectovesical pouch** — a peritoneal recess between the rectum and the bladder
  - **Sigmoid mesocolon** — at the level of S3 vertebra, the peritoneum becomes the mesentery of the sigmoid colon, which is therefore intraperitoneal

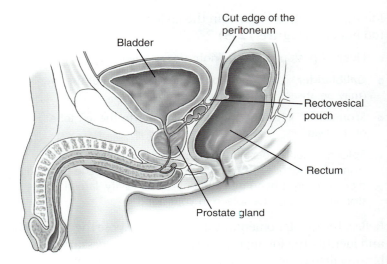

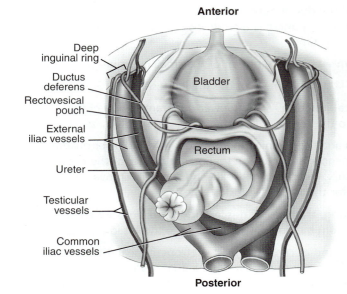

Figure 12-6 Male pelvic peritoneum

Pelvic Peritoneum — Female

- The instructions on this page aim to help you, the student, understand the continuation of the peritoneum into the pelvic cavity (do *not* dissect the pelvic organs at this time)

- Gently lift loops of the small intestine out of the pelvic basin to identify the following **(Figure 12-7)**:

  - **Vesicouterine pouch** — a peritoneal recess between the bladder and uterus
  - **Rectouterine pouch** — a peritoneal recess between the rectum and uterus
  - **Paravesical fossae** — peritoneal recesses lateral to the bladder
  - **Pararectal fossae** — peritoneal recesses lateral to the rectum
  - **Sigmoid mesocolon** — at the level of S3 vertebra, the peritoneum becomes the mesentery of the sigmoid colon, which is therefore intraperitoneal

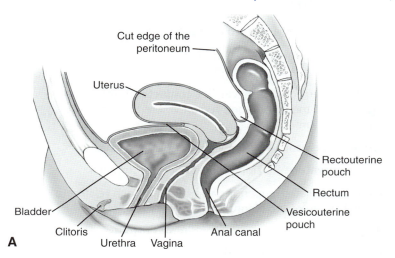

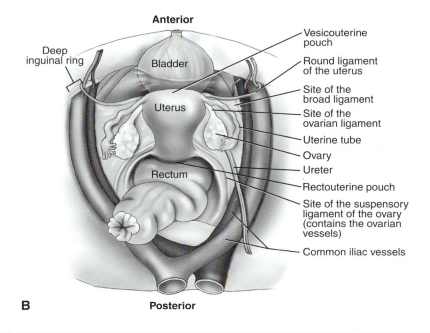

Figure 12-7 Female pelvic peritoneum

Foregut — Stomach

■ Identify the following **(Figures 12-8** and **12-9)**:

- **Esophagus** — the terminal end empties into the cardia of the stomach

- **Cardia** — territory of the **cardiac sphincter**, formed by the right crus of the diaphragm; region where the esophagus enters the stomach

- **Greater curvature** — inferior border of the stomach

- **Lesser curvature** — superior border of the stomach

- **Fundus** — dilated, superior part of the stomach related to the left dome of the diaphragm

- **Body** — region between the fundus and pylorus

- **Pylorus** — funnel-shaped, terminal region of the stomach; surrounds the **pyloric sphincter**

- **Gastric rugae** — use scissors to make an incision through the anterior wall of the stomach to reveal the longitudinal gastric rugae (folds)

- **Pyloric sphincter** — make a sagittal incision through the pylorus to observe the pyloric sphincter (thick band of smooth muscle)

- **Gastric canal** — the direct communication between the cardia and pylorus of the stomach

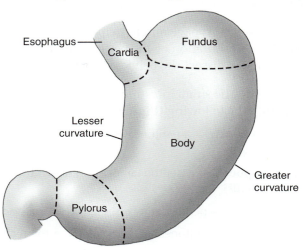

Figure 12-8 Stomach regions

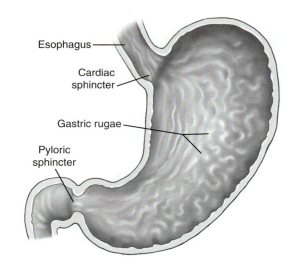

Figure 12-9 Coronal section of the stomach

Vasculature — Locating the Celiac Trunk

- To access the branches of the celiac trunk, follow these instructions:

  - Cut the sixth and seventh right costal cartilages near the xiphisternal junction to open the dissection field; you may partially incise the diaphragm (**Figure 12-10**)
  - Lift the liver superiorly and push the transverse colon inferiorly (**Figure 12-11**)
  - Use forceps and your fingers to shred the lesser omentum to reveal branches of the celiac trunk

- The arterial supply to the GI tract arises from three principal unpaired branches of the abdominal aorta (**Figure 12-12**):

  - Celiac trunk
  - Superior mesenteric artery
  - Inferior mesenteric artery
    - These branches supply the foregut, midgut, and hindgut, respectively

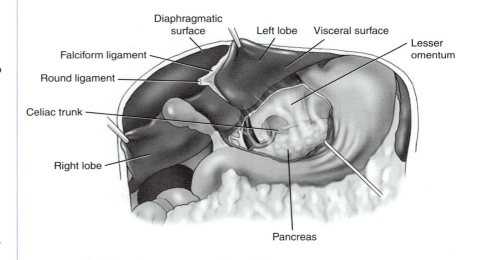

Figure 12-11 Celiac trunk topography

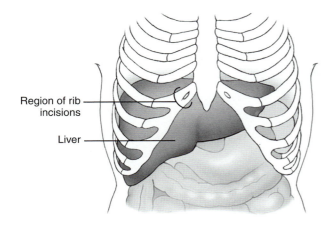

Figure 12-10 Rib dissection to reveal the celiac trunk

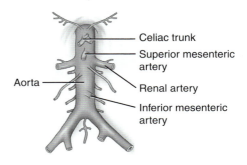

Figure 12-12 Branches of the abdominal aorta

Vasculature — Branches of the Celiac Trunk

- **Celiac trunk** — the principal arterial supply to the foregut; the first unpaired branch from the abdominal aorta; located at the level of T12 vertebra **(Figure 12-13)**

- To dissect the branches of the celiac trunk, you will dissect the lesser omentum to reveal the arteries (and veins) to the foregut organs
  - To avoid cutting the vessels, use pointed forceps and your fingers (do *not* use a scalpel or scissors)
  - Lift up and hold the liver elevated from the lesser omentum, which will be shredded to reveal the branches of the celiac a.
  - The origin of the celiac trunk will be dissected later, once the organs that overlie the abdominal aorta are dissected

- Identify the three primary branches of the celiac trunk, along with their successive branches:
  - **Common hepatic a.** — branch to the liver
  - **Left gastric a.** — branch to the lesser curvature of the stomach
  - **Splenic a.** — branch to the spleen

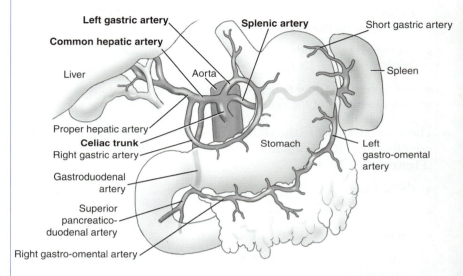

Figure 12-13 Branches of the celiac trunk

Innervation — Nerves of the Stomach and Duodenum

■ Identify the following **(Figure 12-14)**:

- **Celiac ganglia** — bilateral network of autonomic nerve fibers that surrounds the celiac trunk; each ganglia is approximately the size of a quarter and distributes its plexuses of nerves to their destinations along the blood vessels
  - Site of synapse of the preganglionic sympathetic fibers from the greater splanchnic nerves (T5–T9 spinal cord segments)
  - Use scissors to cut the ganglia to see the origin of the celiac trunk
  - Dissection of the celiac trunk is challenging because it is surrounded by the very tough celiac ganglia

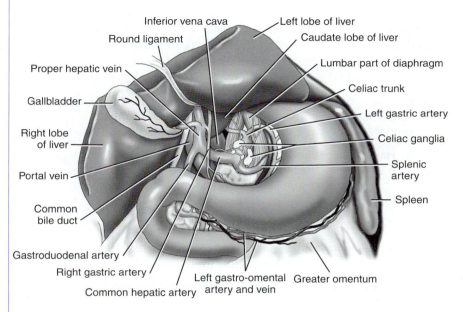

Figure 12-14 Celiac ganglia

Celiac Trunk — Common Hepatic Artery and Its Branches

■ Dissect through the free border of the lesser omentum to reveal and identify the common hepatic a.; follow it proximally and distally to find the other branches (you may want to dissect all of the vessels in their entirety before identifying them); identify the following branches **(Figure 12-15)**:

- **Common hepatic a.** — branch to the liver, gallbladder, stomach, duodenum, and pancreas; gives origin to the proper hepatic, right gastric, and right gastroduodenal aa.
  - **Hepatic a. proper** — dissect the hepatic a. proper, which is superior to the bile duct and lateral to the origin of the right gastric a.; supplies the liver and gallbladder
    - **Right gastric a.** — courses to the lesser curvature of the stomach on its right-hand side
    - **Left and right hepatic aa.** — course to the left and right sides of the liver, respectively
    - **Cystic a.** — a small branch of the right hepatic a. to the gallbladder
  - **Gastroduodenal a.** — free and elevate the duodenum distal to the pylorus; turn the pyloric end of the stomach to the left, and trace the gastroduodenal a. downward posterior to the first part of the duodenum, where it ends by dividing into the following two branches:
    - **Right gastro-omental a.** — right side of the greater curvature of the stomach; dissect through the greater omentum to reveal this artery
    - **Superior pancreaticoduodenal a.** — to dissect the superior pancreaticoduodenal a., lift up the stomach to reveal the duodenum and pancreas; the arteries course along the medial border of the duodenum; the pair of terminal branches consists of the anterior and posterior pancreaticoduodenal aa.

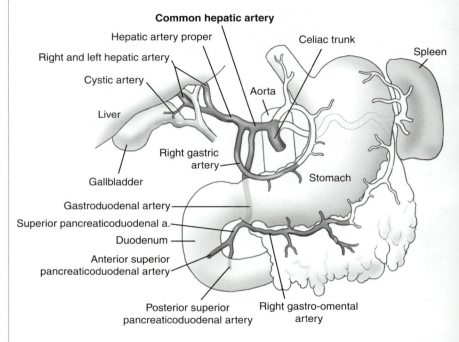

Figure 12-15 Common hepatic artery branches of the celiac trunk

Celiac Trunk — Left Gastric and Splenic Arteries

- Continue to dissect the celiac trunk to identify the remaining two branches; use blunt dissection through the related peritoneal ligaments and omenta **(Figure 12-16)**:

  - **Left gastric a.** — branch to the stomach and distal end of the esophagus; follow to the left side of the lesser curvature of the stomach, where the artery anastomoses with the right gastric a.; complete the dissection of both arteries to reveal their anastomosis

    - **Esophageal a.** — attempt to identify an arterial branch from the left gastric a. to the esophagus

  - **Splenic a.** — lift up the stomach to dissect the splenic a.; branch to the spleen and pancreas, and stomach; shaped like a corkscrew as it courses over/through/under the pancreas to reach the spleen; courses within the splenorenal ligament

    - **Short gastric aa.** — arise from the splenic a., near the hilum of the spleen; supplies the fundus of the stomach

    - **Left gastro-omental a.** — arises from the splenic a., near the hilum of the spleen; supplies the greater curvature of stomach; anastomoses with the right gastro-omental a.; complete the dissection of both arteries to reveal their anastomosis

- If necessary, trim the greater omentum from the greater curvature of the stomach; leave the gastro-omental vessels attached to the stomach and leave the greater omentum attached to the transverse colon

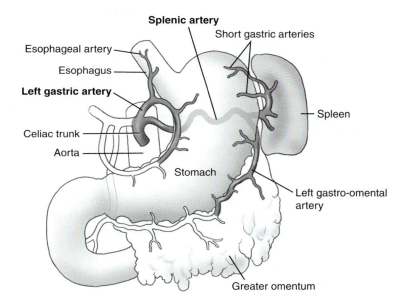

Figure 12-16 Left gastric and splenic artery branches of the celiac trunk

Foregut — Duodenum

- The duodenum is the first segment of the small intestine; C shaped and about 20–25 cm (12 inches) long; curves around the head of the pancreas; most of the duodenum is retroperitoneal (see Figure 12-2)

- To locate the **duodenum**:
  - Lift the transverse colon superiorly **(Figure 12-17)**
  - Grasp and move the small intestine to the left lower side (quadrant) of the abdomen
  - Use blunt dissection (fingers) to shred the transverse mesocolon to reveal the duodenum; avoid damaging blood vessels by dissecting in a superior to inferior plane

- Identify the following **(Figure 12-18)**:
  - **Superior (first) part** — 5 cm long; contiguous with the stomach; lies anterolateral to L1 vertebra; the proximal region is mobile but the distal region and remainder of the duodenum are retroperitoneal
  - **Descending (second) part** — 7–10 cm long; descends to the right of L1–L3 vertebrae; curves around the head of the pancreas; the bile and pancreatic ducts enter its posteromedial wall
  - **Horizontal (third) part** — 6–8 cm long; crosses L3 vertebra; crossed by the superior mesenteric a. and v.
  - **Ascending (fourth) part** — 5 cm long; ascends on the left of L3–L2 vertebrae; contiguous with the jejunum

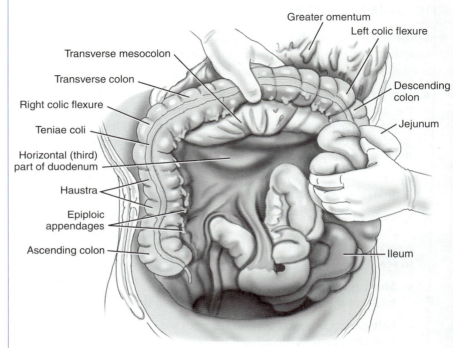

Figure 12-17 Duodenum in situ

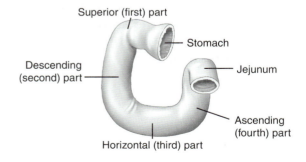

Figure 12-18 Regions of the duodenum

Duodenojejunal Junction

- Lift the transverse colon superiorly onto the rib cage and move the small intestine to the lower left side of the abdomen

- Following the intestinal tube proximally, identify the following (**Figures 12-19** and **12-20**):

  - **Duodenojejunal junction** — region where the immobile (retroperitoneal) duodenum ends and the mobile (intraperitoneal) jejunum begins; demarcated by the suspensory ligament of the duodenum

  - **Suspensory ligament of the duodenum** — attaches the duodenum to the right crus of the diaphragm

  - **Duodenal fossa** — fossa formed by folds of peritoneum created by the retroperitoneal-to-intraperitoneal transition of the first two parts of the duodenum; insert your finger into the fossa (left side of the duodenojejunal junction) to feel the ascending (fourth) portion of the duodenum

  - **Transverse mesocolon** — mesentery of the transverse colon; bluntly dissect the transverse mesocolon at the duodenal fossa to reveal the retroperitoneal part of the pancreas; avoid damaging blood vessels by dissecting in a superior to inferior plain

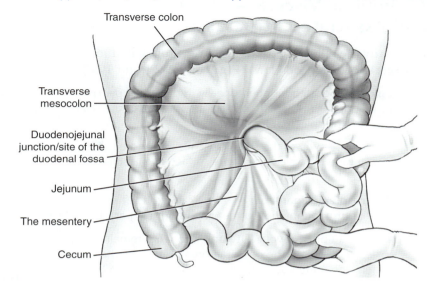

Figure 12-19 Duodenojejunal junction

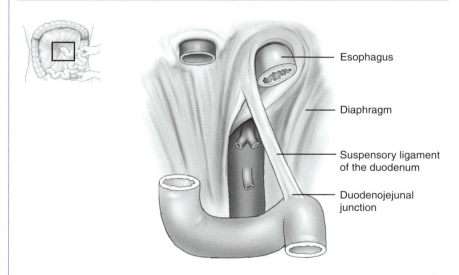

Figure 12-20 Suspensory ligament of the duodenum

Abdominal Viscera — Spleen and Associated Structures

- Identify the following (move the liver, stomach, and other viscera to get a good view) **(Figures 12-21** and **12-22)**:

  - **Spleen** — located intraperitoneally in the left upper quadrant; rests superior to the left colic flexure; the tail of the pancreas touches the spleen at its hilum

    - **Hilum** — where the splenic vessels exit and enter; peritoneum covers the entire surface of the spleen, except at this point

  - **Gastrosplenic ligament** — on the cadaver's left side, push your right hand inferior to the diaphragm to grasp the spleen

    - Push a finger of your left hand into what remains of the lesser sac, from the omental foramen toward the cadaver's left side, until your fingers make contact with a barrier; this barrier is the **gastrosplenic ligament**; contains the short gastric and left gastro-omental vessels

  - **Splenorenal ligament** — stretches between the spleen and left kidney; contains the splenic vessels

- Shift the stomach superiorly; use forceps and your fingers to dissect the splenic a. and its accompanying splenic v.

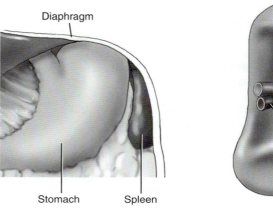
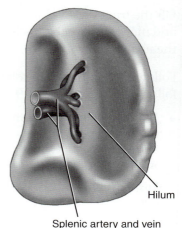

Figure 12-21   Spleen

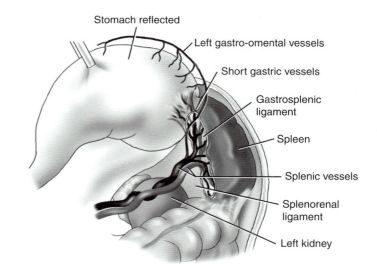

Figure 12-22   Splenic ligaments (stomach reflected superiorly)

Liver

■ Identify the following **(Figures 12-23** and **12-24)**:

- **Right lobe of the liver** — largest of the four lobes; located to the right of the grooves filled by the gallbladder and inferior vena cava (not easily seen at this time); from its inferior, visceral surface hangs the gallbladder

- **Left lobe of the liver** — located to the left of the falciform and round ligaments, and the groove for the ligamentum venosum (not easily seen at this time)

- **Diaphragmatic surface** — region of the liver in contact with the diaphragm

- **Visceral surface** — region of the liver in contact with viscera (stomach, duodenum, colon, right kidney)

- **Subphrenic recess** — slip your hands between the right and left lobes of the liver and the diaphragm; your hands fill the subphrenic recesses; you cannot touch the fingers of one hand to the other hand because of ligaments (reflections of the peritoneum from the liver to the diaphragm)

GAFS p 287   ACGA p 397   NAHA Plates 287–288

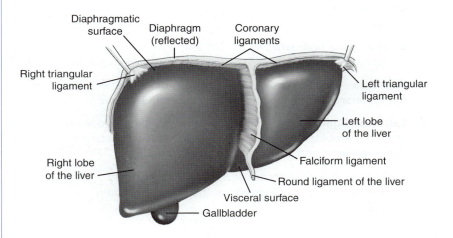

Figure 12-23   Anterior view of the liver (diaphragm reflected)

Liver Continued

Liver—cont'd

- **Coronary ligaments** — reflections of peritoneum from the diaphragm to superior and posterior surfaces of the liver
  - **Triangular ligaments** — the left and right triangular ligaments are sharp lateral margins of the coronary ligaments
- **Bare area** — region on the superior surface of the liver between the coronary and triangular ligaments; lacks peritoneum
- **Falciform ligament** — reflections of the parietal peritoneum around the obliterated umbilical v.; attaches the liver to both the diaphragm and anterior abdominal wall
  - The free (inferior) border of the falciform ligament contains the round ligament of the liver (obliterated umbilical v.)

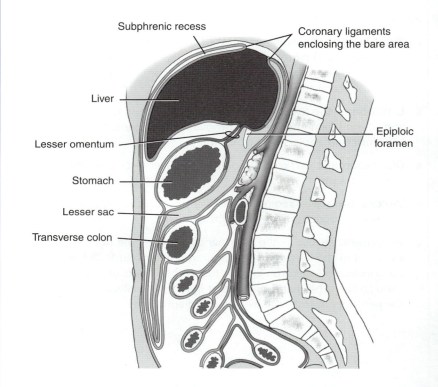

Figure 12-24 Sagittal section through the liver

Liver — Inferior (Visceral) Surface

- Lift the liver superiorly to identify the following structures on its inferior surface **(Figure 12-25)**:

  - **Right lobe** — located to the right of the grooves filled by the gallbladder and inferior vena cava
  - **Left lobe** — located to the left of the falciform ligament, round ligaments, and groove for the ligamentum venosum
  - **Quadrate lobe** — located anteriorly; bordered by the gallbladder, porta hepatis, and round ligament of the liver
  - **Caudate lobe** — located posteriorly; bordered by the groove for the ligamentum venosum, groove for inferior vena cava, and porta hepatis

- Cut a wedge off the left lobe of the liver to identify the following structures:

  - **Intrahepatic portal triads** — continuation of the structures in the porta hepatis; branches of the bile duct, portal v., and hepatic a.
  - **Intrahepatic vv.** — return blood to the inferior vena cava

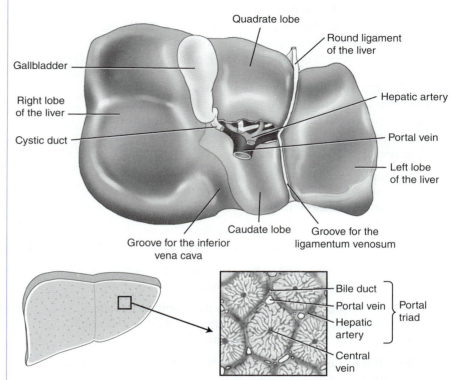

Figure 12-25 Inferior surface of the liver

Porta Hepatis

- Lift the liver superiorly; push the stomach inferiorly to identify the **porta hepatis**, located between the left and right lobes of the liver, within the hepatoduodenal ligament (the free edge of the lesser omentum); contains the common bile duct, hepatic a. proper, and the portal v.

- Use forceps and your fingers to bluntly dissect or use the open scissor technique to remove the remaining peritoneum from the region of the **hepatoduodenal ligament** to identify the following contents (**Figures 12-26** and **12-27**):

  - **Common bile duct** — green and usually on the superficial right side of the porta hepatis; dissect this duct toward the liver and gallbladder to reveal the cystic duct
    - **Cystic duct** — duct from the gallbladder, which joins the **common hepatic duct** to form the common bile duct
      - Follow the common hepatic duct to the liver to locate the **right** and **left hepatic ducts**
  - **Hepatic a. proper** — branch from the common hepatic a., after the latter gives rise to the gastroduodenal a. and right gastric aa., on the superficial left side of the porta hepatis
  - **Portal v.** — deep and posterior to the common bile duct and hepatic a. proper; the largest of the three structures

GAFS pp 286, 290, 303   NAHA Plates 273–275, 288, 290

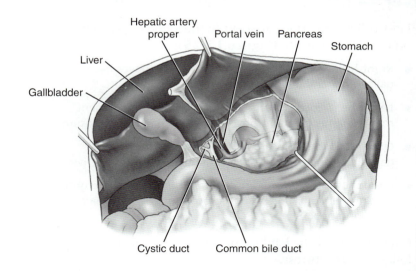

Figure 12-26   Porta hepatis in situ

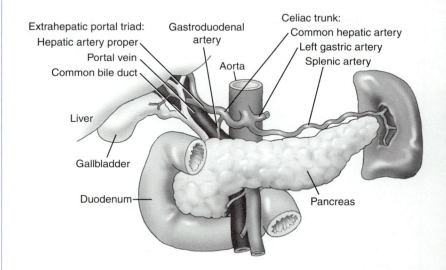

Figure 12-27   Structures associated with the porta hepatis

Unit 3 • Lab 12   Peritoneum and Foregut

Vasculature — Celiac Trunk Review

- Lift the liver superiorly; push the stomach out of the way (superiorly or inferiorly, depending on its size and shape)

- With the foregut dissected, it is easier to review the celiac trunk and its branches

- Identify the following **(Figure 12-28)**:
  - Common hepatic a.
  - Left gastric a.
  - Splenic a.

- Find the union of the three arteries; the point of union is the **celiac trunk** (dissection of the celiac trunk is challenging because it is surrounded by very tough tissue called the celiac ganglia [autonomic ganglia])

GAFS pp 295, 297, 307–309   NAHA Plates 272, 274, 300–301

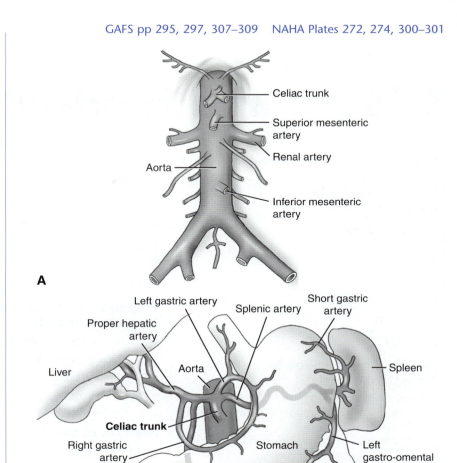

Figure 12-28 The celiac trunk. **A,** Abdominal aorta. **B,** Branches of the celiac trunk

Unit 3 • Lab 12   Peritoneum and Foregut

Lab 13

Midgut and Hindgut

Prior to dissection, you should familiarize yourself with the following structures:

PANCREAS
- Head
- Uncinate process
- Neck
- Body
- Tail
- Main pancreatic duct
- Accessory pancreatic duct

MIDGUT

(Supplied by the Superior Mesenteric Vessels)
- Duodenum (four parts)
  - Major and minor duodenal papillae (inside the duodenum)
    - Proximal to the major papilla — foregut
    - Distal to the major papilla — midgut
  - Pancreaticoduodenal ampulla (outside the duodenum)
  - Duodenal sphincter (surrounds the ampulla)
- Jejunum
  - Circular folds
- Ileum
  - Ileocecal junction/valve
  - Peyer's patches of lymphoid tissue
- Cecum
  - Vermiform appendix
- Ascending colon
- Right colic (hepatic) flexure
- Transverse colon (proximal two thirds)

HINDGUT

(Supplied by the Inferior Mesenteric Vessels)
- Transverse colon (distal one third)
- Left colic (splenic) flexure
- Descending colon
- Sigmoid colon
  - Semilunar folds

Features of the Colon
- Omental (epiploic) appendices
- Haustra
- Taenia coli mm.
- Rectum

PORTAL SYSTEM
- Portal v.
  - Splenic v.
  - Superior mesenteric v.
  - Gastric vv.
  - Gastro-omental vv.
  - Inferior mesenteric v.
  - Superior rectal v.

ARTERIES AND LYMPHATICS
- Aorta
  - Superior mesenteric a.
    - Anterior and posterior inferior pancreaticoduodenal aa.
    - Jejunal aa.
      - Vasa recta
    - Ileal aa.
      - Arcades
    - Ileocolic a.
      - Appendicular a.
    - Right colic a.
    - Middle colic a.
    - Marginal a.
    - Associated lymph nodes and lymphatics
  - Inferior mesenteric a.
    - Left colic a.
    - Sigmoid aa.
    - Marginal a.
    - Superior rectal a.
    - Associated lymph nodes and lymphatics

Lab 13 Dissection Overview

The purpose of this laboratory session is to learn the anatomy of the midgut and hindgut through dissection. You will do so through the following suggested sequence:

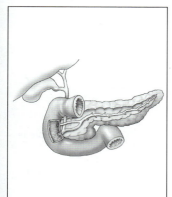

1. Dissect the pancreas and associated structures.

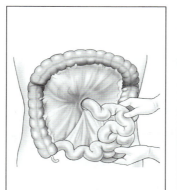

2. Identify the jejunum, ileum, and associated mesentery.

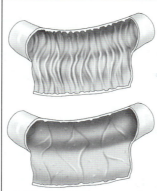

3. Distinguish between the internal surface of the jejunum and ileum.

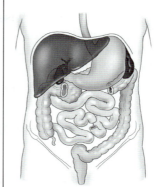

4. Identify the vermiform appendix and the regions and features of the large intestine.

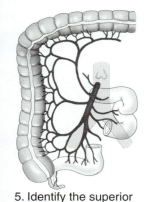

5. Identify the superior mesenteric artery, its branches, associations, and lymph nodes.

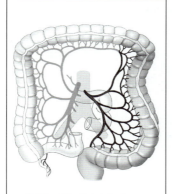

6. Identify the inferior mesenteric artery, its branches, associations, and lymph nodes.

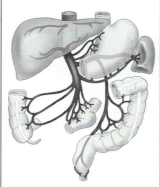

7. Study the portal system of veins.

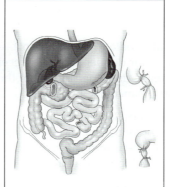

8. Remove the GI tract between the duodenojejunal junction and rectum to better study the posterior abdominal wall.

Duodenum and Pancreas

- Use forceps to dissect and identify the following (**Figure 13-1**):

  - **Duodenum** — dissected in laboratory session 12; lift the transverse colon and reopen the window cut through the transverse mesocolon

    - Follow the common bile duct inferiorly to the posterior surface of the head of the pancreas

    - Bluntly dissect the common bile duct from the surrounding pancreatic tissue

    - Estimate the extent of the descending (second) part of the duodenum

    - With scissors, open the duodenum, opposite to the junction of the second part with the common bile duct; wipe the lumen and wall clean to identify the following:

      - **Circular folds** — invaginations (flaps) of the mucosal lining

      - **Major duodenal papilla** — elevation where the pancreatic and common bile ducts enter the duodenal lumen

      - **Minor duodenal papilla** (may be absent) — 2 cm superior to the major duodenal papilla; receives the accessory pancreatic duct (persistence of the proximal duct of the dorsal pancreatic bud)

  - **Pancreaticoduodenal ampulla** — outside of the second part of the duodenum; the bulbous junction of the common bile and pancreatic ducts; it opens into the lumen of the duodenum via the major duodenal papilla

  - **Duodenal sphincter** — circularly arranged smooth muscle fibers in the wall of the pancreaticoduodenal ampulla

  - **Main pancreatic duct** — use the ampulla as your guide to dissect the pancreatic tissue to reveal the main pancreatic duct

    - Accessory pancreatic duct — superior and parallel to the main pancreatic duct; usually smaller in diameter than the main pancreatic duct

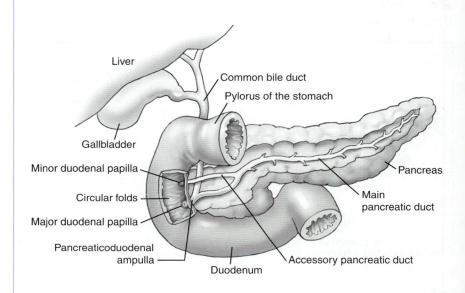

Figure 13-1   Duodenum

Midgut — Jejunum and Ileum

- Lift up the greater omentum and transverse colon to expose the small intestine and identify the following (**Figures 13-2** and **13-3**):

  - **Jejunum** — begins at the duodenojejunal junction and ends at the ileum
    - Pull the small intestine into the left lower quadrant of the abdomen
    - Follow the small intestine proximally to identify the duodenojejunal junction
    - The jejunum forms the proximal three fifths of the small intestine

  - **Ileum** — its beginning is not anatomically demarcated; instead, its end is distinct, at the cecum
    - Pull the small intestine into the left upper quadrant to expose the distal end of the ileum and the cecum
    - Follow the small intestine distally to identify the ileocecal junction
    - The ileum forms the distal two fifths of the small intestine

  - **The mesentery** — a fan-shaped, double fold of peritoneum by which coils of jejunum and ileum are attached to the posterior abdominal wall
    - Provides support for the small intestine and contains the mesenteric vessels (arteries, veins, and lymphatics) and nerves from the posterior abdominal wall to the small intestine

- Reflect, using forceps, the mesentery from the small intestine to expose the mesenteric vessels and nerves (see Figure 13-3)

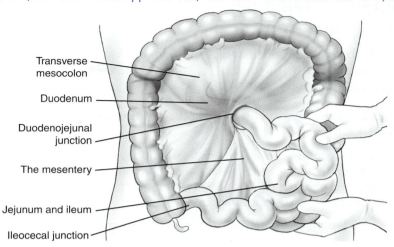

Figure 13-2 Jejunum and ileum

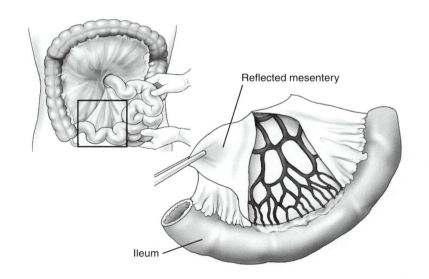

Figure 13-3 Mesentery of the jejunum and ileum

Midgut — Jejunum and Ileum Continued

Midgut — Jejunum and Ileum—cont'd

- Use scissors to cut open and clean segments (several centimeters) of the jejunum, proximal ileum, and distal ileum

- Identify the following internal features (**Figures 13-4** and **13-5**):
  - **Circular folds** — invaginations (flaps) in the mucosal layer of the gut that increase its surface area to accommodate the passage of digesting food; the jejunum may be distinguished from the ileum by appearance:
    - **Jejunum** (proximal) — circular folds are numerous
    - **Ileum** (distal) — circular folds in the proximal ileum are less numerous; they gradually disappear toward the distal ileum

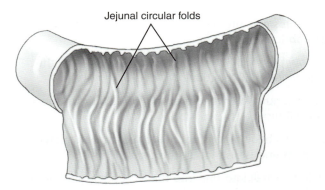

Figure 13-4 Internal features of the jejunum

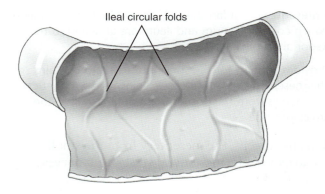

Figure 13-5 Internal features of the ileum

Midgut — Large Intestine

■ Lift up the greater omentum and transverse colon to identify the following **(Figures 13-6** and **13-7)**:

- **Ileocecal junction** — the union of the ileum and cecum; internally, a sphincter muscle separates the small and large intestines; intraperitoneal

- **Cecum** — beginning of the large intestine; extends inferiorly at the ileocecal junction into the right iliac fossa; intraperitoneal

- **Vermiform appendix** — opens into the cecum, inferior to the ileocecal junction; can occupy many different positions and varies in size; intraperitoneal

- **Ascending colon** — extends from the cecum to the transverse colon; ends at the **right colic (hepatic) flexure**; retroperitoneal

- **Transverse colon** — extends from the right colic flexure to the left colic (splenic) flexure

  - Suspended by the transverse mesocolon so it is intraperitoneal

  - **Phrenicocolic ligament** — mesentery attaching the left colic flexure to the diaphragm

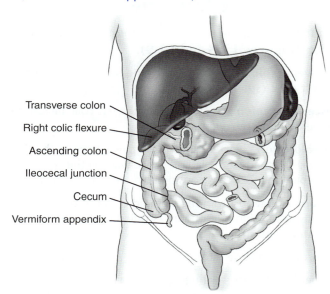

Figure 13-6 Large intestine

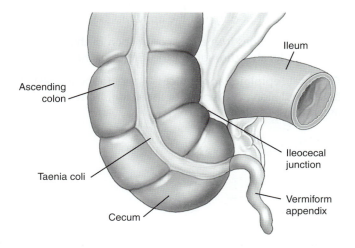

Figure 13-7 Cecum and appendix

Hindgut — Large Intestine

- Continue following the transverse colon to identify the following **(Figures 13-8** and **13-9)**:

  - **Transverse colon** — extends from the right colic flexure to the **left colic (splenic) flexure**
  - **Descending colon** — extends from the left colic flexure to the pelvic brim; retroperitoneal
  - **Sigmoid colon** — extends from the pelvic brim to the rectum; attached to the lateral pelvic wall via the sigmoid mesocolon, hence it has considerable mobility; intraperitoneal
  - **Rectum** — extends from the sigmoid colon to the anal canal; partially covered in peritoneum (studied further in another laboratory session)
  - Features of the large intestine (midgut and hindgut):
    - **Taenia coli mm.** — three longitudinal bands of smooth muscle; the anterior and posterior bands are easy to identify on the colon (the middle muscle is deep to the mesentery and more difficult to observe, except at the cecum)
      - The three bands converge at the bottom of the cecum, at the point of origin of the appendix (see Figure 13-7)
    - **Haustra** — bulges formed by contraction of the taenia coli mm.; located throughout the length of the colon
    - **Omental (epiploic) appendices** — sacs (appendages) of fat located along the length of the colon, from the ascending to sigmoid colon

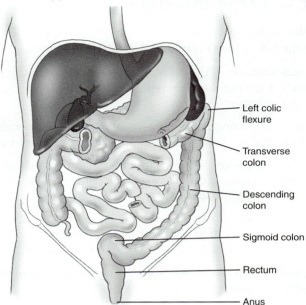

Figure 13-8   Large intestine

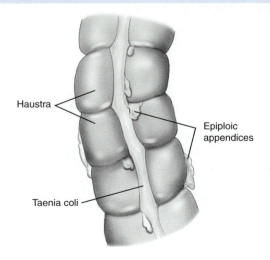

Figure 13-9   Structures of the large intestine

Midgut — Superior Mesenteric Artery

- Lift up the greater omentum and transverse colon, and push aside the small intestine, to identify the following (Figure 13-10):

  - **Superior mesenteric a.** — the second unpaired artery arising from the abdominal aorta, just inferior to the celiac trunk, at the level of L1 vertebra

  - **Superior mesenteric v.** — courses along the right side of the superior mesenteric a.

    - Palpate to the right of the duodenojejunal junction for the superior mesenteric a. and v. (see Figure 13-10B)

    - Use forceps to bluntly dissect through the mesentery to expose the superior mesenteric a. and v.; both vessels emerge from beneath the pancreas and cross over distally to a portion of the small intestine and the third part of the duodenum

    - The midgut also receives blood supply from the celiac trunk via anastomoses among the **anterior** and **posterior superior pancreaticoduodenal aa.**; use forceps to follow, dissect, and identify the anterior and posterior superior pancreaticoduodenal aa.; lift up the head of the pancreas to follow the arteries distally

  - **Superior mesenteric plexus** — plexus of autonomic nerves that surround the superior mesenteric a.

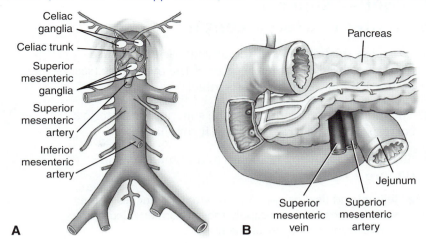

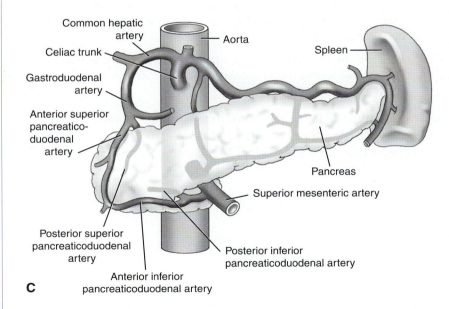

Figure 13-10 Superior mesenteric artery. **A**, Abdominal aorta. **B**, Superior mesenteric artery and vein in situ. **C**, Arteries associated with the pancreas

Midgut — Superior Mesenteric Artery Continued

Midgut — Superior Mesenteric Artery—cont'd

- To expose the branches of the mesenteric vessels, use forceps to shred the anterior layer of the mesentery (see Figure 13-11); keep the vessels intact

- The names of the branches of the superior mesenteric a. correspond to the structures that it supplies

- Identify the following branches to the small intestine **(Figure 13-11)**:

  - **Jejunal** and **ileal aa.** — 15 to 18 arterial branches of the superior mesenteric a.; supply the jejunum and ileum; pass between the two layers of the mesentery

  - **Arterial arcades** — arteries form arches within the mesentery that eventually form straight terminal branches (vasa recta) to the jejunum and ileum
    - Shred the mesentery that is attached to a segment of the proximal jejunum and distal ileum to identify the arterial arcades and vasa recta

- *Note:* Compared to the jejunum, the ileum has more arterial arcades that are stacked upon one another; consequently, the vasa recta of the ileum are shorter than those of the jejunum (see Figure 13-11)

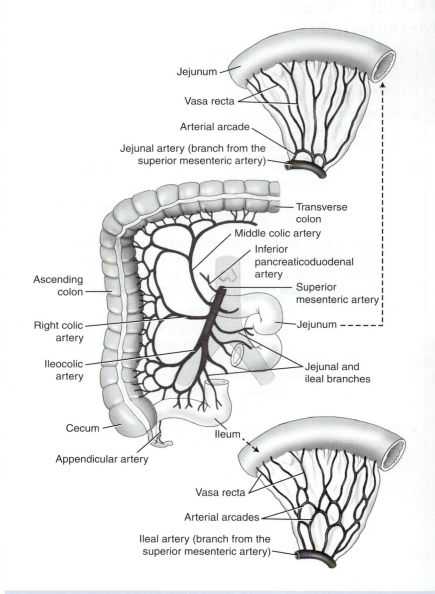

Figure 13-11 Jejunal and ileal arteries

Midgut — Superior Mesenteric Artery—cont'd

- Use blunt dissection through the peritoneum or mesocolon and scrape excess fat to continue revealing the branches of the superior mesenteric a. to identify the following branches to the proximal portion of the colon **(Figure 13-12)**:

  - **Ileocolic a.** — terminal branch of the superior mesenteric a.; supplies the cecum, appendix, and distal portion of the ileum; anastomoses with ileal branches and the right colic a.
    - **Appendicular a.** — terminal branch of the ileocolic a.; supplies the appendix
  - **Right colic a.** — origin is variable, in that it may arise from the superior mesenteric a., the ileocolic a., or the middle colic a.; supplies the ascending colon; anastomoses with the ileocolic and middle colic aa.
  - **Middle colic a.** — supplies the right half of the transverse colon; anastomoses with the right colic a. and the left colic a. (branch of the inferior mesenteric a.)
  - **Marginal a.** — anastomoses of the colic aa.
  - *Note:* Tributaries of the superior mesenteric v. drain the same regions supplied by the superior mesenteric a.
  - **Superior mesenteric lymph nodes** — look for lymph nodes in the mesentery; named according to the organ that they drain

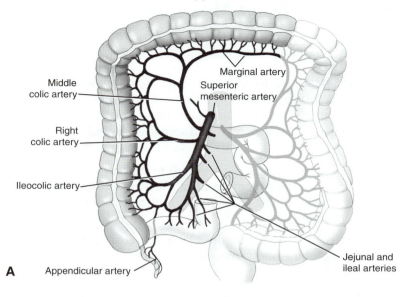

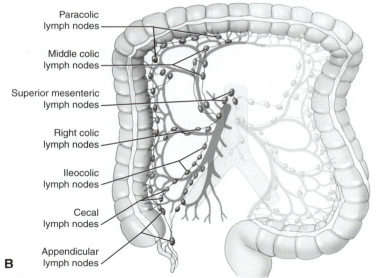

Figure 13-12 Superior mesenteric artery and its branches. **A,** Branches of the superior mesenteric artery. **B,** Superior mesenteric lymph nodes

Hindgut — Inferior Mesenteric Artery

- The inferior mesenteric a. is the third unpaired vessel arising from the abdominal aorta, at the level of L3 vertebra

- Push the small intestine into the upper right quadrant of the abdomen to identify the following branches to the distal portion of the colon; use blunt dissection through the peritoneum or mesocolon and scrape excess fat **(Figure 13-13)**:

  - **Inferior mesenteric a.** — use forceps to dissect over the inferior end of the abdominal aorta, about 3 cm superior to the aortic bifurcation; usually arises to the left of the midline of the aorta

    - **Left colic a.** — supplies the descending colon and the left portion of the transverse colon; anastomoses with the middle colic a. (from the superior mesenteric a.)

    - **Sigmoid aa.** — within the sigmoid mesocolon; usually four to five branches that form arches; supply blood to the sigmoid colon

    - **Superior rectal a.** — supplies the proximal portion of the rectum; usually a large vessel (the terminal branch of the inferior mesenteric a.)

    - **Marginal a. (of Drummond)** — anastomoses of the colic aa. around the mesenteric margin of the large intestine

      - Begins at the ileocecal junction, where anastomoses occur from the cecal branches of the superior mesenteric a., to the superior rectal a. of the inferior mesenteric a.

  - **Inferior mesenteric lymph nodes** — look for lymph nodes in the mesentery; named according to the organ that they drain

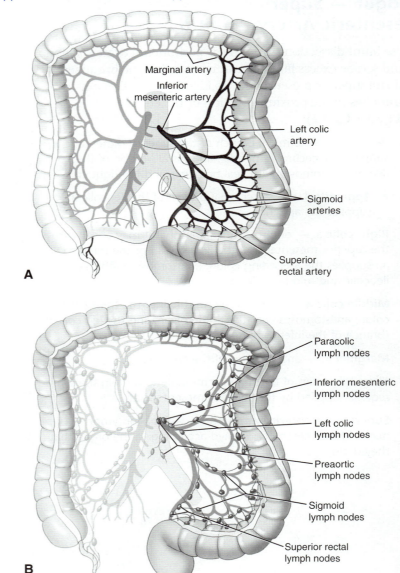

Figure 13-13 Inferior mesenteric artery and its branches. **A,** Branches of the inferior mesenteric artery. **B,** Inferior mesenteric lymph nodes

Portal System of Veins

GAFS pp 239–240, 303–306   ACGA pp 410–412, 415–418   NAHA Plates 309–313

■ Drains poorly oxygenated, but nutrient-rich, venous blood from the gastrointestinal (GI) tract to the liver (expect variation)

- The three principal tributaries are the superior mesenteric v., inferior mesenteric v., and splenic v.

■ Lift up the great omentum and transverse colon and push the small intestine inferiorly to identify the following veins, tinted blue, usually accompanying the previously dissected arteries **(Figure 13-14)**:

- **Portal v.** — relocate the portal v. in the porta hepatis; usually 5 cm long; formed posterior to the neck of the pancreas via the union of the superior mesenteric v. and the splenic v.

- **Superior mesenteric v.** — drains blood from the midgut; located to the right of the superior mesenteric a.

- **Splenic v.** — courses inferior to the splenic a. and posterior to the pancreas
  - Clean and follow the splenic v. and superior mesenteric v. to their union at the portal v.

- **Inferior mesenteric v.** — usually drains into the splenic v.; to the left of the superior mesenteric v. (expect variation)

- **Right** and **left gastric vv.** — drain blood from the right and left sides of the lesser curvature of the stomach to the portal v.; course with the corresponding arteries

- **Gastro-omental vv.** — drain blood from the greater curvature of the stomach to the superior mesenteric v.; course with the corresponding arteries

- **Superior rectal v.** — drains the rectum to the inferior mesenteric v.; courses with the corresponding artery; do not attempt to follow the superior rectal a. and v. distally (they will be dissected in a future laboratory session)

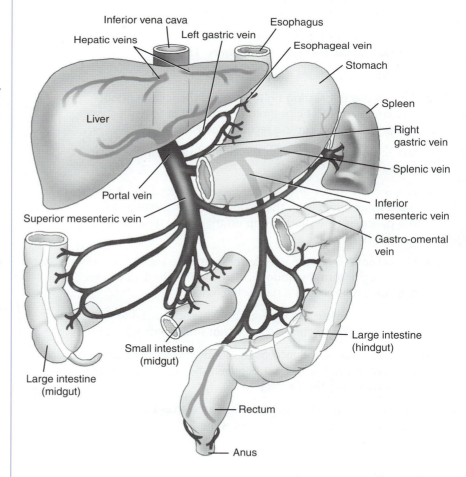

Figure 13-14   Portal venous system

Removal of the Gastrointestinal Tract

- To improve study of the posterior abdominal wall, you will remove most of the GI tract; however, you will leave intact the celiac trunk and its associated organs (foregut)

- Follow these instructions to remove the GI tract:
  - Locate the **duodenojejunal junction** and the **rectum**; use your fingers to free up a segment of each part of the gut
  - Tie two pieces of string tightly around the duodenojejunal junction, about 2–3 cm apart **(Figure 13-15)**
  - Free the rectum from the peritoneum
  - Tie two pieces of string tightly around the rectum about 2–3 cm apart; this helps limit the amount of feces that will escape when you cut the rectum (see Figure 13-15B)
  - Use scissors to cut through the GI tract between the adjacent pairs of ties
  - Use scissors to cut the superior mesenteric a. about 2 cm distal to its origin from the abdominal aorta, inferior to the pancreas (the short stump on the aorta will serve as a handy reference)
  - Use scissors to cut the inferior mesenteric a. about 2 cm distal to its origin from the abdominal aorta (the short stump on the aorta will serve as a handy reference)
  - Use scissors to cut the superior mesenteric v. distal to its union with the splenic v. (or superior mesenteric v.)
  - Use your fingers and forceps to bluntly dissect the peritoneal attachments of the GI tract between the pairs of string ties while removing the GI tract
  - Leave as much mesentery (and its vasculature) as possible attached to the excised small intestine

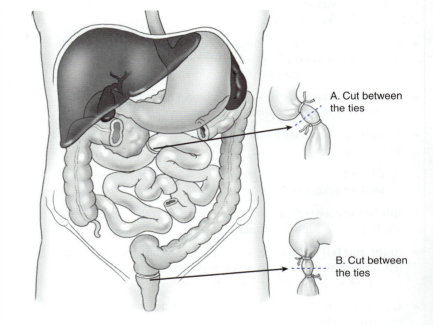

Figure 13-15 Removal of the GI tract. Transection of the duodenojejunal junction *(A)*. Transection of the rectum *(B)*

Posterior Abdominal Wall

Lab 14

Prior to dissection, you should familiarize yourself with the following structures:

MUSCLES
- Psoas major m.
- Psoas minor m.
- Iliacus m.
- Quadratus lumborum m.
  - Iliolumbar ligament
- Diaphragm
  - Right and left crura
  - Central tendon
  - Vena caval hiatus
  - Esophageal hiatus
  - Aortic hiatus
  - Medial and lateral arcuate ligaments
  - Median arcuate ligament

NERVES
- Subcostal n. (T12)
- Iliohypogastric n. (L1)
- Ilioinguinal n. (L1)
- Genitofemoral n. (L1–L2)
- Lateral femoral cutaneous n. (L2–L3)
- Obturator n. (L2–L4)
- Femoral n. (L2–L4)
- Lumbosacral trunk (L4–L5)

ARTERIES
- Abdominal aorta
  - Inferior phrenic a.
  - Celiac trunk
  - Superior mesenteric a.
  - Suprarenal aa. (superior, middle, and inferior)
  - Renal aa.
  - Gonadal (testicular/ovarian) aa.
  - Inferior mesenteric a.
  - Lumbar aa.
  - Median sacral a.
  - Common iliac aa.
    - External iliac aa.
    - Internal iliac aa.

VEINS
- Inferior vena cava
  - Renal vv.
    - Suprarenal vv.
    - Left gonadal v.
- Right gonadal v.
- Lumbar vv.
- Middle sacral v.
- Common iliac vv.
- External iliac vv.
- Internal iliac vv.

LYMPHATICS
- Cisterna chyli
- Lymph nodes
  - Preaortic lymph nodes
  - Common iliac lymph nodes
  - External iliac lymph nodes
  - Internal iliac lymph nodes

KIDNEY
- Perirenal fascia
- Fibrous capsule
- Renal cortex
- Renal medulla
  - Renal columns
  - Renal pyramids
  - Renal papillae
- Minor and major calyces
- Renal pelvis
- Ureter
- Hilum

Lab 14 Dissection Overview

The purpose of this laboratory session is to learn the anatomy of the posterior abdominal wall through dissection. You will do so through the following suggested sequence:

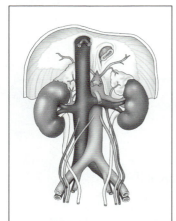

1. Identify the major structures of the posterior abdominal wall.

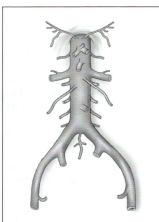

2. Identify the branches of the abdominal aorta.

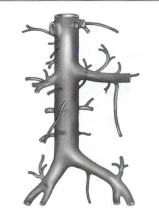

3. Identify the branches of the inferior vena cava.

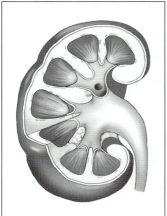

4. Dissect the kidneys and ureter.

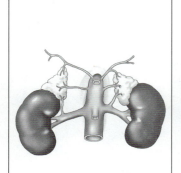

5. Dissect the adrenal glands and associated blood supply.

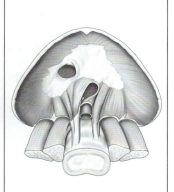

6. Dissect the diaphragm.

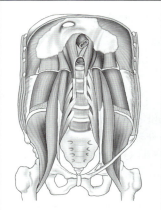

7. Dissect along the muscles of the posterior abdominal wall.

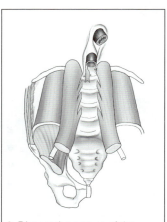

8. Dissect the nerves of the lumbar plexus that course along the posterior abdominal wall.

Table 14-1 Muscles of the Posterior Abdominal Wall

Muscle	Proximal Attachment	Distal Attachment	Action	Innervation
Psoas major m.	Lateral surfaces of the bodies of T12–L5 vertebrae, transverse processes of the lumbar vertebrae, and the intervertebral discs between T12–L5 vertebrae	Lesser trochanter of the femur	Flexes the thigh at the hip joint	Anterior rami of spinal nerves L1–L3
Psoas minor m.	Lateral surface of the bodies of T12–L1 vertebrae and the intervening intervertebral disc	Pectineal line of the pelvic brim and iliopubic eminence	Weakly flexes the lumbar region of the vertebral column	Anterior rami of spinal nerve L1
Quadratus lumborum m.	Transverse process of the L5 vertebra, iliolumbar ligament, and iliac crest	Transverse processes of L1–L5 vertebrae and the inferior border of rib 12	Depresses and stabilizes rib 12; can laterally flex the trunk	Anterior rami of spinal nerves T12–L4
Iliacus m.	Upper two thirds of the iliac fossa, anterior sacroiliac and iliolumbar ligaments, and upper lateral surface of the sacrum	Lesser trochanter of the femur	Flexes the thigh at the hip joint	Femoral n. (L2–L4)

Posterior Abdominal Wall — Overview

- Remove the remaining peritoneum and extraperitoneal fat, using blunt dissection and scraping, to identify the following **(Figure 14-1)**:

  - **Kidneys** — lateral to vertebrae T12–L3; use scissors and your fingers to remove the parietal peritoneum and perirenal fat from over and around the kidneys, respectively

  - **Ureters** — use forceps to free the ureters from the parietal peritoneum and fat; extend from the renal pelvis to the urinary bladder, you will not be able to follow the ureters to the bladder at this time

  - **Adrenal (suprarenal) glands** — positioned on the superior pole of each kidney; pale in color and somewhat triangular shaped

  - **Abdominal aorta** — use forceps to dissect through the parietal peritoneum to reveal the aorta (and neighboring vena cava and branches); the abdominal aorta courses longitudinally to the left of the midsagittal line, on the anterior surface of the vertebral bodies

  - **Inferior vena cava** — courses longitudinally to the right of the midsagittal line, also on the anterior surface of the vertebral bodies

  - **Iliac crest** — palpate its internal surface

  - **Diaphragm** — move the liver and stomach to different positions to see the diaphragm

  - **Lymphatics**
    - **Lymph nodes** — named according to where they are located:
      - ◆ **Preaortic lymph nodes**
      - ◆ **External iliac lymph nodes**
      - ◆ **Internal iliac lymph nodes**

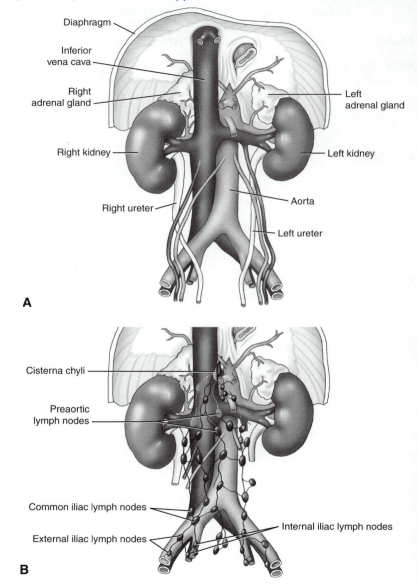

Figure 14-1 **A**, Overview of the posterior abdominal wall. **B**, Lymphatics of the posterior abdominal wall

Posterior Abdominal Wall — Abdominal Aorta

- Use forceps to reveal and identify the following **(Figure 14-2)**:
  - **Abdominal aorta** — courses longitudinally to the left of the midsagittal line, on the anterior surface of the vertebral bodies; the bifurcation of the abdominal aorta is at L4 vertebra
    - **Inferior phrenic aa.** — paired arteries that arise immediately inferior to the diaphragm; first paired branches from the abdominal aorta; give superior suprarenal aa. to the suprarenal glands
    - **Celiac trunk** — T12 vertebral level; unpaired artery; supplies the foregut
    - **Superior mesenteric a.** — L1 vertebral level; unpaired artery; supplies the midgut
    - **Inferior mesenteric a.** — L3 vertebral level; unpaired artery; supplies the hindgut
    - **Middle suprarenal a.** — paired arteries from the abdominal aorta, near the level of the celiac trunk; supplies the suprarenal glands
    - **Renal aa.** — L1 vertebral level; paired arteries that originate between the superior and inferior mesenteric aa.; the left renal a. is shorter than the right renal a.; multiple arteries are frequently encountered (expect variation)
      - Give rise to the **inferior suprarenal aa**.
    - **Gonadal (testicular/ovarian) aa.** — L2 vertebral level; paired arteries that arise inferior to the renal aa. and superior to the inferior mesenteric a.; cross anterior to the ureters and external iliac vessels
    - **Lumbar aa.** — four paired arteries that course laterally across the sides of vertebrae L1–L4; segmental blood supply of the lumbar region
    - **Median sacral a.** — unpaired artery that arises from the abdominal aorta at its bifurcation into the common iliac aa.
    - **Common iliac aa.** — paired arteries from the distal end of the aorta at the L4 vertebral level; each bifurcates into the **external** and **internal iliac aa**.

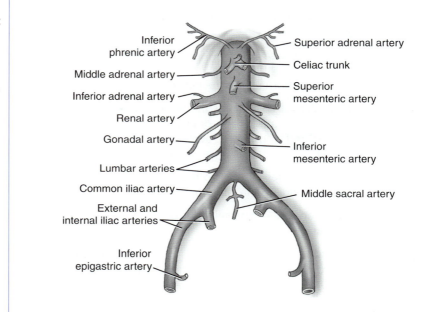

Figure 14-2 Branches of the abdominal aorta

Posterior Abdominal Wall — Inferior Vena Cava

- Use forceps to reveal and identify the following **(Figure 14-3)**:

Inferior vena cava

- **Right renal v.** — shorter than the left renal v.
  - **Right suprarenal v.** — drains the right adrenal gland; only one suprarenal v. drains each adrenal gland compared to the three adrenal aa. that supply each gland
- **Left renal v.** — crosses anterior to the aorta and just inferior and posterior to the superior mesenteric a.
  - **Left suprarenal v.** — one vein also drains the left adrenal gland
  - **Left gonadal (testicular/ovarian) v.** — drains the left gonad into the inferior border of the left renal v.
- **Right gonadal v.** — drains the right gonad into the inferior vena cava
- Lumbar vv.
- Middle sacral v.
- Common iliac vv.

- *Note:* The superior and inferior mesenteric vv. are not tributaries to the inferior vena cava; rather, they are tributaries to the portal venous system

- *Note:* You may not see the inferior phrenic vv. and hepatic vv. because the liver will be in the way

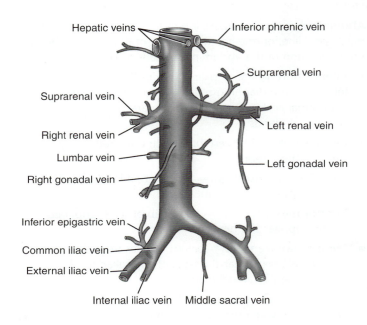

Figure 14-3 Branches of the inferior vena cava

Kidneys and Adrenal Glands In Situ

- Identify the following **(Figure 14-4)**:

  - **Kidneys** — right and left; observe that the right kidney is slightly lower than the left kidney, due to the presence of the liver in the upper right quadrant of the abdomen

  - **Perirenal fat** — each kidney is embedded in a substantial layer of fat; with your fingers, shell out the kidneys from the perirenal fat

  - **Adrenal glands** — each adrenal gland is separated from the superior pole of each kidney by a layer of connective tissue; use forceps or your fingers to separate the adrenal glands from the kidneys, *but* leave the adrenal blood vessels intact

  - **Ureters** — cross the psoas major m. and course deep to the gonadal vessels en route to the true pelvis (urinary bladder); use forceps to delineate both ureters; do not cut the ureters

- To remove the right kidney, cut its artery and vein; lift the kidney from the posterior abdominal wall by scooping out the kidney with your fingers; leave the ureter attached to the right kidney

GAFS pp 320–326   ACGA pp 377–378   NAHA Plates 329, 332

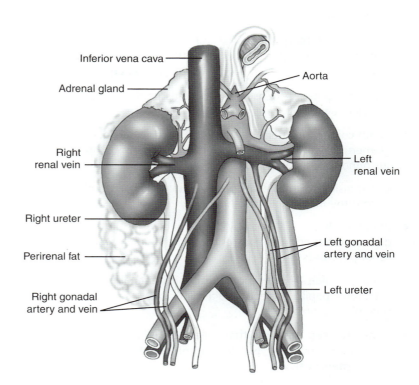

Figure 14-4   Kidneys in situ

Kidneys and Adrenal Glands In Situ Continued

Kidneys and Adrenal Glands
In Situ—cont'd

- Using a scalpel, bisect the freed right kidney, coronally, to identify the following internal structures (scrape excess fat from the area of the renal pelvis) **(Figure 14-5)**:

  - **Fibrous capsule** — dense connective tissue that surrounds each kidney; easily stripped away

  - **Renal cortex** — outer one third of the kidney; location of glomeruli; a continuous band of pale tissue that completely surrounds the renal medulla
    - Extensions of the renal cortex **(renal columns)** project into the inner aspect of the kidney

  - **Renal medulla** — divided by the renal columns into discontinuous aggregations of triangular-shaped tissue called **renal pyramids**

  - **Renal papillae** — inner, pointed tip of the renal pyramids; each renal papilla projects into a minor calyx, one papilla to one minor calyx

  - **Minor calyces** — "cups" that collect urine from the papilla of each renal pyramid; two to four minor calyces unite to form a **major calyx**

  - **Renal pelvis** — formed by union of the major calyces

  - **Ureter** — the continuation of the renal pelvis; connects the kidney to the urinary bladder

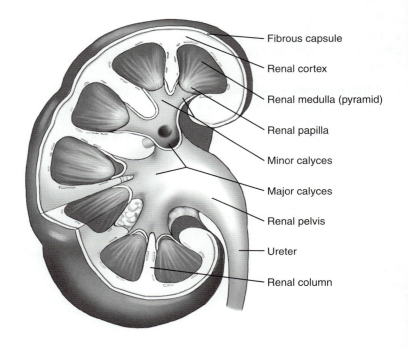

Figure 14-5 Coronal section of the kidney

Adrenal Glands

- Identify the following **(Figure 14-6)**:
  - **Adrenal glands** — superior to each kidney
  - **Adrenal (suprarenal) vessels** — fairly thin; may be difficult to identify
    - **Superior suprarenal a.** — arises from the inferior phrenic a.
    - **Middle suprarenal a.** — arises from the aorta
    - **Inferior suprarenal a.** — arises from renal a.
    - **Suprarenal v.** — usually drains to the renal v.; only one vein compared to three arteries; the veins are asymmetric

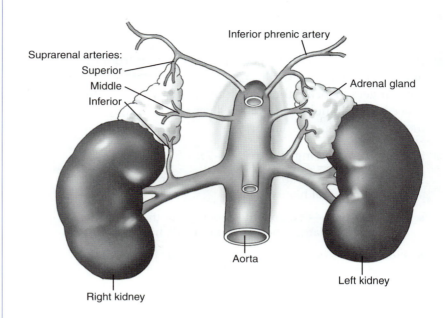

Figure 14-6 Arterial supply of the adrenal glands

Diaphragm

- A dome-shaped muscle that separates the thoracic cavity from the abdominal cavity

- If not already cut, cut the peritoneal reflections from the diaphragm muscle to the liver; to cut those reflections, use your fingers to locate them and scissors to cut them; this procedure will mobilize (free) the liver so that it may be moved away from the diaphragm

- Identify the following **(Figure 14-7)**:

  - **Central tendon** — observe the opening for the inferior vena cava **(vena caval hiatus)**
  - **Muscular part** — observe the openings for the esophagus **(esophageal hiatus)** and the aorta **(aortic hiatus)**
  - **Right crus** — originates lateral to the aortic hiatus; loops around the esophagus to form the esophageal hiatus, the physiologic sphincter of the esophagus
    - You may observe a muscle slip coursing inferomedially from the right crus of the diaphragm to the duodenojejunal junction — this is the **suspensory ligament of the duodenum**
  - **Left crus** — move the stomach and spleen away from the diaphragm; the left crus is lateral to the aortic hiatus; fleshy fibers contribute to the median arcuate ligament
  - **Med*ian* arcuate ligament** — formed by the right and left crura arching over the aorta
  - **Med*ial* arcuate ligaments** — tendinous thickenings of the diaphragm; form openings for the psoas major mm.
  - **Lateral arcuate ligaments** — tendinous thickenings of the diaphragm; form openings for the quadratus lumborum mm.

GAFS pp 227, 317–319   ACGA p 381   NAHA Plates 195, 263

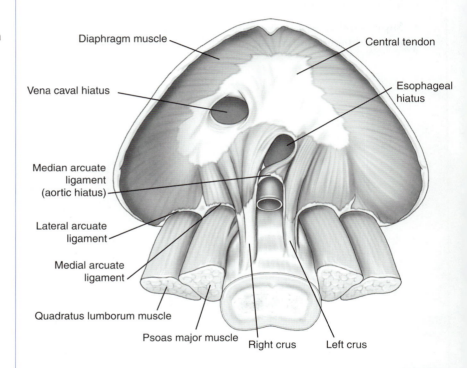

Figure 14-7 Abdominal surface of the diaphragm

Posterior Abdominal Wall — Muscles and Associated Structures

- Use forceps and your fingers to remove the parietal peritoneum and fat from both sides of the posterior abdominal wall to identify the following (try not to cut nerves that are encountered) **(Figure 14-8)**:

  - **Psoas major m.** — long muscle attached to the bodies and transverse processes of L1–L5 vertebrae
    - Overlaps the medial portion of the quadratus lumborum m. and crosses anterior to the sacroiliac joint; passes inferior to the inguinal ligament to insert on the lesser trochanter of the femur
    - Lumbar plexus of nerves exits the intervertebral foramina and emerges through and between the psoas major muscle fibers, where they arise from the lumbar transverse processes
  - **Psoas minor m.** — this thin muscle courses anteriorly on and medial to the psoas major m.; inserts distally on the pecten pubis (the psoas minor m. is sometimes absent)
  - **Quadratus lumborum m.** — quadrilateral-shaped muscle that is lateral and deep to the psoas major m.
    - **Iliolumbar ligament** — courses from the ilium to the lumbar vertebrae along the attachment of the quadratus lumborum m.
  - **Iliacus m.** — located in the iliac fossa pelvis; attaches to the iliac fossa and courses distally to the lesser trochanter of the femur (may be covered by a considerable amount of fat)

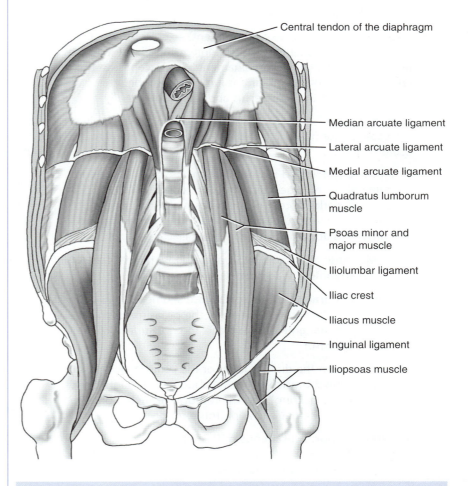

Figure 14-8 Muscles of the posterior abdominal wall

Nerves of the Posterior Abdominal Wall

- Use forceps to remove residual fat from the posterior abdominal wall to identify the following **(Figure 14-9)**:

  - Dissect all of the following nerves along the entire course; then return to the nerves in the listed sequence to identify them by name; expect variation

  - **Subcostal n.** (T12 spinal cord segment) — scrape/dissect through the peritoneum and fascia inferior to rib 12; emerges inferior to the lateral arcuate ligament and descends on the anterior surface of the quadratus lumborum m. before passing through the transversus abdominis m. laterally

  - **Lumbar plexus** — emerges laterally from the muscle belly of the psoas major m.; locate the following nerves lateral to the psoas major m.:

    - **Iliohypogastric** and **ilioinguinal nn.** (both L1 spinal cord segment) — diverge from their common trunk at the lateral, superior border of the psoas major m.; course across the quadratus lumborum m. prior to crossing the transversus abdominis m. above the iliac crest

      ◆ May arise as a single nerve and split within the layers of the abdominal wall musculature

    - **Genitofemoral n.** (L1–L2 spinal cord segments) — located on the anterior surface of the psoas major m. (the only nerve that emerges from the anterior surface of the psoas major m.)

      ◆ Divides on the distal portion of the psoas major m. into the **genital branch** (exits the abdomen through the deep inguinal ring) and the **femoral branch** (courses with the external iliac a. on route to the thigh)

    - **Lateral femoral cutaneous n.** (L2–L3 spinal cord segments) — located along the lateral border of the psoas major m., where the psoas major m. crosses the iliac crest

      ◆ Crosses the iliacus m. before passing deep to the inguinal ligament en route to the thigh

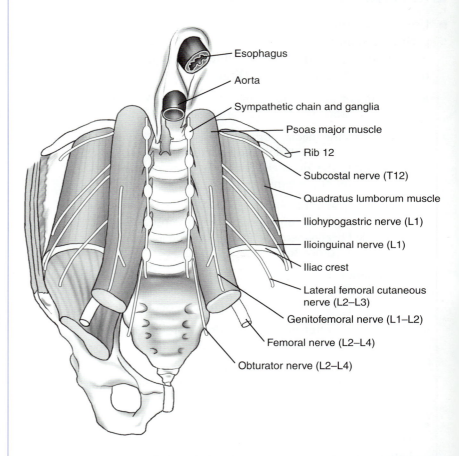

Figure 14-9 Nerves of the posterior abdominal wall

Nerves of the Posterior Abdominal Wall—cont'd

- **Femoral n.** (L2–L4 spinal cord segments) — located deep and lateral to, and often overlapped by, the psoas major m., near its union with the iliacus m.; courses deep to the inguinal ligament en route to the thigh

- **Obturator n.** (L2–L4 spinal cord segments) — probe the fat deep and medial to the inferior portion of the psoas major m. near the sacral promontory to reveal the obturator nerve

- **Lumbosacral trunk** (L4–L5 spinal cord segments) — medial and deep to the obturator n.; descends along the front of the sacrum medial to the psoas major m. to join with the ventral rami of S1–S3 in the pelvis

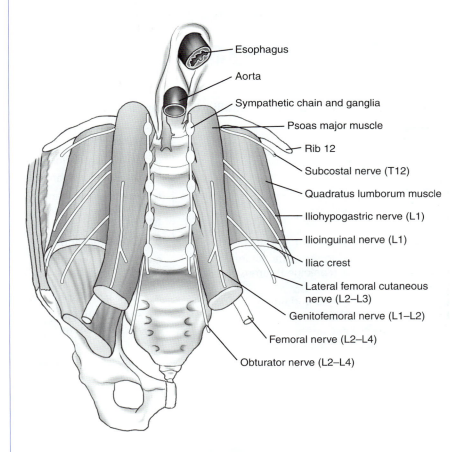

Figure 14-9   Nerves of the posterior abdominal wall

Lab 15

Gluteal Region and Ischioanal Fossa

Prior to dissection, you should familiarize yourself with the following structures:

OSTEOLOGY
- Os coxae
  - Obturator foramen
  - Ilium
    - Iliac crest
    - Posterior superior iliac spine
  - Ischium
    - Ischial spine and tuberosity
    - Greater and lesser sciatic foramina
    - Ischiopubic (conjoined) ramus
  - Pubis
    - Pubic symphysis and arch
    - Superior pubic ramus
    - Inferior pubic ramus
    - Ischiopubic (conjoint) ramus

LIGAMENTS
- Sacrotuberous ligament
- Sacrospinous ligament
- Anococcygeal ligament

MUSCLES
- Gluteus maximus m.
- Obturator internus m.
- Piriformis m.
- External anal sphincter m.
- Pelvic diaphragm
  - Levator ani m.
    - Puborectalis m.
    - Pubococcygeus m.
    - Iliococcygeus m.
  - Coccygeus m.

ISCHIOANAL (ISCHIORECTAL) FOSSA
- Internal pudendal aa. and vv.
  - Inferior rectal n. and vessels
- Pudendal nn.
- Inferior gluteal nn., aa., and vv.
- Obturator fascia over pudendal canal
- External anal sphincter
- Sciatic n.

Lab 15 Dissection Overview

The purpose of this laboratory session is to learn the anatomy of the gluteal region and ischioanal fossa through dissection. You will do so through the following suggested sequence:

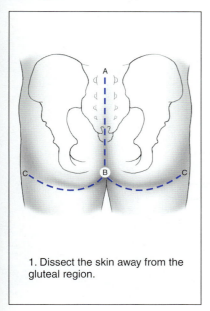

1. Dissect the skin away from the gluteal region.

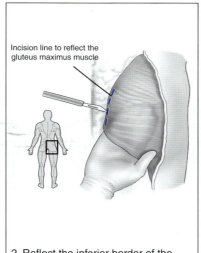

2. Reflect the inferior border of the gluteus maximus muscle in a lateral direction to reveal the ischioanal fossa.

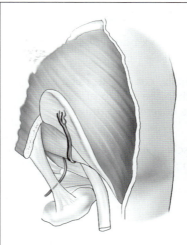

3. Identify the arteries, veins, and nerves in the gluteal region.

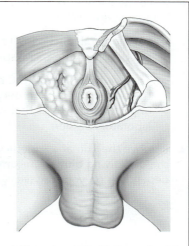

4. Dissect and identify the pudendal canal, levator ani muscles, and other structures of the ischioanal fossa.

Gluteal Region — Skin Incisions

■ Follow these instructions to dissect the gluteal region (avoid entering the posterior region of the thigh):

- Place the cadaver prone to make the following skin incisions, using a scalpel **(Figure 15-1)**:
  - Lumbosacral junction *(A)* to the coccyx bone *(B)*; cut deeply to the sacral spines
  - The coccyx bone *(B)* to C bilaterally; cut only as deep as the skin; avoid cutting deeper than the skin to protect important structures that will be covered in a future laboratory session
- Remove the skin and superficial fascia as one piece to expose the underlying gluteus maximus m.; this may take a while, depending on your cadaver

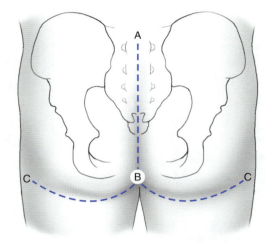

Figure 15-1 Skin incisions of the gluteal region

Gluteal Region

- Identify the following structures on both sides **(Figure 15-2)**:
  - **Gluteus maximus m.** — study its attachments along the iliac crest, sacrum, sacrotuberous ligament, and coccyx (this muscle also attaches to the iliotibial tract) and femur
    - Expose the inferior (free) border of the gluteus maximus m. by lifting up the inferior border
      - You may need to use a scalpel to free the inferior border from the deep fascia
    - Once the inferior border is freed, slide your hand deep to the gluteus maximus m. to separate the muscle from deeper muscles
    - With your hand deep to the gluteus maximus m., use your other hand to cut its sacral attachment with a scalpel, starting inferiorly and proceeding superiorly (this approach will preserve the neurovascular supply to the gluteus maximus m.); be careful to avoid cutting your hand with the scalpel
    - Cut the gluteus maximus m. from the superficial surface of the **sacrotuberous ligament**, *without* cutting that ligament
    - Reflect the gluteus maximus m. laterally only as far as necessary to uncover the sciatic n. and piriformis m. (studied further in another laboratory session)

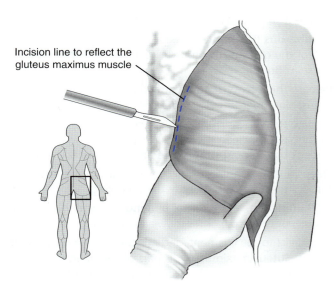

Figure 15-2 Gluteus maximus muscle

Gluteal Region Continued

Gluteal Region—cont'd

- Lift up the cut (medial) attachment of the gluteus maximus m. to reveal and identify the following **(Figure 15-3)**:
  - **Sacrotuberous ligament** — deep and parallel to the inferior border of the gluteus maximus m.; a firm band that may feel as dense as bone
    - Palpate the inferior (lateral) attachment of the ligament to the ischial tuberosity
    - Palpate the superior (medial) attachment of the ligament to the sacrum; clean the entire length of the ligament with forceps by scraping the surface and edges of the muscle
    - Deep to the ligament is a neurovascular bundle; use forceps to reveal and identify the following:
      - **Pudendal n.** and **internal pudendal a. and v.** — emerge inferior to the piriformis m., via the greater sciatic foramen
    - Superficial to the ligament, and attached to the deep surface of the gluteus maximus m., is part of the neurovascular supply to that muscle. Use forceps to dissect the inferior gluteal n., a., and v.
  - **Ischial spine** — attachment for the sacrospinous ligament, which is deep to the sacrotuberous ligament
    - Use your finger to probe around the pudendal n. and internal pudendal a. and v. to locate a pointed bone — the ischial spine, to which is attached the sacrospinous ligament
    - The pudendal n. and internal pudendal a. and v. course between the sacrospinous and sacrotuberous ligaments (the lesser sciatic foramen)
  - **Sacrospinous ligament** — attached to the sacrum and ischial spine
  - **Piriformis m.** — attached to the sacrum and greater trochanter of the femur; the sciatic n., pudendal n., internal pudendal a., and inferior gluteal n., a., and v. exit the pelvis inferior to the piriformis m. via the greater sciatic foramen (studied further in another laboratory session)
  - **Sciatic n.** — formed from ventral primary rami of spinal cord segments L4–S3; also emerges inferior to the piriformis m. via the greater sciatic foramen

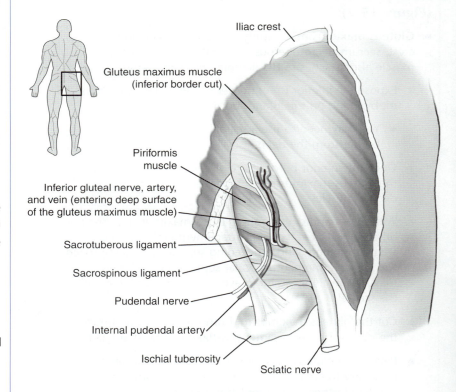

Figure 15-3   Gluteal region

Ischioanal (Ischiorectal) Fossa

- The two ischioanal fossae are located in the anal triangle, which is bounded by oblique lines from the sacrum to both ischial tuberosities and a coronal line from one ischial tuberosity to the other; each triangle is bounded medially by a sagittal line from the sacrum to the perineal body

  - Each ischioanal fossa is shaped like the curved keel of a boat; each fossa is positioned in an anterior-posterior direction; the posterior ends (recesses) communicate across the midline

  - The anterior recess (apex) of each fossa is anterior and superior to the urogenital diaphragm and inferior to the pelvic diaphragm (studied further in another laboratory session)

- With the cadaver prone, separate the legs (use a wooden block between the knees to keep the legs separated); reflect, using a scalpel, the remaining skin from the tip of the coccyx to each ischial tuberosity and across from one tuberosity to the other

- Use forceps and your fingers (not scissors or scalpels) to peel and scrape away the fat in both ischioanal fossae

- Once the fat is removed, identify and dissect further the following (**Figures 15-4** and **15-5**):

  - **Inferior rectal n., a., and v.** — arise from the pudendal n. and internal pudendal a. and v.; lateral to the sacrotuberous ligament (in the gluteal region); emerge medial to the sacrotuberous ligament and course diagonally to the anus; preserve these neurovascular bundles

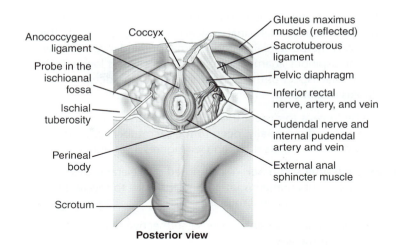

Figure 15-4 Ischioanal fossa (male)

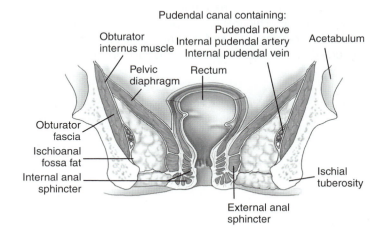

Figure 15-5 Ischioanal fossa (coronal section)

Ischioanal (Ischiorectal) Fossa Continued

Ischioanal (Ischiorectal) Fossa—cont'd

- **Pudendal canal** — the obturator fascia splits into two layers to form the pudendal canal, a sleeve of connective tissue that envelops the pudendal n. and internal pudendal vessels near the sacrospinous ligament; the pudendal canal is located on the medial aspect of the obturator internus m., deep to the gluteus maximus m. and sacrotuberous ligament
    - Use forceps to dissect the full extent of the inferior rectal n., a., and v. laterally, deep to the sacrotuberous ligament and into the gluteal region (see Figures 15-4 and 15-5):
- **External anal sphincter** — composed of skeletal muscle; scrape the subcutaneous fat around the anus to reveal the wisps of circumferential muscle
- **Anococcygeal ligament** — dense connective tissue that spans from the anus to the coccyx
- **Pelvic diaphragm** — closes the pelvic outlet by spanning the space between the pubis anteriorly and the coccyx posteriorly, and from one side of the pelvis to the other
    - **Levator ani m.** — a broad, thin, curved muscle sheet that is deep to the ischioanal fat; shaped like a funnel; combines with the coccygeus m. to form the pelvic diaphragm (studied in more detail in a future laboratory session)

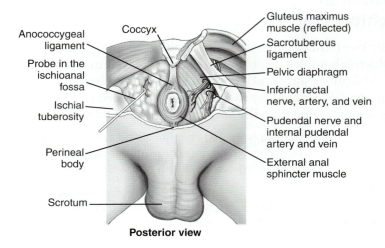

Figure 15-4 Ischioanal fossa (male)

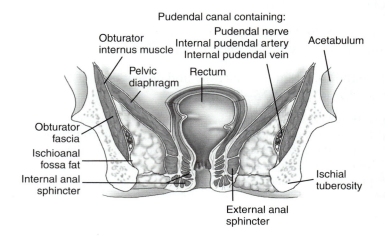

Figure 15-5 Ischioanal fossa (coronal section)

Urogenital Triangle

Lab 16

Prior to dissection, you should familiarize yourself with the following structures:

MALE (go to page 207)
- Perineum — urogenital and anal triangles
- External genitalia
  - Penis — crura, body, glans, penile raphe, prepuce
  - Scrotum
  - Testis — epididymis, tunica vaginalis, tunica albuginea, seminiferous tubules, epididymal sinus, gubernaculum testis
  - Spermatic cord
    - Ductus deferens, testicular a., pampiniform plexus of vv., autonomic nn., genital branch of the genitofemoral n.
- Superficial perineal space (see Table 16-1)
  - Roots of the external genitalia
    - Bulb/corpus spongiosa penis
    - Crura/corpora cavernosa penis
  - Bulbospongiosus m.
  - Ischiocavernosus mm.
  - Spongy urethra
  - Perineal nn., aa., and vv.
    - Posterior scrotal n., a., and v.
  - Superficial transverse perineal mm.
- Deep perineal space (see Table 16-2)
  - Perineal membrane

FEMALE (go to page 218)
- Perineum — urogenital and anal triangles
- External genitalia
  - Labia majora and minora
  - Mons pubis
  - Clitoris — crura, body, and glans
  - Urethra
  - Vagina
  - Vestibule
- Superficial perineal space (see Table 16-1)
  - Roots of the external genitalia
    - Bulb of the vestibule
    - Crura/corpora cavernosa clitoris
  - Bulbospongiosus m.
  - Ischiocavernosus mm.
  - Spongy urethra
  - Perineal nn., aa., and vv.
    - Posterior labial n., a., and v.
  - Superficial transverse perineal mm.
  - Greater vestibular glands
  - Vagina
- Deep perineal space (see Table 16-2)
  - Perineal membrane (urogenital diaphragm)

Lab 16 Dissection Overview

The purpose of this laboratory session is to learn the anatomy of the urogenital triangle through dissection. You will do so through the following suggested sequence:

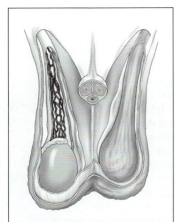

1. Dissect the spermatic cord and scrotal sac (male cadavers).

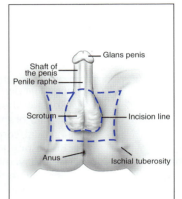

2. Dissect the scrotum to reveal the superficial perineal space.

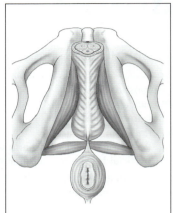

3. Dissect the muscles and erectile tissue in the superficial perineal space.

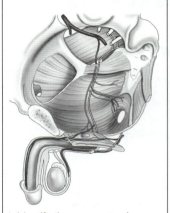

4. Identify the neurovascular branches of the internal pudendal vessels and pudendal nerves.

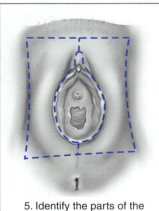

5. Identify the parts of the female perineum.

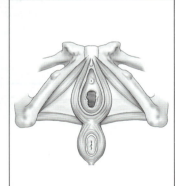

6. Dissect the muscles and erectile tissue of the superficial perineal space.

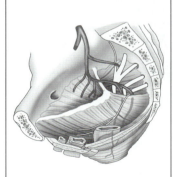

7. Identify the neurovascular branches of the internal pudendal vessels and pudendal nerves.

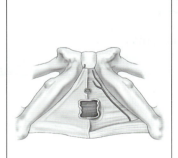

8. Discuss with your laboratory instructor if the deep perineal space is to be dissected.

Table 16-1 Contents of the Superficial Perineal Space

Male

1. Roots of external genitalia
   a. Bulb*/corpus spongiosum penis
   b. Crura†/corpora cavernosa penis
2. Bulbospongiosus m. — covers the bulb of the penis
3. Ischiocavernous m. — covers the crura
4. Spongy urethra
5. Perineal nerves, arteries, and veins
   a. Posterior scrotal n., a., and v.
   b. Muscular branches
6. Superficial transverse perineal mm.
7. —
8. —

Female

1. Roots of external genitalia
   a. Bulb of the vestibule
   b. Crura†/corpora cavernosa clitoris
2. Bulbospongiosus m. — covers the vestibular bulbs
3. Ischiocavernous m. — covers the crura
4. Spongy urethra
5. Perineal nerves, arteries, and veins
   a. Posterior labial n., a., and v.
   b. Muscular branches
6. Superficial transverse perineal mm.
7. Greater vestibular glands and ducts
8. Vagina

*Changes name distal to the suspensory ligament to the corpus spongiosum penis
†Change names distal to the suspensory ligament to the corpora cavernosa penis/clitoris

Table 16-2 Contents of the Deep Perineal Space

Male

1. Membranous urethra
2. Deep transverse perineal mm.
3. Sphincter urethrae m.
4. Internal pudendal a.
   a. Artery to the bulb
   b. Deep a. of the penis — no paired v.
   c. Dorsal a. of the penis
   d. Muscular branches
5. Internal pudendal v. and branches
6. Branches of the pudendal n. — dorsal n. and muscular branches of the perineal n.
7. Bulbourethral glands and ducts
8. —

Female

1. Membranous urethra
2. Deep transverse perineal mm.
3. Sphincter urethrovaginalis m.
4. Internal pudendal a.
   a. Artery to the bulb
   b. Deep a. of the clitoris — no paired v.
   c. Dorsal a. of the clitoris
   d. Muscular branches
5. Internal pudendal v. and branches
6. Branches of the pudendal n. — dorsal n. and muscular branches of the perineal n.
7. —
8. Vagina

Table 16-3 Structures of the Abdominal Wall, Scrotum, and Spermatic Cord

Layers of the Abdominal Wall	Corresponding Layers in the Scrotum and Spermatic Cord
1. Skin	1. Skin
Superficial fascia	
2. Fatty (Camper's)	2. Disappears because the scrotum contains no fat
3. Membranous (Scarpa's)	3. Dartos muscle and fascia
4. External oblique m.	4. External spermatic fascia
5. Internal oblique m.	5. Cremaster muscle and fascia
6. Transversus abdominis m.	6. No contribution
7. Transversalis fascia	7. Internal spermatic fascia
8. Extraperitoneal fatty tissue	8. Areolar connective tissue
9. Peritoneum	9. Tunica vaginalis

MALE

Spermatic Cord and Scrotum Overview

- The spermatic cord and scrotum are surrounded by fascial coverings that are continuous with and derived from the abdominal wall (see Table 16-3)

- To study the spermatic cord, place the cadaver supine **(Figure 16-1)**:
  - **Scrotal sac** — hangs inferior to the pubis and the root of the penis
    - Use a scalpel to make cutaneous, vertical incisions along the left and right sides of the scrotum to fully reveal the spermatic cord on both sides

- Visually identify the following:
  - **Spermatic cord** — begins at the deep inguinal ring, lateral to the inferior epigastric vessels, and ends in the scrotum at the posterior border of the testis

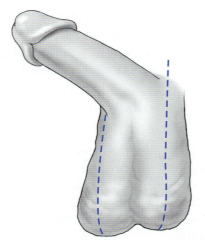

Figure 16-1   Scrotal incisions

MALE

Scrotum — Tissue Layers

- Use forceps to reveal and identify the following **(Figure 16-2)**:

  - **Superficial scrotal (Dartos) fascia** — very thin layer that is continuous with Scarpa's fascia; devoid of fat; forms the scrotal septum; use forceps to dissect into the fascia to find the following:

    - **Posterior scrotal nn. and vessels** — originate from branches of the perineal branch of the pudendal n. and perineal branches of the internal pudendal vessels

      - These neurovascular structures may be difficult to find (dissected in a future laboratory session)

    - **Anterior scrotal nn. and vessels** — branches from the ilioinguinal n. and external pudendal vessels from the femoral vessels

- With a scalpel, cut through the external spermatic fascia at the superficial inguinal ring; extend the cut to the testis, open the cut external spermatic fascia of the spermatic cord to identify the following contents (the layers of the anterior abdominal wall cover the spermatic cord because the testis carried the layers during its descent from the posterior abdominal wall to the scrotum; of the layers in the list that follows, you probably will not be able to identify the internal spermatic fascia):

  - **External spermatic fascia** — outer layer of spermatic fascia; continuous with the external oblique aponeurosis; deep to the Dartos fascia

  - **Cremasteric fibers/fascia** — middle layer of spermatic fascia; composed of loose connective tissue and thin fibers of cremasteric m. derived from the internal oblique m.; deep to the external spermatic fascia; best seen by looking for muscle strands while holding the cord in front of a light source

  - **Internal spermatic fascia** — innermost layer of spermatic fascia; continuous with the transversalis fascia; deep to the cremasteric fibers/fascia

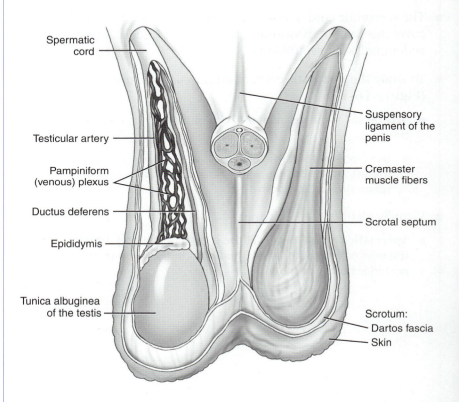

Figure 16-2 Spermatic cord and scrotum

MALE

Spermatic Cord — Contents

■ Use forceps to reveal and identify the following structures within the spermatic cord **(Figure 16-3)**:

- **Ductus deferens** — muscular tube that conveys sperm from the epididymis to the ejaculatory duct
  - Palpate this firm, tubular structure (the hardest structure) within the spermatic cord
- **Testicular a.** — arises from the aorta; in the spermatic cord, the artery courses with the pampiniform plexus of veins
- **Pampiniform plexus of veins** — venous network that drains into the right or left testicular vv.
- **Sympathetic nerve fibers** — on the wall of the testicular a.
- **Genital branch of the genitofemoral n.** — motor supply to the cremaster m.; may not be evident
- **Testis** — primary sex organ in the male
- **Tunica vaginalis** — fibrous drape that surrounds the testis; extension of parietal peritoneum that forms a sleeve around much of the testis

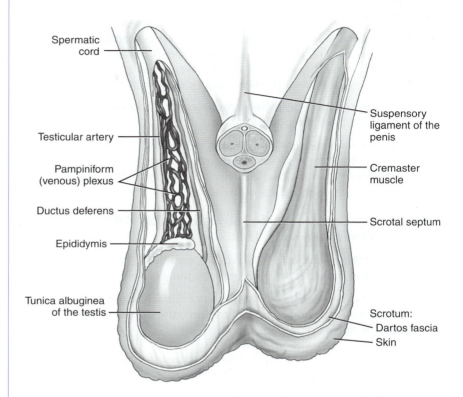

Figure 16-3 Coronal section through the anterior wall of the scrotal sac; penis cut in cross-section for reference

MALE

Testis

- Use forceps to reveal and identify the following **(Figures 16-4 and 16-5)**:

  - **Tunica vaginalis** — derived from the parietal peritoneum; covers most of the testis; has a parietal layer (fused with the internal spermatic fascia) and visceral layer (bound to the anterolateral surface of the testis and epididymis)
    - Covers the anterior, medial, and lateral surfaces of the testis, but not the posterior surface
  - **Gubernaculum testis** — connective tissue band between the inferior pole of the testis and the scrotum; remnant of the embryologic ligament that attached the inferior pole of the testis to the inferior surface of the scrotal sac

- With scissors, open the tunica vaginalis to inspect the interior of the serous sac of the testis

  - **Sinus of the epididymis** — lift up the epididymis; the sinus is a space that separates the testis from the body of the epididymis
  - **Epididymis** — attached to the posterior surface of the testis; observe its **head, body,** and **tail regions**; the ductus deferens begins at the tail of the epididymis

- With a scalpel, cut the testis longitudinally into left and right portions but leave the epididymis intact

  - **Tunica albuginea** — deep to the visceral layer of the tunica vaginalis; tough, white layer of connective tissue that is the capsule of the testis; observe the numerous pyramidal **lobules** of the testis that are created by septa from the tunica albuginea
  - **Seminiferous tubules** — fine, threadlike tubes that produce sperm

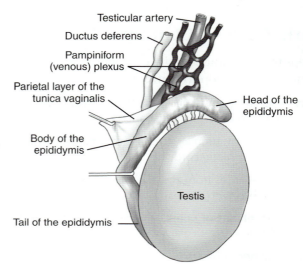

Figure 16-4 Lateral view of the testis and epididymis

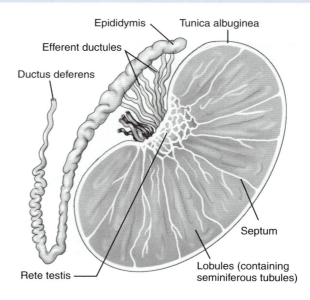

Figure 16-5 Coronal section of the testis

MALE

Overview of the Urogenital Triangle

- Place a block between the knees to expose the perineum

- The perineum is a diamond-shaped area between the thighs; it is divided into two triangles by a line from one ischial tuberosity to the other ischial tuberosity **(Figure 16-6)**:
  - **Urogenital (UG) triangle** — anterior triangular region bounded by the ischial tuberosities, ischiopubic (conjoint) rami, and pubic symphysis
  - **Anal triangle** — posterior triangular region bounded by the two ischial tuberosities and the coccyx bone

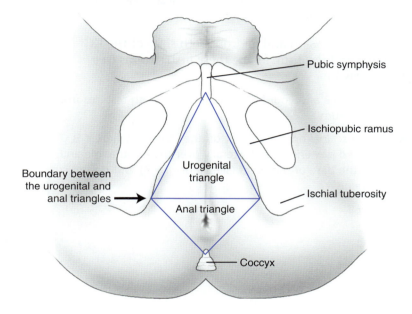

Figure 16-6 Male perineum

MALE

Dissection of the Urogenital Triangle

- Visually identify the following structures **(Figure 16-7)**:
  - **Shaft of the penis** — the body of the penis
  - **Glans penis** — the head or tip of the penis
  - **Penile raphe** — located on the ventral surface of the penis (erect in the anatomic position)

- To remove the skin and fat from both sides of the UG triangle and scrotum, follow these instructions (see Figure 16-7):
  - Use forceps and your fingers to separate both testicles from the scrotum
  - With a scalpel or scissors, cut off the scrotum where it is attached posteriorly and laterally over the UG triangle and from the base of the penis (see Figure 16-7), but do *not* cut the penis

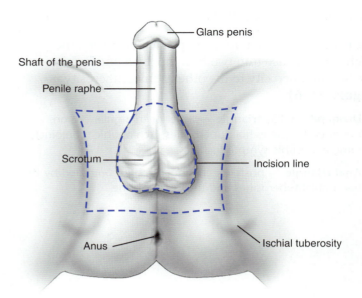

Figure 16-7 Skin incision in the male perineum

GAFS pp 403, 420–428, 439–451   ACGA pp 457, 473–475   NAHA Plates 381, 385

MALE

Shaft of the Penis

- Use a scalpel to cut the penis in cross section, about 2 cm from its root **(Figure 16-8)**

- Use forceps to reveal and observe the following structures on the cross-section of the cut penis (homologous to the clitoris of the female) **(Figure 16-9)**:

  - **Superficial penile fascia** — continuous with Scarpa's and Dartos fasciae; devoid of fat tissue
    - **Superficial dorsal v.** — drains to the external pudendal v.
  - **Deep penile fascia** — also called Buck's fascia
  - **Deep dorsal v.** — courses deep to the pubic symphysis to drain into the prostatic plexus of veins (studied further in another laboratory session)
  - **Dorsal a.** — originates from the internal pudendal a.
  - **Dorsal n.** — originates from the pudendal n.
  - **Tunica albuginea** — connective tissue sheath surrounding the erectile tissues; forms the **septum penis**, which separates the corpora cavernosa
  - **Corpora cavernosa (two)** — paired dorsal erectile tissue bodies
  - **Corpus spongiosum** — ventral erectile tissue that contains the **spongy urethra**
  - **Deep a.** — in the center of each of the two corpora cavernosa; branch of the internal pudendal a.; no accompanying veins

- Retain the detached penile cross-section for review

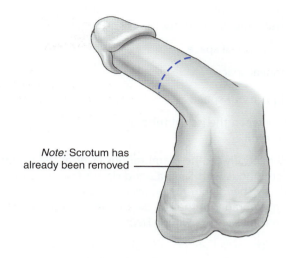

Figure 16-8   Transection of the penile shaft

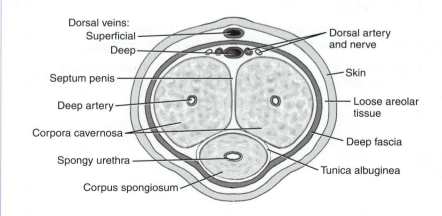

Figure 16-9   Cross-section of the penis

Unit 3 • Lab 16   Urogenital Triangle

MALE

Perineum and Superficial Perineal Space — Description

- The perineum contains the external genitalia and is divided into two anatomic compartments **(Figure 16-10)**:
  - Superficial perineal space
  - Deep perineal space

- Superficial perineal space
  - Located between the ischial tuberosities and ischiopubic (conjoint) rami
  - Bounded inferiorly by the membranous layer of the superficial fascia (continuous with Scarpa's and dartos fasciae) and superiorly by the inferior fascia, also called the inferior perineal membrane, of the UG diaphragm; this space extends into the scrotal sac (see Figure 16-10)
    - Palpate the area between the bulb and crura of the penis; your finger is stopped by the inferior fascia of the UG diaphragm

- **Deep perineal space**
  - Located between the ischial tuberosities, ischiopubic (conjoint) rami, and inferior arch of the pubic symphysis
  - Consists of two muscles and their superior and inferior fasciae (UG diaphragm)

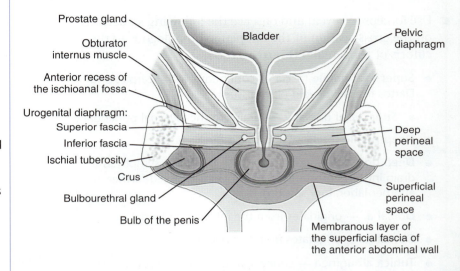

Figure 16-10 Coronal section of the male perineum

MALE

Superficial Perineal Space — Contents

- Follow these instructions to reveal the three muscles of the superficial perineal space (ischiocavernosus, bulbospongiosus, and superficial transverse perineal mm.):

  - Use a scalpel to remove the remaining skin and superficial fascia that may extend inferiorly from the anterior abdominal wall to the penis (this will require a variety of dissection techniques and instruments); note the fundiform ligament on the dorsal surface of the penis while you dissect the deeper fibrous **suspensory ligament of the penis** (not shown)

- Use forceps to reveal and identify the following muscles of the superficial perineal space **(Figure 16-11)**:

  - **Ischiocavernosus mm.** — paired muscles that cover each crus of the **corpora cavernosa**

    - Follow the paired corpora cavernosa laterally and posteriorly proximally to their respective attachment on each ischiopubic (conjoint) ramus

    - These fixed (nonpendulous) parts of the penis are called **crura** (legs); both crura are covered superficially (inferiorly) by an ischiocavernosus m.

  - **Bulbospongiosus m.** — covers the midline corpus spongiosus and **bulb of the penis**

- Follow the corpus spongiosum and bulb of the penis posteriorly to find the perineal body and the inferior fascia of the UG diaphragm

  - The perineal body is a midline thickening where the bulbospongiosus, superficial transverse perineal, deep transverse perineal, and external anal sphincter mm. converge, between the bulb of the penis and the anus

  - **Superficial transverse perineal m.** — crosses transversely between the medial aspects of the ischial tuberosities and the perineal body

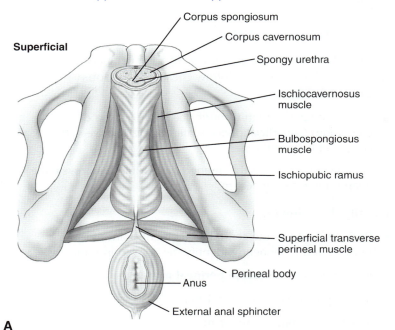

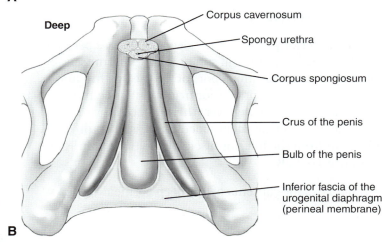

Figure 16-11 Superficial perineal space of the male. **A,** Muscles overlie the erectile tissue. **B,** Erectile tissue; muscle removed from the erectile tissue

Unit 3 • Lab 16 Urogenital Triangle

MALE

Deep Perineal Space

- To identify some of the structures in the deep perineal space (see Figure 16-10), follow these instructions **(Figure 16-12)**:

    - Make a scalpel incision through the inferior fascia of the UG diaphragm (superficial perineal membrane), between the crura and bulb of the penis

    - Use forceps to spread the opened inferior fascia to reveal the deep transverse perineal m.

- Identify the following:

    - **Perineal body** — the central attachment point of the muscles in the perineum; identify the converging muscles:

        - **Superficial transverse perineal mm.**
        - **Deep transverse perineal mm.**
        - **External anal sphincter m.**
        - **Levator ani m.**

- *Note:* The anterior portion of the deep transverse perineal m. is also called the urethral sphincter m.; this muscle surrounds the membranous portion of the urethra and acts as a voluntary sphincter for urination; difficult to dissect without destroying everything in both the superficial and deep perineal spaces, unless the bulb of the penis is cut from the inferior fascia of the UG diaphragm (see Figure 16-12B)

- See Table 16-2 for contents of the deep perineal space

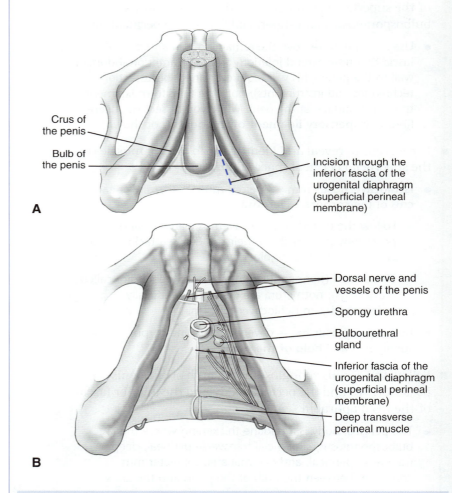

Figure 16-12 Deep perineal space. **A,** Incision in the inferior fascia of the urogenital (UG) diaphragm. **B,** Structures associated with the deep perineal space

MALE

Review — Branches of the Internal Pudendal Artery and Pudendal Nerve

- Review this page and note the compartmentalization of the artery, vein, and nerve distribution **(Figure 16-13)**

- Blood supply to the UG region:
  - **Internal pudendal a. and v.** (remember the presence of the portal–caval anastomosis between the superior rectal v. and the middle/inferior rectal vv.)
    - **Inferior rectal a. and v.**
    - **Perineal a. and v.**
      - Posterior scrotal a. and v.
    - **Deep a. of the penis** — no accompanying veins
    - **Dorsal a. and v. of the penis**
  - **External pudendal a. and v.**
    - **Anterior scrotal a. and v.**

- Innervation to the UG region:
  - **Pudendal n.**
    - **Inferior rectal n.**
    - **Deep perineal n.**
    - **Dorsal n. of the penis**
    - **Superficial perineal n.**
    - **Posterior scrotal nn.**
  - **Ilioinguinal n. (L1)**
    - **Anterior scrotal nn.**

- Return to the cadaver to follow the course and distribution of the internal pudendal a. and v. and the pudendal n.

- *Note:* Similarly named veins accompany each artery

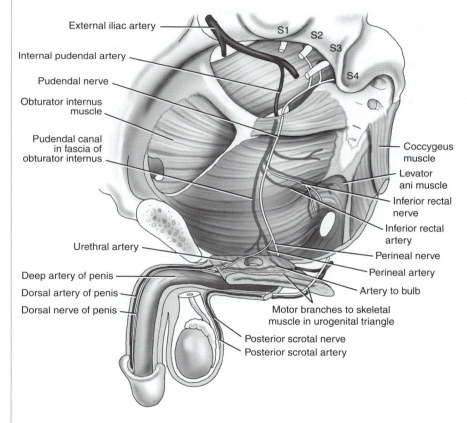

Figure 16-13 Branches of the internal pudendal a. and pudendal n. (From Drake R, Vogl W, Mitchell A: Gray's Anatomy for Students. Philadelphia: Elsevier, 2005, Figs. 5.76, 5.77)

FEMALE

Overview of the Urogenital Triangle

- Turn the cadaver supine and place a block between the knees to expose the perineum

- The perineum is a diamond-shaped area between the thighs; it is divided into two triangles by a line from one ischial tuberosity to the other ischial tuberosity **(Figure 16-14)**:

  - **UG triangle** — anterior triangular region bounded by the ischial tuberosities, ischiopubic (conjoined) rami, and pubic symphysis

  - **Anal triangle** — posterior triangular region bounded by the two ischial tuberosities and the coccyx bone

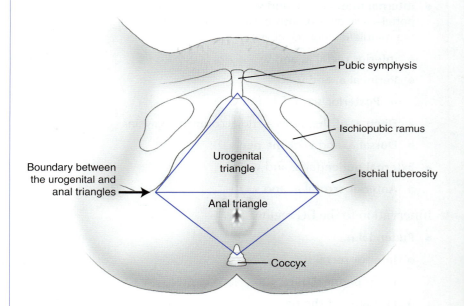

Figure 16-14 Female perineum

FEMALE

External Genitalia — Perineum

■ Visually identify the following **(Figure 16-15)**:

- **Mons pubis** — skin and adipose tissue superficial to the pubic symphysis; point of attachment for the round ligament of the uterus

- **Labia majora** — two large folds of skin filled with adipose tissue; they are joined anteriorly by the anterior labial commissure; pubic hair lines this region of the perineum

- **Labia minora** — two thin delicate folds of adipose-free, hairless skin that lie between the labia majora and enclose the vestibule of the vagina; lie on each side of the opening of the urethra and vagina

- **Vestibule** — space between the labia minora

- **Clitoris** — located between the anterior ends of the labia minora; composed of erectile tissue (and its muscle), like the penis, and capable of erection

- **External urethral orifice** — opening for the urethra; anterior to the vaginal orifice

- **Vaginal orifice** — opening for the vagina; positioned between the external urethral orifice and the anus

- **Anus** — opening for the rectum; posterior to the vaginal orifice

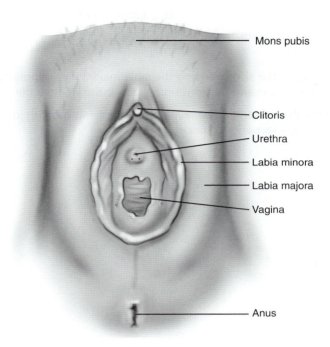

Figure 16-15 Female external genitalia

FEMALE

Dissection of the Urogenital Triangle

■ Make the following incisions, using a scalpel **(Figure 16-16)**:

- Cut circumferentially around the lateral surface of the labia minora
  - Remove the skin overlying the labia majora and minora to remove skin and fat from both sides of the UG triangle
- Reflect the skin and fat to reveal the underlying muscles in the superficial perineal space

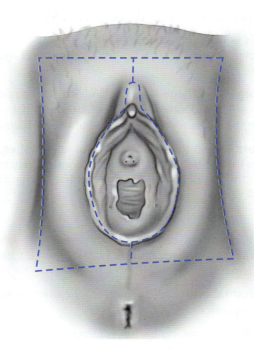

Figure 16-16 Dissection of the labia majora and minora

FEMALE

Perineum and Superficial Perineal Space — Description

- The perineum contains the external genitalia and is divided into two anatomic compartments **(Figure 16-17)**:
  - Superficial perineal space
  - Deep perineal space

- **Superficial perineal space**
  - Located between the ischial tuberosities and ischiopubic (conjoint) rami
  - Bounded inferiorly by the membranous layer of the superficial fascia (continuous with Scarpa's and dartos fasciae) and superiorly by the inferior fascia of the UG diaphragm, also called the inferior perineal membrane (see Figure 16-17)
    - Palpate the area between the bulb and crura of the clitoris; your finger is stopped by the inferior fascia of the UG diaphragm

- **Deep perineal space**
  - Located between the ischial tuberosities, ischiopubic (conjoint) rami, and inferior arch of the pubic symphysis
  - Consists of two muscles and their superior and inferior fasciae (UG diaphragm)

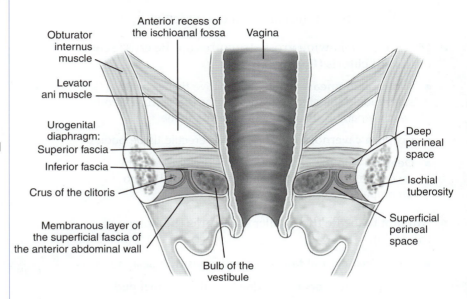

Figure 16-17 Coronal section of the female perineum

FEMALE

Shaft of the Clitoris

- Inclusion of this dissection of the clitoris will be indicated by your instructor

- Use a scalpel to cut the clitoris in cross-section

- Observe the following gross structures on the cross-section of the cut clitoris **(Figure 16-18)**:
  - **Tunica albuginea** — white, connective tissue sheath surrounding the erectile tissues; forms the septum clitoris, which separates the corpora cavernosa tissue
  - **Corpora cavernosa (two)** — paired erectile tissue bodies
  - **Deep a.** — in the center of each of the two corpora cavernosa; branches of the internal pudendal a. (no accompanying vein)

- Attempt to locate the smaller structures (homologous to the male):
  - **Superficial clitoral fascia** — continuous with Scarpa's fascia
    - **Superficial dorsal v.** — drains to the external pudendal v.
  - **Deep clitoral fascia**
  - **Deep dorsal v.** — courses deep to the pubic symphysis (studied further in a future laboratory session)
  - **Dorsal a.** — originates from the internal pudendal a.; no paired veins
  - **Dorsal n.** — originates from the pudendal n.
  - **Greater vestibular glands** — located posterior to each vestibular bulb beneath the bulbospongiosus m.; do not try to locate these glands

- Retain the detached clitoral cross-section for review

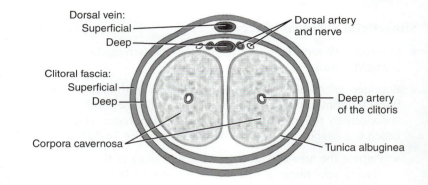

Figure 16-18 Cross-section of the clitoris

FEMALE

Superficial Perineal Space — Contents

- Use forceps to reveal and identify the following muscles of the superficial perineal space **(Figure 16-19)**:

  - **Ischiocavernosus mm.** — paired muscles that cover each crus of the **corpora cavernosa**
    - Follow the paired corpora cavernosa laterally and posteriorly to their respective attachment on each ischiopubic (conjoint) ramus
    - These fixed (nonpendulous) parts of the clitoris are called **crura** (legs); both crura are covered superficially (inferiorly) by a thin muscle called the ischiocavernosus m.

  - **Bulbospongiosus m.** — covers the **bulb of the vestibule**
    - Clean the area between the crura and vaginal orifice to locate the bulbospongiosus m. fibers on the lateral surface of the labia minora
    - Follow the bulbospongiosus m. posteriorly to its attachment to the perineal body and the inferior fascia of the UG diaphragm
    - The perineal body is a midline thickening where the bulbospongiosus, superficial transverse perineal, deep transverse perineal, and external anal sphincter mm. converge

  - **Superficial transverse perineal m.** — crosses transversely between the medial aspect of the ischial tuberosities and the perineal body

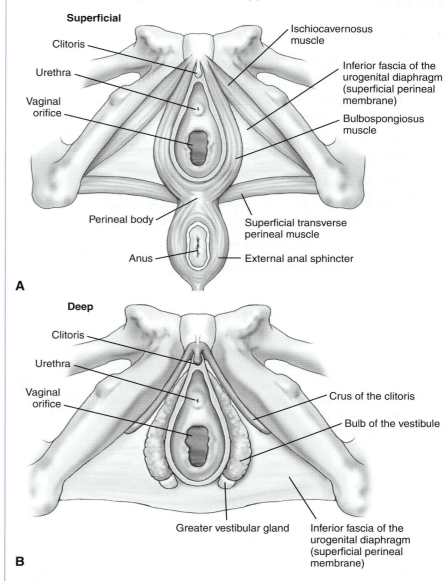

GAFS pp 440–446   ACGA pp 477–481   NAHA Plates 378–379

Figure 16-19 Superficial perineal space of the female. **A**, Muscles overlie the erectile tissue. **B**, Structures associated with the deep perineal space

FEMALE

Deep Perineal Space

- To identify some of the structures in the deep perineal space, take the following steps **(Figure 16-20)**:
  - Make a scalpel incision through the inferior fascia of the UG diaphragm, between the crura and bulb
  - Use forceps to spread the opened inferior fascia to reveal the deep transverse perineal muscle

- Identify the following:
  - **Perineal body** — the central attachment point of the muscles of the perineum; identify the converging muscles:
    - **Deep transverse perineal mm.**
      - Sphincter urethrovaginalis
    - **Superficial transverse perineal mm.**
    - **External anal sphincter m.**
    - **Levator ani m.**

- *Note:* The anterior portion of the deep transverse perineal m. contains both the urethral sphincter and vaginal sphincter mm.; the sphincter urethrovaginalis is difficult to dissect without destroying everything in the superficial and deep perineal spaces

- See Table 16-2 for contents of the deep perineal space

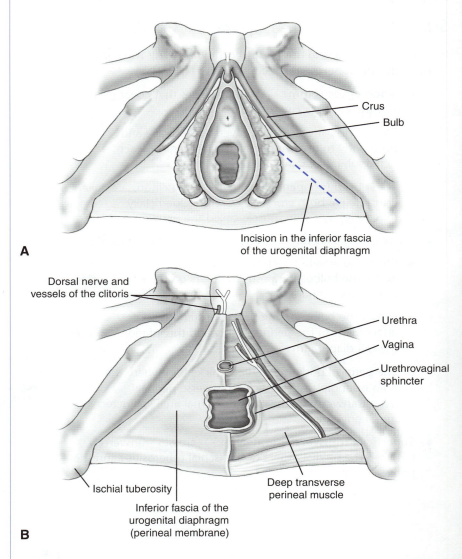

Figure 16-20 Deep perineal space. **A,** Incision in the inferior fascia of the urogenital (UG) diaphragm. **B,** Structures associated with the deep perineal space

FEMALE

Review — Branches of the Internal Pudendal Artery and Pudendal Nerve

- Review this page and note the compartmentalization of the artery, vein, and nerve distribution **(Figure 16-21)**

- Blood supply to the UG region:
  - **Internal pudendal a. and v.** (remember the presence of the portal–caval anastomosis between the superior rectal v. and the middle/inferior rectal vv.)
    - Inferior rectal a. and v.
    - Perineal a. and v.
      - Posterior labial a. and v.
    - Deep a. of the clitoris — no accompanying vein
    - Dorsal a. and v. of the clitoris
  - **External pudendal a. and v.**
    - Anterior labial a. and v.

- Review the innervation to the UG region:
  - Pudendal n.
    - Dorsal n. of the clitoris
    - Inferior rectal n.
    - Deep perineal n.
    - Superficial perineal n.
    - Posterior labial nn.
  - Ilioinguinal n.
    - Anterior labial n.

- Return to the cadaver to follow the course and distribution of the internal pudendal a. and v. and the pudendal n.

- *Note:* Similarly named veins accompany each artery

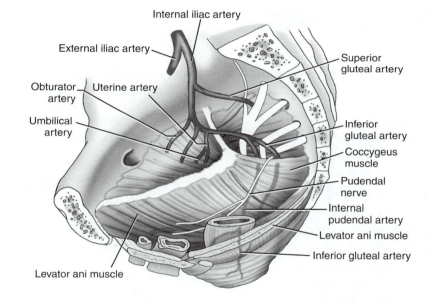

Figure 16-21 Branches of the internal pudendal artery and pudendal nerve. (From Drake R, Vogl W, Mitchell A: Gray's Anatomy for Students. Philadelphia: Elsevier, 2005, Figs. 5.76, 5.77)

Lab 17

Pelvis and Reproductive Systems

Prior to dissection, you should familiarize yourself with the following structures:

OSTEOLOGY
- Pelvic brim
  - False pelvis
  - True pelvis
- Pelvic inlet and outlet

FEMALE PELVIC STRUCTURES
- Pubovesical ligament
- Transverse cervical (cardinal) ligament
- Uterosacral ligament
- Broad ligament
  - Mesometrium
  - Mesovarium
  - Mesosalpinx
- Ligament of the ovary
- Suspensory ligament of the ovary
- Round ligament of the uterus
- Vesicouterine pouch
- Rectouterine pouch

FEMALE PELVIC ORGANS
- Bladder
  - Trigone
  - Obliterated urachus
- Uterus — fundus, body, uterine horn, uterine cavity, internal os, cervix, isthmus, external os
- Vagina — rugae; anterior, two lateral, and posterior fornices; hymen
- Uterine tube — fimbriae, isthmus, ampulla
- Ovary

MALE PELVIC STRUCTURE
- Rectovesical pouch

MALE PELVIC ORGANS
- Bladder
  - Trigone
  - Obliterated urachus
- Prostate gland
- Seminal vesicle
- Ductus deferens

MUSCLES
- Urogeniral diaphragm
- Pelvic diaphragm
  - Levator ani m.
    - Puborectalis m.
    - Pubococcygeus m.
    - Iliococcygeus m.
  - Coccygeus m.
- Piriformis m.
- Obturator internus m.

NERVES
- Lumbosacral trunk (L4, L5)
- Sacral plexus (ventral rami of S1–S4)
  - Sciatic n.
  - Pudendal n.
- Superior and inferior gluteal nn.

ARTERIES AND VEINS
- Common iliac a. and v.
  - External iliac a. and v.
    - Inferior epigastric a. and v.
  - Internal iliac a. and v.
    - Iliolumbar aa. and vv.
    - Lateral sacral a. and v.
    - Obturator a. and v.
    - Superior gluteal a. and v.
    - Inferior gluteal a. and v.
    - Obliterated umbilical a. and v.
      - Branch to the ductus deferens (male)
    - Inferior vesical aa. and vv. (male)
    - Uterine and vaginal aa. and vv. (female)
    - Superior vesical a.
    - Vaginal aa. (female)
    - Middle rectal a. and vv.
    - Internal pudendal a. and v.
      - Inferior rectal a. and v.

Lab 17 Dissection Overview

The purpose of this laboratory session is to learn the anatomy of the pelvis and reproductive systems through dissection. You will do so through the following suggested sequence:

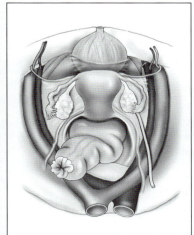

1. Dissect the structures of the pelvis.

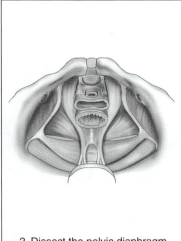

2. Dissect the pelvic diaphragm.

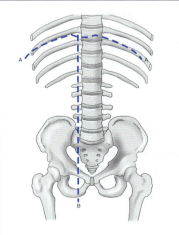

3. Bisect the cadaver to better study the pelvic structures.

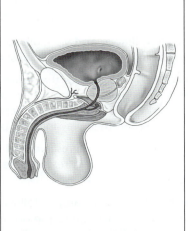

4. Study the pelvis and perineum in sagittal section in the male cadaver.

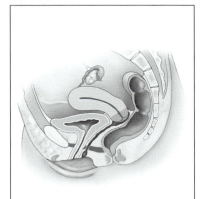

5. Study the pelvis and perineum in sagittal section in the female cadaver.

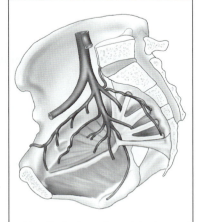

6. Identify the branches of the internal iliac artery (male and female).

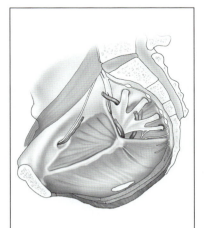

7. Identify the nerves of the pelvic cavity.

BOTH SEXES

Pelvis — Overview

- Bluntly dissect and peel the overlying peritoneum and use the scraping technique to remove extraperitoneal fat; then identify the following **(Figures 17-1 and 17-2)**:

  - **Common iliac a. and v.** — bifurcate at the sacroiliac joint into the internal and external iliac aa. and vv., respectively

  - **Ureters** — paired tubes that drain urine from the kidneys; course inferiorly along both sides of the posterior abdominal wall to the pelvic brim; cross anterior to the common/external iliac vessels on their way into the pelvis to the urinary bladder

  - **Urinary bladder** — a reservoir for urine; located in the true pelvis, retroperitoneal; rests on the pelvic floor, posterior to the pubic symphysis

  - **Ductus deferens (male)** — follow the ductus deferens from the deep inguinal ring to the posterior surface of the bladder; crosses over the ureter; push the bladder anteriorly and the rectum posteriorly to follow to the prostate gland as far as possible

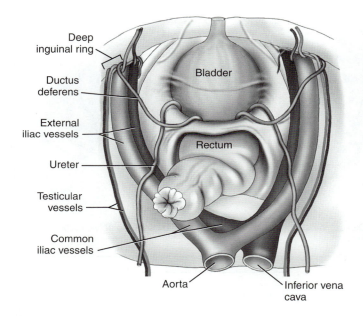

Figure 17-1 Superior view of the male pelvis

Pelvis — Overview—cont'd

- **Round ligament of the uterus (female)** — follow the round ligament from the deep inguinal ring to the anterior and superior surface of the uterus; the round ligament is located between the layers of the broad ligament

- **Gonadal aa. (testicular/ovarian)** — follow their course along the posterior abdominal wall, from the abdominal aorta to the deep inguinal ring (male) or from the abdominal aorta to the ovaries (female); use forceps to reveal these vessels but do not cut or break them

- **Left gonadal v. (testicular/ovarian)** — observe its course from the deep inguinal ring to the left renal v. in males or from the left ovary to the left renal v. in females

- **Right gonadal v. (testicular/ovarian)** — observe its course from the deep inguinal ring to the inferior vena cava in males or from the right ovary to the inferior vena cava in females

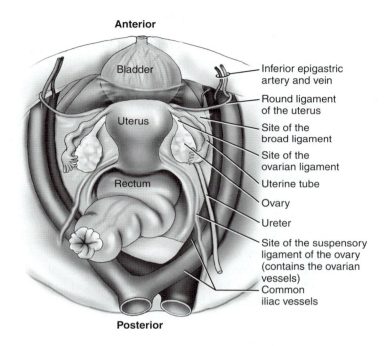

Figure 17-2 Superior view into the female pelvis

FEMALE

Pelvic Peritoneum — Broad Ligament

- Move the uterus and rectum to different positions to identify the following components of the broad ligament **(Figure 17-3)**:

- *Note:* If the uterus is absent (hysterectomy), go to another female cadaver that has a uterus to observe the following structures:

  - **Broad ligament** — a drape of pelvic peritoneum over the female reproductive organs; has anterior and posterior sheets

  - **Mesosalpinx** — the mesentery of the uterine (fallopian) tube; most superior part of the broad ligament, between the uterine tube and ovary; bilateral

  - **Mesovarium** — the mesentery of the ovary; posterior (perpendicular) extension of the broad ligament; to reveal the mesovarium, pull the ovary posteriorly 90 degrees to the plane of the mesosalpinx and broad ligament; bilateral

    - The remainder of the broad ligament is inferior to the ovary and mesosalpinx

  - **Round ligament of the uterus** — courses from the anterolateral surface of the uterine wall, inferior to the origin of the uterine tube, to the deep inguinal ring and ends by attaching to the mons pubis; bilateral

  - **Ovarian ligament** — courses from the posterolateral surface of the uterine wall, inferior to the origin of the uterine tube, to the medial pole of the ovary (remnant of the gubernaculum); contains the ovarian branches of the uterine a. and v.; bilateral

  - **Suspensory ligament of the ovary** — courses from the pelvic brim to the lateral pole of the ovary; formed by the peritoneum where it drapes the ovarian vessels; bilateral

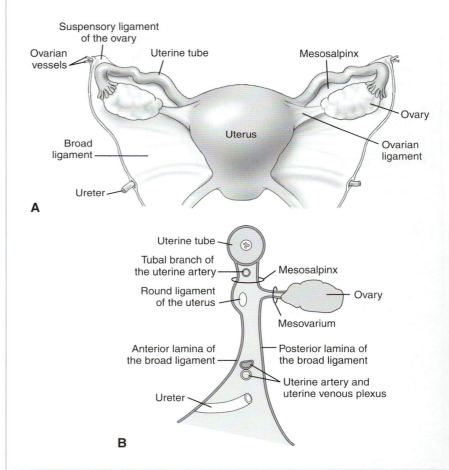

Figure 17-3 Female pelvic peritoneum. **A**, Posterior view of the broad ligament and uterus. **B**, Sagittal section through the uterine tube (lateral to the uterus) and broad ligament

BOTH SEXES

Pelvic Diaphragm

- This is a challenging dissection; dry the pelvic floor with paper towels; peel and shred the pelvic peritoneum from around the pelvic organs

- The openings of the bony pelvis are closed by muscles bilaterally; identify the following **(Figure 17-4)**:
  - Lateral: **obturator internus m.** — covers the obturator foramen and is pierced by the obturator n., a., and v., which pass through the **obturator canal**
  - Center: **pelvic diaphragm**
  - Posterior: **piriformis m.**

- Identify the following structures (see Figure 17-4):
  - **Tendinous arch** — inferior to the opening of the obturator canal, the obturator internus fascia thickens and forms a tendinous arch between the ischial spine and pubic bone; the tendinous arch serves as the lateral attachment for the iliococcygeus part of the levator ani m.
  - **Pelvic diaphragm** — a funnel-shaped muscle that forms the floor of the pelvic outlet; the pelvic organs are anchored to the middle of the pelvic diaphragm; composed of two paired muscles (levator ani m. and coccygeus m.) that fuse at the midline:
    - **Levator ani m.** — consists of three contiguous parts that are named by their attachments (it will be difficult to isolate individual components):
      - **Puborectalis m.** — medial part
      - **Pubococcygeus m.** — intermediate part
      - **Iliococcygeus m.** — lateral part (arises from the tendinous arch of the obturator internus fascia)

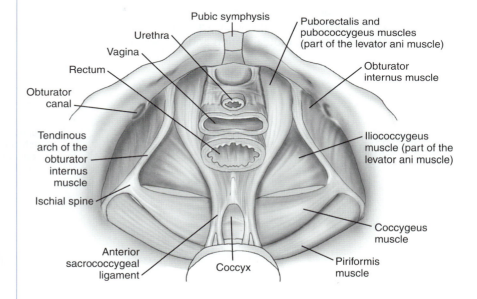

Figure 17-4 Superior view of the female pelvis (pelvic organs are shown cut; do not cut the organs)

Pelvic Diaphragm Continued

Unit 3 • Lab 17 Pelvis and Reproductive Systems

Pelvic Diaphragm—cont'd

- **Coccygeus (ischiococcygeus) m.** — arises from the ischial spines and from the posterior part of the pelvic diaphragm; attaches to the coccyx

- **Piriformis m.** — closes the pelvic outlet posterior to the pelvic diaphragm

    - Arises from the sacrum and attaches to the femur
    - The gap between the piriformis m. and pelvic diaphragm is the primary passageway for nerves and vessels from the pelvis to the gluteal region and perineum

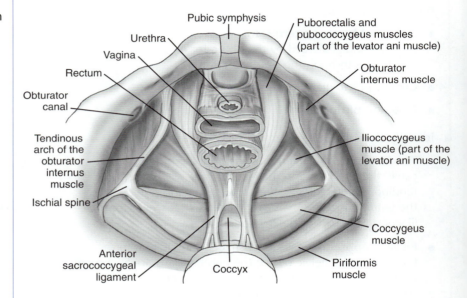

Figure 17-4 Superior view of the female pelvis (pelvic organs are shown cut; do not cut the organs)

BOTH SEXES

Hemisection

- After this part of the dissection, your cadaver will be divided into three segments; these steps are taken to enlarge the field of dissection to improve your understanding of the pelvic wall

- *Note:* Not all courses bisect the cadaver; follow the instructions from your course director

- To prepare the cadaver to be bisected, follow these instructions **(Figure 17-5)**:
  - If not already done, cut the coronary and triangular ligaments of the liver
  - Using scissors, cut the inferior vena cava between the liver and diaphragm
  - Reflect the liver to the left
  - With a scalpel, cut horizontally through intercostal space 9 superior to the diaphragm (*A* to *A*) on both sides of the vertebral bodies
  - Use a hand saw to cut through the T9 intervertebral disc across the plane marked *A*
  - Use a scalpel to cut any soft tissue necessary to divide your cadaver into superior and inferior segments
  - Cut (with a hand saw or bandsaw) through the pubic symphysis in a parasagittal plane (*B*), up to the horizontal cut (*A*)
    - If you are going to use a handsaw, first use a scalpel to cut through the soft tissues and then use the saw for cutting through bone
  - **Male pelvis** — go to page 234
  - **Female pelvis** — go to page 236

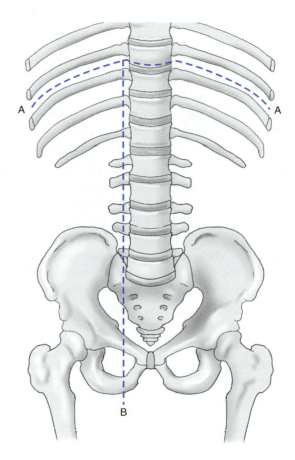

Figure 17-5 Scalpel and saw cuts for hemisection

MALE

Pelvis

- Rotate the hemisected pelvis so that a side view of the larger side of the pelvis is obtained to identify the following structures **(Figure 17-6)**:

    - **Bladder** — superior and posterior to the pubic symphysis

        - **Ureters** — enter the lateral sides of the bladder; use forceps to dissect along the ureter to find its entry into the posterolateral surface of the bladder

        - **Trigone** — internal triangular space between the two ureteral orifices and the internal urethral orifice (you will see only half of the trigone)

    - **Seminal vesicles** — inferior and posterior to the bladder; push the bladder anteriorly and use forceps to dissect (only one will be present on the hemisected pelvis)

    - **Ductus deferens** — use forceps to follow the ductus deferens from the deep inguinal ring across the external iliac vessels and obturator n. and vessels to join the duct of the seminal vesicle to become the ejaculatory duct; push the bladder anteriorly to do so

    - **Prostate gland** — dark, solid organ between the bladder and urogenital diaphragm; normally about the size of a walnut; push the bladder anteriorly to reveal the prostate gland

        - **Ejaculatory ducts** — you may see the ejaculatory ducts leading to the prostatic urethra; they are formed by the union of the ductus deferens and the duct of the seminal vesicle

    - **Urethra** — divided into three regions based on location; delineate the three regions:

        - **Prostatic urethra** — travels through the prostate gland

        - **Membranous urethra** — travels through the urogenital diaphragm

        - **Spongy urethra** — travels through the bulb and corpus spongiosum penis

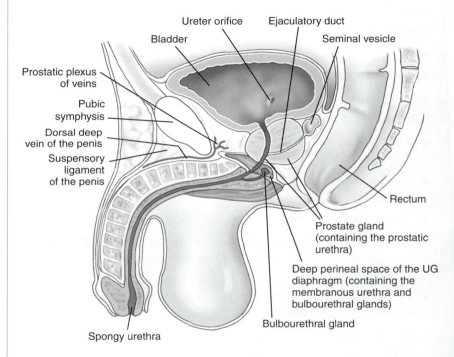

Figure 17-6 Sagittal section of the male pelvis

Pelvis—cont'd

- **Urogenital diaphragm** — the thin, solid septum between the prostate gland superiorly and the bulb of the penis inferiorly, and between the perineal body posteriorly and the pubic bone anteriorly; use forceps to delineate the superior and inferior fascia; contains the **bulbourethral glands**, **membranous urethra**, and **urethral sphincter m**.

- **Deep dorsal v. of the penis** — use forceps to follow and dissect this vein from the dorsum of the penis to deep to the pubic symphysis, where it enters the prostatic plexus of veins

GAFS pp 365, 397–410   ACGA pp 453–458   NAHA Plate 361

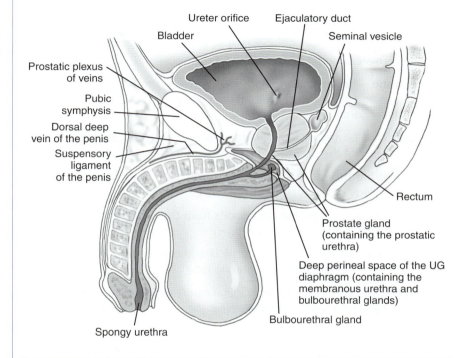

Figure 17-6   Sagittal section of the male pelvis

FEMALE

Pelvis

- Rotate the hemisected pelvis so that a side view of the larger side of the pelvis is obtained to identify the following structures **(Figure 17-7)**:

  - **Bladder** — superior and posterior to the pubic symphysis

  - **Ureters** — enter the lateral sides of the bladder; use forceps to dissect along the ureter to find its entry into the posterolateral surface of the bladder

  - **Trigone** — internal triangular space between the two ureteral orifices and the internal urethral orifice (you will see only half of the trigone)

  - **Uterus** — posterior to the bladder; identify the fundus, body, and cervix of the uterus, as well as the following:

    - **Uterine tubes** — extend laterally from the upper part of the body of the uterus

    - **Fimbria** — finger-like projections from the distal end of the uterine tube; the end is open

    - **Ovaries** — almond-shaped; the lateral pole is cupped by the fimbriated end of the uterine tube

  - **Cervix** — protrudes into the vaginal canal; **external os** opens into the vagina; use forceps to reveal the cervical canal and external os

    - **Vagina** — anterior wall, posterior wall, and two lateral fornices; use forceps to reveal the fornices

    - **Urethra** — between the clitoris and vagina; use forceps to reveal the urethra

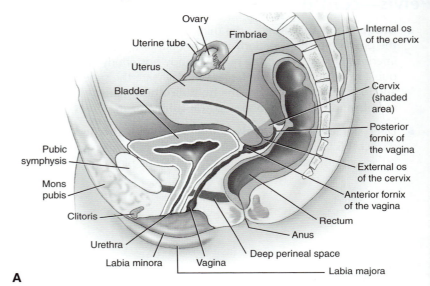
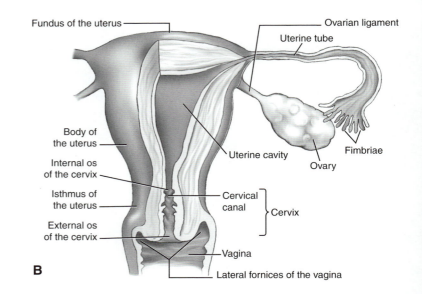

Figure 17-7 Female pelvis. **A**, Sagittal section. **B**, Coronal section through the uterus.

Pelvis—cont'd

- Connective tissue supports of the uterus (see Figure 17-7C)

  - Pubovesical ligament — fascia that extends from the cervix to the anterior pelvic wall

  - **Transverse cervical (cardinal) ligament** — thickening of the pelvic fascia around the uterine a. and v.; push the uterus away from the lateral pelvic wall; use forceps to locate the ureter and follow it inferiorly toward the bladder to locate the uterine a., which crosses over (superior to) the ureter; continue dissecting the uterine a. to find its branches to the uterus, uterine tube, and vagina

  - Uterosacral ligament — fascia that extends from the cervix to the posterior pelvic wall

GAFS pp 410–416   ACGA pp 460–465   NAHA Plates 365–371

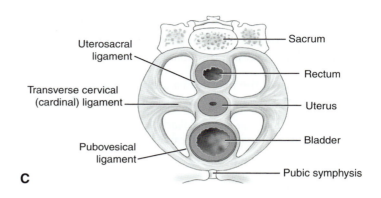

Figure 17-7, cont'd C, Cross-section of the female pelvis

BOTH SEXES

Pelvic Vasculature

- Use forceps to bluntly dissect and peel the peritoneum and extraperitoneal fat covering the iliac vessels and nerves

- Use forceps to dissect the pelvic vasculature, following these instructions:

  - Remove branches of the internal iliac vv. to more clearly demonstrate the arterial distribution

  - Identify the following **(Figure 17-8)**:

    - **Common iliac a.** — divides into two divisions at the level of the sacroiliac joint:

      - **Internal iliac a.** — anterior and posterior divisions that supply the pelvis and perineum

      - **External iliac a.** — courses deep to the inguinal ligament, after which it becomes the femoral a.

    - **Lymph nodes** — distributed along both the external and internal iliac aa.

- **Male pelvis** — go to page 239

- **Female pelvis** — go to page 241

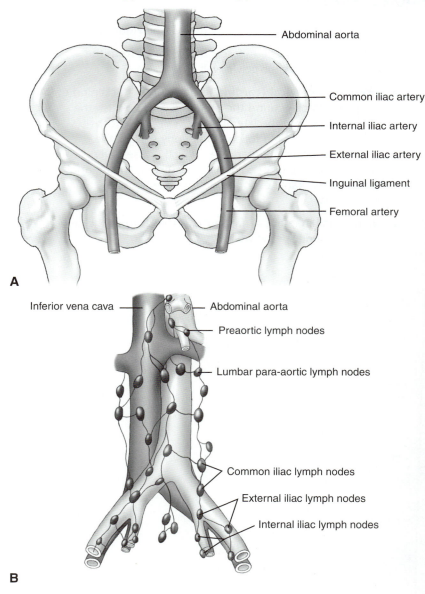

Figure 17-8 Common iliac vessels. **A,** Common iliac artery. **B,** Lymphatics

MALE

Pelvic Vasculature — Internal Iliac Artery (Anterior Division)

- Use forceps and hemostats to peel away the peritoneum and extraperitoneal fat covering the iliac vessels and nerves from the half of the pelvis that does not have the bulk of the pelvic organs attached

- Use forceps to reveal and identify the following branches **(Figure 17-9)**:

  - **Anterior division of the internal iliac a.**

    - **Umbilical a.** — continuation of the anterior division to the anterior abdominal wall; becomes the **medial umbilical ligament (obliterated umbilical a.)**; may give off three to four **superior vesical aa.**

    - **Obturator a.** — courses through the obturator canal

    - **Inferior vesical a.** — trace to the posteroinferior part of the bladder, prostate gland, and seminal vesicles (not present in females)

    - **Middle rectal a.** — to the rectum

    - **Internal pudendal a.** — exits the pelvis through the greater sciatic foramen to enter the gluteal region, inferior to the piriformis m.; enters the perineum by traveling through the lesser sciatic foramen

    - **Inferior gluteal a.** — exits the pelvis, between S2 and S3 nn. usually; courses through the greater sciatic foramen to enter the gluteal region, inferior to the piriformis m.

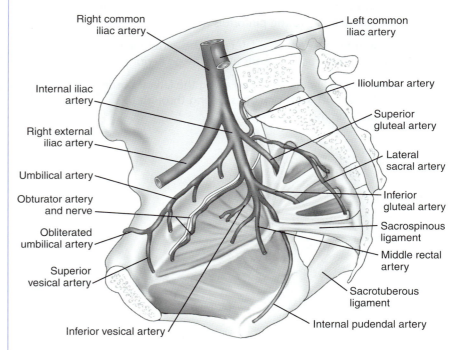

Figure 17-9 Branches of the right internal iliac artery of the male

MALE

Pelvic Vasculature — Internal Iliac Artery (Posterior Division)

GAFS pp 428–434 ACGA pp 441–442 NAHA Plates 398–399

■ Use forceps to reveal and identify the following branches **(Figure 17-10)**:

- **Posterior division of the internal iliac a.**

  - **Superior gluteal a.** — exits the pelvis between the lumbosacral trunk (L4, L5) and S1 nn. usually; courses through the greater sciatic foramen to enter the gluteal region, anterior to the piriformis m.

  - **Iliolumbar a.** — located lateral to the vertebrae near the lumbosacral trunk; ascends along the posterior pelvic wall

  - **Lateral sacral aa.** — located along the lateral border of the sacrum, with branches exiting through the sacral foramina

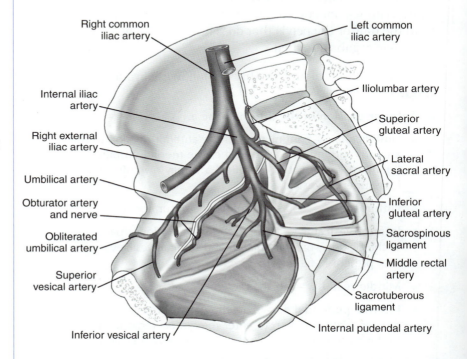

Figure 17-10 Branches of the right internal iliac artery of the male

FEMALE

Pelvic Vasculature — Internal Iliac Artery (Anterior Division)

- Use forceps and hemostats to peel away the peritoneum and extraperitoneal fat covering the iliac vessels and nerves from the half of the pelvis that does not have the bulk of the pelvic organs attached

- Use forceps to reveal and identify the following branches **(Figure 17-11)**:

    - **Anterior division of the internal iliac a.**

    - **Umbilical a.** — continues to the anterior abdominal wall, becomes the **medial umbilical ligament (obliterated umbilical a.)**; may give off three to four **superior vesical aa**.

    - **Obturator a.** — courses through the obturator canal

    - **Uterine a.** — trace it to the isthmus of the uterus; located within the cardinal ligament; divides into a large superior branch to the body and fundus of the uterus and a smaller branch to the cervix, vagina, and inferior region of the bladder; anastomoses with the ovarian and vaginal aa.; crosses superior to the ureter, near the lateral fornix of the vagina

        - **Vaginal a.** — often is a branch of the uterine a.; trace to the vagina and posteroinferior surface of the urinary bladder

    - **Middle rectal a.** — to the lateral wall of the rectum

    - **Internal pudendal a.** — exits the pelvis through the greater sciatic foramen, inferior to the piriformis m.

    - **Inferior gluteal a.** — exits the pelvis between S2 and S3 nn.; courses through the inferior part of the greater sciatic foramen to enter the gluteal region inferior to the piriformis m.

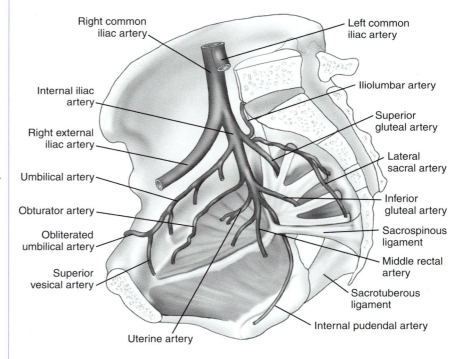

Figure 17-11 Branches of the right internal iliac artery of the female

FEMALE

Pelvic Vasculature — Internal Iliac Artery (Posterior Division)

■ Use forceps to reveal and identify the following branches **(Figure 17-12)**:

- **Posterior division of the internal iliac a**.

  - **Superior gluteal a.** — exits the pelvis between the lumbosacral trunk (L4–L5) and S1 superiorly through the greater sciatic foramen and enters the gluteal region above the piriformis m.

  - **Iliolumbar a.** — located lateral to the vertebrae near the lumbosacral trunk; ascends along the posterior pelvic wall

  - **Lateral sacral aa.** — located along the lateral border of the sacrum, with branches exiting through the sacral foramina

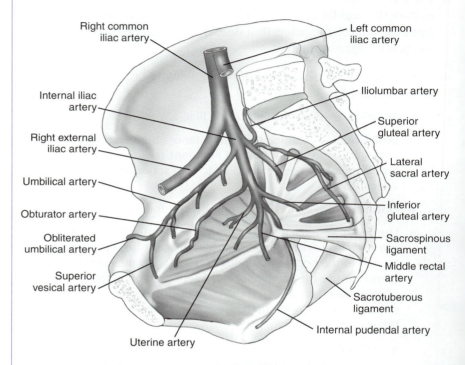

Figure 17-12 Branches of the right internal iliac artery of the female

BOTH SEXES

Pelvic Innervation

- Use forceps to move the dissected arteries to gain access to the nerves of the pelvic wall, which you will dissect with forceps to identify the following **(Figure 17-13)**:

  - **Lumbosacral trunk** (joined L4, L5 spinal cord segments) — contributes to the sacral plexus; located at the lateral side of the sacral promontory

  - **S1, S2, S3 nn.** — anterior rami from the spinal cord levels of S1–S3 that emerge from the sacral foramina, inferior to the lumbosacral trunk, with which they merge to form the sciatic n.

  - **Sciatic n.** (L4–S3 spinal cord segments) — exits the pelvis through the greater sciatic foramen and enters the gluteal region anterior to the piriformis m.

  - **Pudendal n.** (S2, S3, S4 spinal cord segments) — arises from the inferior surface of S4 n.; courses deep to the coccygeus m. to enter the perineum

  - **Superior gluteal n.** — courses with the superior gluteal a.; exits the pelvis between the lumbosacral trunk and S1 n. usually

  - **Inferior gluteal n.** — courses with the inferior gluteal a.; exits the pelvis between S1 and S2 nn. usually

  - **Obturator n.** — courses with the obturator a. and v. to the obturator canal

  - **Sympathetic trunk** — the sympathetic chain and its ganglia are medial to the sacral foramina

- *Note:* The arteries, veins, and nerves exit the pelvis en route to the gluteal region (and beyond) by passing between the coccygeus and piriformis mm.

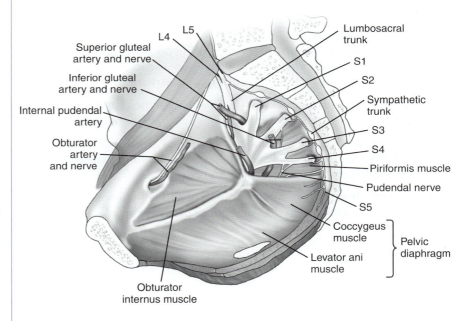

Figure 17-13 Nerves of the right pelvic wall

Pelvic Autonomics

- Use forceps to remove residual endopelvic fat and pelvic peritoneum and identify the following (pelvic extensions of the sympathetic and parasympathetic nn. reach the pelvic viscera by plexuses in sequence, the superior and inferior hypogastric plexuses) **(Figure 17-14)**:

  - **Superior hypogastric plexus** — lies inferior to the bifurcation of the aorta; branches from the superior hypogastric plexus descend into the pelvis along the common iliac aa., as nerve trunks known as the **left and right hypogastric nn.**
  - **Inferior hypogastric plexus** — each inferior hypogastric n. surrounds the corresponding internal iliac a. and its branches
  - **Pelvic splanchnic nn.** — preganglionic parasympathetic fibers derived from S2–S4 sacral nn.; contribute to the inferior hypogastric nerve plexus (difficult to reveal)
  - **Visceral plexus** — extension of the right and left inferior hypogastric plexuses in the walls of the pelvic viscera

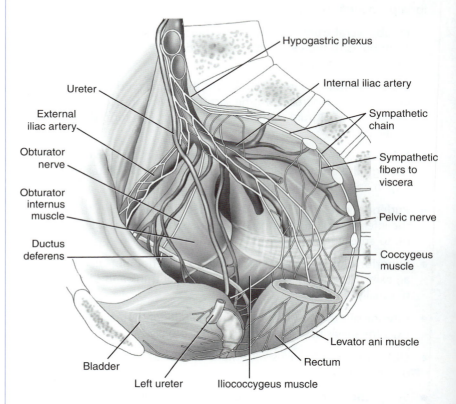

Figure 17-14 Pelvic autonomics

Unit 3 Abdomen, Pelvis, and Perineum Overview

At the end of Unit 3, you should be able to identify the following structures on cadavers, skeletons, and/or radiographs:

Osteology

- Sternum
  - Xiphoid process
- Ribs (12 pairs)
  - Costal margin and costal cartilage
- Sacrum
  - Promontory
  - Anterior and posterior sacral foramina
  - Ala
  - Sacral canal
  - Sacral hiatus
- Os coxae
  - Acetabulum
  - Ischiopubic (conjoint) ramus
  - Obturator foramen
  - Greater sciatic notch/foramen
  - Pelvic brim, inlet, and outlet
  - False and true pelvis
  - Linea terminalis (arcuate line, pecten pubis, and pubic crest)
  - Ilium
    - Iliac crest and fossa
    - Anterior superior iliac spine
    - Posterior superior/inferior iliac spine
    - Arcuate line
  - Ischium
    - Ischial ramus (ischiopubic ramus)
    - Ischial tuberosity and spine
    - Lesser sciatic notch/foramen
  - Pubis
    - Pubic tubercle
    - Pubic crest
    - Superior pubic ramus
      Pecten pubis/pectineal line
    - Pubic symphysis and arch
    - Inferior pubic ramus (ischiopubic ramus)

Muscles and Associated Structures

- Rectus abdominis m.
  - Tendinous intersections
  - Rectus sheath
  - Arcuate line
- Pyramidalis m.
- External oblique m.
  - Inguinal ligament
    - Lacunar ligament
    - Pectineal ligament
  - Superficial inguinal ring
    - Medial and lateral crura
    - Intercrural fibers
- Internal oblique m.
  - Cremaster m.
  - Transversus abdominis m.
  - Conjoined tendon
  - Deep inguinal ring
- Linea alba
  - Umbilicus
- Linea semilunaris
- Inguinal canal
  - Spermatic cord (male)
  - Round ligament of the uterus (female)
- Inguinal triangle
- Quadratus lumborum m.
- Pelvic diaphragm
  - Levator ani m.
    - Puborectalis m.
    - Pubococcygeus m.
    - Iliococcygeus m.
  - Coccygeus m.
- Piriformis m.
- Gluteus maximus and medius mm.
- Obturator internus m.
- External anal sphincter

Muscles and Associated Structures—cont'd

- Diaphragm
  - Right and left crura
  - Central tendon
  - Vena caval hiatus
  - Esophageal hiatus
  - Aortic hiatus
  - Medial and lateral arcuate ligaments
  - Median arcuate ligament
- Psoas major and minor mm.
- Iliacus m.

Arteries

- Aortic arch
  - Subclavian a.
  - Internal thoracic a.
    - Superior epigastric a.
    - Musculophrenic a.
- Aorta
  - Inferior phrenic a.
    - Superior suprarenal aa.
  - Lumbar aa.
  - Median sacral a.
  - Celiac trunk
    - Left gastric a.
      - Esophageal a.
    - Splenic a.
      - Left gastro-omental a.
      - Short gastric aa.
    - Common hepatic a.
      - Hepatic a. proper
        - Right gastric a.
        - Left and right hepatic aa.
        - Cystic a.
      - Gastroduodenal a.
        - Supraduodenal a.
        - Anterior superior pancreaticoduodenal a.
        - Posterior superior pancreaticoduodenal a.
        - Right gastro-omental a.
  - Superior mesenteric a.
    - Anterior and posterior inferior pancreaticoduodenal aa.
    - Jejunal aa., vasa recta
    - Ileal aa., arcades
    - Ileocolic a.
      - Appendicular a.
    - Right colic a.
    - Middle colic a.
    - Marginal a.
  - Inferior mesenteric a.
    - Left colic a.
    - Sigmoid aa.
    - Superior rectal a.
    - Marginal a.
  - Middle suprarenal a.
  - Renal a.
    - Inferior suprarenal a.
  - Gonadal aa. (ovarian/testicular)
  - Common iliac a.
    - Internal iliac a.
      - Iliolumbar a.
      - Lateral sacral a.
      - Obturator a.
      - Superior and inferior gluteal aa.
      - Umbilical a.
        - Branch to the ductus deferens (male)
        - Superior vesical a.
      - Inferior vesical a. (male)
      - Uterine and vaginal aa. (female)
      - Middle rectal a.
      - Internal pudendal a.
        - Inferior rectal a.
        - Perineal a.
        - Posterior labial a. (female) or scrotal a. (male)
        - Artery to the bulb of the vestibule (female) or penis (male)
        - Dorsal a. of the clitoris (female) or penis (male)
        - Deep a. of the clitoris (female) or penis (male)
      - External iliac a.
        - Inferior epigastric a.
        - Deep circumflex iliac a.
- External iliac a.
  - Femoral a.
    - Superficial epigastric a.
    - Superficial circumflex iliac a.

Veins

- Inferior vena cava
  - Inferior phrenic vv.
  - Lumbar vv.
  - Right and left hepatic vv.
  - Renal v.
    - Left suprarenal v.
    - Left ovarian v. (female) or testicular v. (female)
  - Right suprarenal v.
  - Right ovarian v. (female) or testicular v. (male)
  - Common iliac v.
    - Median sacral v.
    - Iliolumbar v.
    - Internal iliac v.
      - Superior gluteal vv.
      - Inferior gluteal vv.
      - Obturator vv.
      - Lateral sacral vv.
      - Vesical vv.
      - Deep dorsal v. of the clitoris (female) or penis (male)
      - Uterine vv. (female)
      - Superior vesical v.
      - Middle rectal v.
      - Internal pudendal v.
        - Deep vv. of the clitoris (female) or penis (male)
        - Inferior rectal v.

- ◆ Posterior labial vv. (female) or scrotal vv. (male)
- ◆ Vein of the bulb of the vestibule (female) or penis (male)
- • Common iliac v.
- • External iliac v.
  - ◆ Inferior epigastric v.
  - ◆ Deep circumflex iliac v.
- ■ Portal venous system
  - • Portal v.
    - ◆ Umbilical part
      - ■ Ligamentum venosum
        - ■ Round ligament of the liver
    - ◆ Cystic v.
    - ◆ Paraumbilical vv.
    - ◆ Left gastric v.
    - ◆ Right gastric v.
  - • Superior mesenteric v.
    - ◆ Jejunal and ileal vv.
    - ◆ Right gastro-omental vv.
    - ◆ Pancreatic vv.
    - ◆ Ileocolic vv.
    - ◆ Right and middle colic vv.
  - • Splenic v.
    - ◆ Pancreatic vv.
    - ◆ Short gastric vv.
    - ◆ Left gastro-omental vv.
    - ◆ Inferior mesenteric v.
      - ■ Left colic v.
      - ■ Sigmoid vv.
      - ■ Superior rectal v.
- ■ Lateral thoracic v.
  - • Thoracoepigastric v.

Lymphatics

- ■ Thoracic duct
- ■ Cisterna chyli
- ■ Lumbar and intestinal lymphatics
- ■ Preaortic lymph nodes
- ■ Lumbar lymph nodes
- ■ Superior mesenteric lymph nodes
- ■ Inferior mesenteric lymph nodes
- ■ Common iliac lymph nodes
- ■ External iliac lymph nodes
- ■ Internal iliac lymph nodes

Autonomic Nerves

- • Sympathetic part
- • Thoracic ganglia
  - • Greater splanchnic n.
  - • Lesser splanchnic n.
  - • Least splanchnic n.
- • Lumbar ganglia
- • Sacral ganglia
- ■ Parasympathetic part
  - • Pelvic splanchnic nn.
- ■ Peripheral autonomic plexuses/ganglia
  - • Celiac ganglia and plexuses
  - • Aorticorenal ganglia and plexus
  - • Superior mesenteric ganglia and plexuses
  - • Renal plexus
  - • Inferior mesenteric plexus
  - • Superior hypogastric plexus
    - • Hypogastric n.
  - • Inferior hypogastric plexus
  - • Uterovaginal plexus (female)
  - • Prostatic plexus (male)

Spinal Nerves

- ■ Intercostal nn. (ventral rami)
  - • Lateral cutaneous nn.
  - • Anterior cutaneous nn.
- ■ Subcostal n.
- ■ Iliohypogastric and ilioinguinal nn.
- ■ Genitofemoral n.
  - • Genital and femoral branches
- ■ Lateral femoral cutaneous n.
- ■ Obturator n.
- ■ Femoral n.
- ■ Lumbosacral trunk
- ■ Sacral plexus
  - • Superior and inferior gluteal nn.
  - • Posterior femoral cutaneous n.
  - • Pudendal n.
    - • Inferior rectal nn.
    - • Dorsal n. of the clitoris or penis
    - • Perineal nn.
      - ◆ Posterior labial and scrotal nn.
  - • Coccygeal n.
    - • Anococcygeal n.
  - • Sciatic n.

Anterior Abdominal Wall (Internally)

- ■ Median fold (urachus)
- ■ Medial folds (obliterated umbilical aa.)
- ■ Lateral folds (inferior epigastric vessels)
- ■ Medial and lateral inguinal fossae
- ■ Superior epigastric vessels
- ■ Obliterated umbilical v.
  - • Ligamentum teres
- ■ Falciform ligament
- ■ Umbilicus

Layers of the Anterolateral Abdominal Wall

- ■ Skin
- ■ Superficial fascia
  - • Fatty (Camper's fascia) layer
  - • Membranous (Scarpa's fascia) layer
- ■ External oblique m./aponeurosis
- ■ Internal oblique m./aponeurosis
- ■ Transversus abdominis m./aponeurosis
- ■ Transversalis fascia
- ■ Extraperitoneal fat
- ■ Parietal peritoneum

Ligaments
- Sacrotuberous ligament
- Sacrospinous ligament
- Iliolumbar ligament
- Anococcygeal ligament

Peritoneum
- Mesentery
  - Root of the mesentery
- Mesocolon
  - Transverse mesocolon
  - Sigmoid mesocolon
  - Mesoappendix
- Lesser omentum
  - Hepatophrenic ligament
  - Hepatogastric ligament
  - Hepatoduodenal ligament
- Greater omentum
  - Gastrosplenic ligament
  - Splenorenal ligament
- Peritoneal attachments of the liver
  - Coronary ligament
    - Falciform ligament
    - Triangular ligaments
    - Hepatorenal ligament
- Recesses, fossae, and folds
- Peritoneal cavity
  - Greater sac
  - Lesser sac (omental bursa)
    - Omental (epiploic) foramen
  - Paravesical fossa
  - Rectovesical pouch (male)
  - Vesicouterine pouch (female)
  - Rectouterine pouch (female)

Stomach
- Greater and lesser curvatures
- Pylorus and pyloric sphincter
- Body, cardia, and fundus
- Gastric rugae

Small Intestine
- Duodenum (four parts)
  - Major and minor duodenal papillae
  - Duodenojejunal junction
  - Suspensory ligament of the duodenum
  - Pancreaticoduodenal ampulla
  - Duodenal sphincter
  - Circular folds
- Jejunum: circular folds
- Ileum: circular folds
  - Ileocecal junction
  - Peyer's patches of lymphoid tissue

Large Intestine
- Cecum
  - Vermiform appendix
- Ascending colon — right colic (hepatic) flexure
- Transverse colon
- Descending colon — left colic (splenic) flexure
- Sigmoid colon
- Rectum and anus
- Colon
  - Omental (epiploic) appendices
  - Haustra
  - Taenia coli

Abdominal Organs
- Pancreas
  - Head, neck, body, and tail
  - Main and accessory pancreatic ducts
  - Uncinate process
- Spleen
- Liver
  - Diaphragmatic and visceral surfaces
  - Left and right lobes
  - Quadrate and caudate lobes
  - Falciform and round ligaments
  - Porta hepatis
  - Subphrenic recess
  - Bare area
  - Common hepatic duct
    - Cystic duct
    - Common bile duct
- Gallbladder
- Kidney
  - Perirenal fascia and fibrous capsule
  - Hilum, renal sinus, renal pelvis, and ureter
  - Major and minor calyces
  - Renal cortex: renal columns
  - Renal medulla
    - Renal pyramids and papillae
- Bladder
  - Apex, body, and fundus
  - Trigone
  - Internal urethral orifice
  - Median umbilical ligament

Female Internal Genitalia
- Ovary
  - Ligament of the ovary
  - Suspensory ligament of the ovary
- Uterine tube
- Infundibulum
- Fimbria
- Ampulla and isthmus
- Uterus
  - Fundus and body
  - Uterine horn
  - Uterine cavity
  - Internal os
  - Cervix
  - Isthmus
  - External os

- Round ligament of the uterus
- Pubocervical ligament
- Cardinal (transverse cervical) ligament
- Uterosacral (rectouterine) ligament
- Vagina
  - Vaginal fornices
    - Anterior, posterior, and two lateral
- Hymen
- Vaginal rugae

Female External Genitalia

- Mons pubis
- Labia majora
- Labia minora
- Vestibule
  - Bulb of the vestibule
  - Vaginal orifice
  - Greater and lesser vestibular glands
- Clitoris
  - Crus, body, and glans
  - Corpus cavernosum of the clitoris
  - Suspensory ligament of the clitoris
- Female urethra

Male Internal Genitalia

- Testis
  - Tunica vaginalis
    - Parietal and visceral layers
    - Sinus of the epididymis
  - Tunica albuginea
  - Mediastinum of the testis
  - Lobules of the testis
  - Seminiferous tubules
  - Gubernaculum testis
- Epididymis
  - Head, body, and tail

- Spermatic cord
  - External spermatic fascia
  - Cremaster m.
  - Cremasteric fascia
  - Internal spermatic fascia
  - Process vaginalis
  - Pampiniform plexus of vv.
- Ductus deferens
- Seminal vesicle
- Ejaculatory duct
- Prostate gland
- Bulbourethral gland

Male External Genitalia

- Penis
  - Root, body, dorsum, and crus
  - Glans penis
  - Prepuce/foreskin
    - Frenulum
  - Raphe of the penis
  - Corpus cavernosum penis (crus)
  - Corpus spongiosum penis
    - Bulb of the penis
  - Tunica albuginea of corpora cavernosa and corpus spongiosum
  - Septum penis
  - Suspensory ligament of the penis
  - Fundiform ligament of the penis
- Male urethra
  - Prostatic urethra
  - Membranous urethra
  - Spongy urethra
  - External urethral orifice
- Scrotum
  - Raphe of the scrotum
  - Dartos fascia
    - Dartos m.

Perineum

- Triangles
  - Urogenital triangle
  - Anal triangle
- External anal sphincter
- Perineal body (anococcygeal body/ligament)
- Superficial perineal space
  - Superficial perineal fascia
  - Superficial transverse perineal m.
  - Ischiocavernosus m.
  - Bulbospongiosus m.
- Deep perineal space
  - Perineal membrane
  - Deep transverse perineal m.
  - External urethral sphincter
  - Sphincter urethrovaginalis m. (female)
- Ischioanal fossa
  - Fat
  - Pudendal canal
    - Obturator fascia over the pudendal canal
    - Pudendal n.
    - Internal pudendal a. and v.

Urogenital Peritoneum

- Paravesical fossa
- Transverse vesical fold
- Vesicouterine pouch (female)
- Broad ligament of the uterus (female)
  - Mesometrium
  - Mesosalpinx
  - Mesovarium
- Suspensory ligament of the ovary (female)
- Rectouterine fold (female)
- Rectouterine pouch (female)
- Rectovesical pouch (male)
- Pararectal fossa

Unit 4

Head and Neck

The purpose of this unit is to learn the anatomic structure of the head and neck through dissection.

Lab 18 Osteology of the Head and Neck	253
Lab 19 Posterior Triangle of the Neck	267
Lab 20 Anterior and Visceral Triangles of the Neck	278
Lab 21 Scalp, Calvarium, Meninges, and Brain	300
Lab 22 Base of the Skull and Cranial Nerves	317
Lab 23 Orbit	329
Lab 24 Superficial Face	338
Lab 25 Deep Face and Pharynx	358
Lab 26 Nasal Cavity, Palate, and Oral Cavity	373
Lab 27 Larynx	393
Lab 28 Ear	403
Unit 4 Head and Neck Overview	411

Lab 18

Osteology of the Head and Neck

Prior to dissection, you should familiarize yourself with the following structures:

OSTEOLOGY
- Parietal bone
  - Groove for the superior sagittal sinus
  - Grooves for the middle meningeal a.
- Frontal bone
  - Glabella
  - Supraorbital margin
    - Supraorbital foramen
  - Frontal sinus
  - Foramen cecum
- Occipital bone
  - Foramen magnum
  - Basioccipital region
    - Clivus
    - Pharyngeal tubercle
    - Grooves for the inferior petrosal sinuses
  - Occipital condyle
  - Hypoglossal canal
  - Condylar canal
  - Jugular notch (for the jugular foramen)
  - External occipital protuberance
  - Internal occipital crest
  - Internal occipital protuberance
  - Groove for the superior sagittal sinus
  - Grooves for the transverse sinuses
  - Groove for the occipital sinus
- Temporal bone
  - Petrous part
    - Mastoid process
    - Mastoid notch
    - Grooves for the sigmoid sinuses
    - Mastoid foramen
    - Facial canal
    - Carotid canal
    - Canal for the auditory tube
    - Tegmen tympani
    - Hiatus and groove for the greater petrosal n.
    - Internal acoustic meatus
    - Grooves for the inferior petrosal sinuses
    - Jugular notch (for the jugular foramen)
    - Styloid process
    - Stylomastoid foramen
  - External acoustic meatus
  - Groove for the middle meningeal a.
  - Zygomatic process
  - Mandibular fossa
  - Petrotympanic fissure
  - Foramen lacerum
- Sphenoid bone
  - Sella turcica
    - Hypophysial fossa
    - Dorsum sellae
    - Posterior clinoid processes
  - Carotid sulcus
  - Sphenoid sinus
  - Lesser wing
    - Optic canal
    - Anterior clinoid process
    - Supraorbital fissure
  - Greater wing
    - Foramen rotundum
    - Foramen ovale
    - Foramen spinosum
  - Pterygoid process
    - Lateral plate
    - Medial plate
  - Pterygoid notch and fossa
  - Pterygoid hamulus
  - Pterygoid canal
  - Sphenopalatine foramen
  - Inferior orbital fissure
  - Foramen lacerum
  - Sphenoethmoidal recess
- Ethmoid bone
  - Cribriform plate
    - Cribriform foramina
    - Crista galli
    - Perpendicular plate
    - Ethmoidal air cells
    - Anterior and posterior ethmoid foramina

Continued

OSTEOLOGY—cont'd

- Ethmoid bone—cont'd
  - Superior nasal concha
    - Superior meatus
  - Middle nasal concha
    - Middle meatus
  - Ethmoidal bulla
  - Uncinate process
  - Hiatus semilunaris
  - Sphenoethmoidal recess
  - Atrium
  - Inferior nasal concha
    - Inferior meatus
- Lacrimal bone
- Nasal bone
- Vomer
- Zygomatic bone
  - Temporal process
  - Zygomaticofacial foramen
  - Zygomaticotemporal foramen
- Palatine bone
  - Perpendicular plate
    - Sphenopalatine notch
    - Greater and lesser palatine canals
  - Horizontal plate
    - Greater palatine foramen
    - Lesser palatine foramen
- Maxilla
  - Infraorbital foramen and canal
  - Alveolar foramen
  - Maxillary sinus
  - Incisive canal and foramen
  - Pterygomaxillary fissure
  - Anterior nasal spine
  - Palatine process
  - Greater palatine groove
  - Greater palatine foramen
- Mandible
  - Ramus, angle, neck, and body
  - Mental protuberance
  - Mental foramen
  - Oblique line
  - Digastric fossa
  - Superior and inferior mental spines
  - Mylohyoid line
  - Sublingual fossa
  - Mandibular foramen
    - Lingula
    - Mandibular canal
  - Coronoid and condylar processes
  - Mandibular notch
- Hyoid bone
  - Lesser horn
  - Greater horn
- Cranial fossae
  - Anterior
  - Middle
  - Posterior
- Sutures and landmarks
  - Sagittal
  - Coronal
  - Pterion
  - Lambdoidal
  - Squamous
  - Bregma/lambda
- Auditory ossicles
  - Malleus, incus, stapes
- Vertebral column
  - C1 (atlas)
  - C2 (axis)
    - Odontoid process (dens)
  - Transverse foramina
- Sternum
  - Manubrium
    - Jugular notch
- Clavicle
- Scapula
  - Acromion
  - Superior angle of the scapula

Lab 18 Dissection Overview

The purpose of this laboratory session is to learn the osteology of the head and neck through dissection. You will do so through the following suggested sequence:

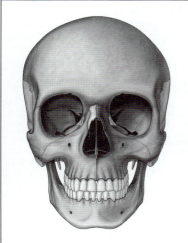

1. Learn skull structures from anterior, lateral, superior, and posterior views.

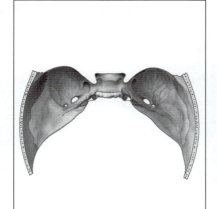

2. Learn the structures associated with the anterior, middle, and posterior cranial fossae.

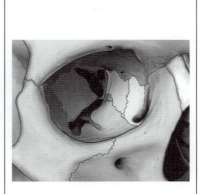

3. Learn the osteology of the orbit.

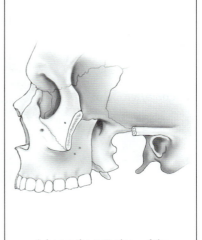

4. Learn the osteology of the pterygopalatine fossa.

Table 18-1 Foramina of the Skull

Bone	Foramen	Corresponding Structure(s)
Sphenoid	Optic canal	Optic n.
	Superior orbital fissure	Ophthalmic, oculomotor, abducens, and trochlear nn.
	Foramen rotundum	Maxillary n.
	Foramen ovale	Mandibular n.
	Foramen spinosum	Middle meningeal vessels
	Foramen venosum	Emissary v.
	Pterygoid canal	Nerve of the pterygoid canal (Vidian n.)
Sphenoid/temporal	Foramen lacerum	Emissary vessels
Temporal	Internal acoustic meatus	Vestibulocochlear and facial nn.
	External acoustic meatus	Sound waves traveling to the tympanic membrane
	Stylomastoid foramen	Facial n.
	Carotid canal	Internal carotid a. and sympathetic nerve plexus
	Hiatus for the greater petrosal n.	Greater petrosal n.
	Hiatus for the lesser petrosal n.	Lesser petrosal n.
	Mastoid foramen	Emissary v.
	Petrotympanic fissure	Chorda tympani n.
Temporal/occipital	Jugular foramen	Internal jugular v.; glossopharyngeal, vagus, and spinal accessory nn.
Occipital	Foramen magnum	Spinal cord and vertebral aa.
	Hypoglossal canal	Hypoglossal n.
	Condylar canal	Emissary v.
Mandible	Mandibular canal	Inferior alveolar n.
	Mental foramen	Mental n.
Ethmoid	Cribriform foramina	Olfactory nn.
Ethmoid/frontal	Anterior ethmoidal foramen	Anterior ethmoid n.
	Posterior ethmoidal foramen	Posterior ethmoid n.
Frontal	Supraorbital foramen	Supraorbital vessels and n.
	Frontal foramen	Supratrochlear vessels and n.
Maxilla	Incisive foramen	Greater palatine vessels and nasopalatine nn.
	Infraorbital foramen	Infraorbital vessels and n.
Maxilla/palatine	Greater palatine foramen	Greater palatine vessels and nn.
Palatine	Lesser palatine foramen	Lesser palatine vessels and nn.

Table 18-1 Foramina of the Skull—cont'd

Bone	Foramen	Corresponding Structure(s)
Palatine, vomer, and sphenoid	Palatovaginal canal	Pharyngeal branch from the pterygopalatine ganglion
Zygomatic	Zygomaticofacial foramen Zygomaticotemporal foramen	Zygomaticofacial vessels and n. Zygomaticotemporal vessels and n.
Parietal	Parietal foramen	Emissary v.

Skull — Anterior View

- *Note:* A human skull is fragile and must be handled with great care; always hold the skull with both hands to ensure the mandible and/or calvarium does not fall and break; when disarticulating the mandible and/or calvarium, do so over a table or countertop to stop the fall in case one of the bones were to slip

- Identify the following structures on a skull from the anterior view **(Figure 18-1)**:

  - **Frontal bone** — forehead bone; observe the glabella, superciliary arch, and supraorbital notch (foramen)
  - **Zygomatic bone** — paired; articulates with the maxilla completing the anterior part of the zygomatic arch
  - **Maxilla** — paired; upper jaw bone; observe the infraorbital foramen, alveolar process, and anterior nasal spine
  - **Nasal bone** — paired; bridge of the nose
  - **Lacrimal bone** — paired; found in the medial anterior floor of each orbit
  - **Nasal cavity** — the piriform aperture is the entrance to the nasal cavity
  - **Mandible** — lower jaw bone; observe the mental foramen, mental protuberance, and the body, angle, and ramus of the mandible

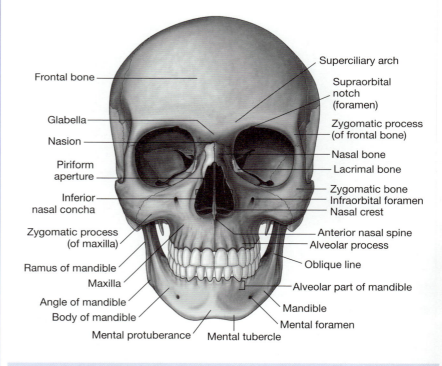

Figure 18-1 Anterior view of skull. (Redrawn from Drake R, Vogl W, Mitchell A: Gray's Anatomy for Students. Philadelphia: Elsevier, 2005, Fig 8.18)

Skull — Lateral View

- Identify the following structures on a skull from the lateral view **(Figure 18-2)**:

  - **Pterion** — junction of the frontal, parietal, sphenoid, and temporal bones
  - **Frontal bone**
  - **Coronal suture** — connects the frontal bone to the parietal bones
  - **Parietal bone**
  - **Lambdoid suture** — connects the occipital bone to the parietal bones
  - **Occipital bone**
  - **Occipitomastoid suture**
  - **Temporal bone** — observe the external auditory meatus, mastoid process, styloid process, and zygomatic process (contributes to the zygomatic arch); zygomatic process of the temporal bone articulates with the zygomatic bone anteriorly
  - **Zygomatic bone** — observe the zygomaticofacial foramen; articulates with the temporal bone via the zygomatic arch
  - **Maxilla** — upper jaw bone
  - **Nasal bone** — bridge of the nose
  - **Lacrimal bone**
  - **Mandible** — lower jaw bone; observe the mental foramen, body, angle, ramus, coronoid process, and condylar process

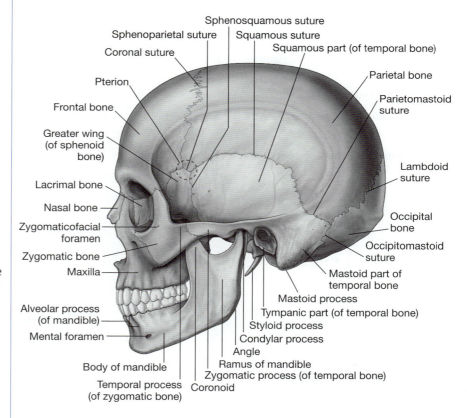

Figure 18-2 Lateral view of skull. (Redrawn from Drake R, Vogl W, Mitchell A: Gray's Anatomy for Students. Philadelphia: Elsevier, 2005, Fig 8.19)

Skull — Posterior View

- Identify the following structures on a skull from the posterior view **(Figure 18-3)**:
  - **Occipital bone** — observe the external occipital protuberance, superior nuchal line, and inferior nuchal line
  - **Parietal bones**
  - **Sagittal suture** — connects adjacent parietal bones
  - **Lambdoid suture** — connects the occipital bone to the parietal bones
  - **Temporal bone** — observe the mastoid process

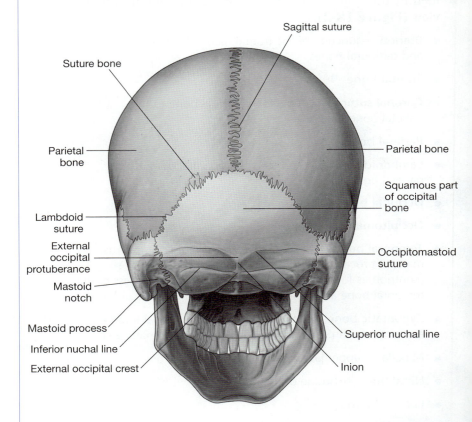

Figure 18-3 Posterior view of skull. (Redrawn from Drake R, Vogl W, Mitchell A: Gray's Anatomy for Students. Philadelphia: Elsevier, 2005, Fig 8.20)

Skull — Inferior View

- Identify the following structures on a skull from the inferior view **(Figure 18-4)**:

  - **Maxilla** — paired; observe the palatine process contributing to the hard palate, incisive canal, and alveolar arch

  - **Palatine bone** — paired; observe the contribution to the hard palate and greater and lesser palatine foramen

  - **Sphenoid bone** — observe the foramen ovale, foramen spinosum, foramen lacerum, lateral pterygoid plate, pterygoid fossa, medial pterygoid plate, and greater wing of the sphenoid bone

  - **Vomer**

  - **Temporal bone** — paired; observe the mandibular fossa, styloid process, stylomastoid foramen, mastoid process, carotid canal, groove for auditory tube, and jugular foramen

  - **Occipital bone** — observe the occipital condyle, hypoglossal canal, foramen magnum, external occipital protuberance, superior and inferior nuchal lines, pharyngeal tubercle, and basilar part of the occipital bone

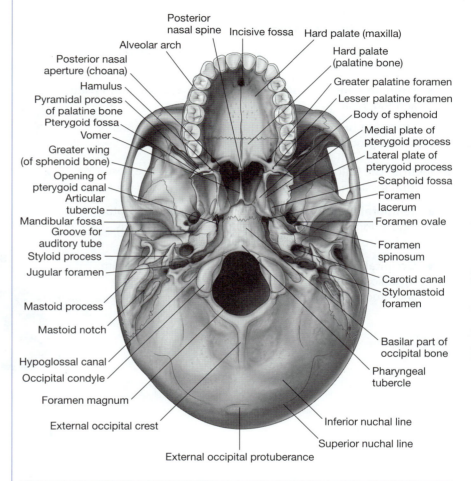

Figure 18-4 Inferior view of skull. (Redrawn from Drake R, Vogl W, Mitchell A: Gray's Anatomy for Students. Philadelphia: Elsevier, 2005, Fig 8.23)

Skull — Anterior and Posterior Cranial Fossae

- Identify the following structures on a skull in the anterior cranial fossa **(Figure 18-5A)**:
  - **Frontal bone** — observe the foramen cecum, orbital plate, and frontal crest
  - **Ethmoid bone** — observe the crista galli and cribriform plate and foramina
  - **Sphenoid bone** — observe the lesser wings and anterior clinoid process

- Identify the following structures on a skull in the posterior cranial fossa (see Figure 18-5B):
  - **Temporal bone** — observe the internal acoustic meatus, jugular foramen, groove for the inferior petrosal sinus, and petrous part of the temporal bone
  - **Occipital bone** — observe the clivus, foramen magnum, hypoglossal canal, internal occipital protuberance, and groove for transverse sinus

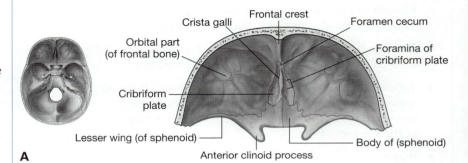

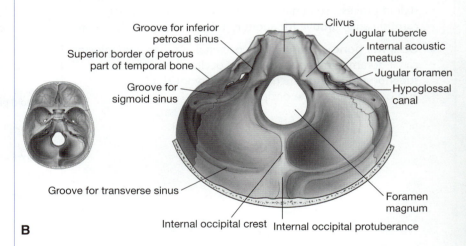

Figure 18-5 **A**, Anterior cranial fossa. **B**, Posterior cranial fossa. (Redrawn from Drake R, Vogl W, Mitchell A: Gray's Anatomy for Students. Philadelphia: Elsevier, 2005, Figs 8.25, 8.27)

Skull — Middle Cranial Fossae

GAFS pp 774–778   ACGA p 18   NAHA Plates 9–11

■ Identify the following structures on a skull in the middle cranial fossa (**Figure 18-6**):

- **Sphenoid bone** — observe the optic canal, foramen rotundum, superior orbital fissure, greater wing, carotid canal, foramen spinosum, foramen ovale, foramen lacerum, dorsum sellae, posterior clinoid process, and hypophysial fossa

- **Temporal bone** — observe the groove for the greater petrosal hiatus and lesser petrosal hiatus

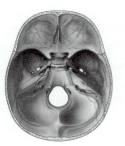

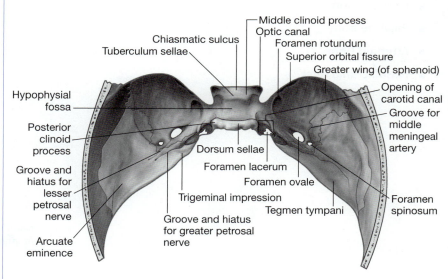

Figure 18-6   Middle cranial fossae. (Redrawn from Drake R, Vogl W, Mitchell A: Gray's Anatomy for Students. Philadelphia: Elsevier, 2005, Fig 8.26)

Skull — Orbit

■ Identify the following structures on a skull in the orbital region **(Figure 18-7)**:

- **Frontal bone** — observe the ethmoidal foramina and supraorbital notch
- **Sphenoid bone** — observe the greater wing, superior orbital fissure, optic canal, and lesser wing
- **Maxilla bone**
- **Zygomatic bone**
- **Lacrimal bone**
- **Palatine bone**
- **Ethmoid bone**
- **Nasolacrimal duct**

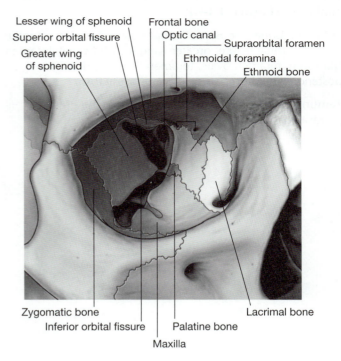

Figure 18-7 Orbit. (Redrawn from Drake R, Vogl W, Mitchell A: Gray's Anatomy for Students. Philadelphia: Elsevier, 2005, Fig 8.70)

Review of the Osteology of the Pterygopalatine Fossa

- With a dry skull and broom straws, probe the various foramina radiating from the pterygopalatine fossa **(Figure 18-8)**:
  - **Infraorbital fissure**
  - **Infraorbital foramen**
  - **Zygomaticofacial foramen**
  - **Zygomaticotemporal foramen**
  - **Posterior superior alveolar foramina**
  - **Pterygomaxillary fissure**
    - Deep to this fissure is the **pterygopalatine fossa**

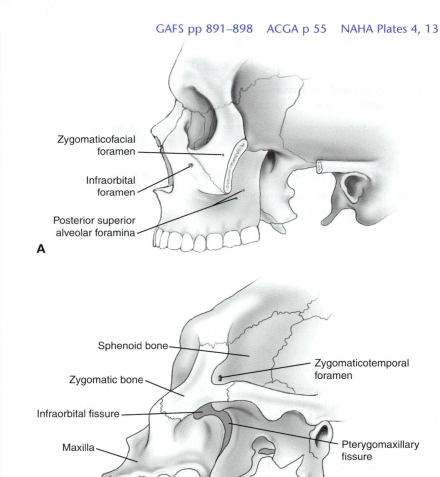

Figure 18-8 Foramina of the skull for branches CN V-2. **A**, Lateral view. **B**, Skull tilted to show an inferior view

Unit 4 • Lab 18   Osteology of the Head and Neck

Pterygopalatine Fossa

- Identify the following on a dry skull **(Figure 18-9)**:

  - **Pterygopalatine fossa** — a small pyramidal space inferior to the orbital apex; the fossa has the following borders:

    - **Posterior** — pterygoid plates of the sphenoid bone
    - **Anterior** — maxilla
    - **Medial** — perpendicular plate of the palatine bone
    - **Lateral** — open to the infratemporal fossa (pterygomaxillary fissure)

  - The pterygopalatine fossa communicates with the following (see Table 26-3A):

    - **Lateral communication** — infratemporal fossa via the pterygomaxillary fissure
    - **Medial communication** — nasal cavity via the sphenopalatine foramen
    - **Anterior communication** — orbit via the medial end of the inferior orbital fissure
    - **Posterior communication** — the foramen rotundum is located in the posterior wall; the latter is traversed by the maxillary n. (CN V-2) (see Table 26-3B)

  - Contents of the pterygopalatine fossa:

    - **Maxillary n. (CN V-2)**
    - **Pterygopalatine ganglion**
    - **Terminal branches of the maxillary a.**

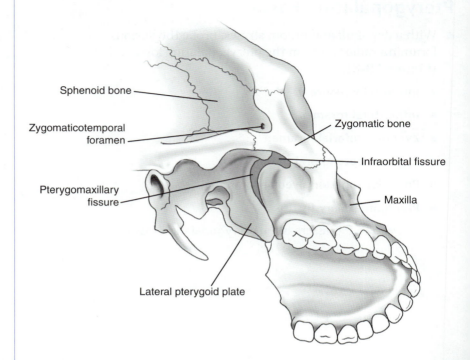

Figure 18-9 Pterygopalatine fossa. Right side of the skull tilted to show an inferior view

Lab 19

Posterior Triangle of the Neck

Prior to dissection, you should familiarize yourself with the following structures:

OSTEOLOGY
- Manubrium
  - Jugular notch
- Clavicle
- Scapula
  - Acromion
- Hyoid bone
- Temporal bone
  - Mastoid process
- Mandible
  - Mental symphysis
  - Mental tubercles
  - Ramus of the mandible

MUSCLES
- Platysma m.
- Sternocleidomastoid m.
- Trapezius m.
- Splenius capitis m.
- Levator scapulae m.
- Scalene mm.
  - Anterior
  - Middle
  - Posterior
- Infrahyoid mm.
  - Omohyoid m.

NERVES
- Spinal accessory n. (CN XI)
- Cervical plexus
  - Great auricular n.
  - Lesser occipital n.
  - Transverse cervical n.
  - Supraclavicular nn.
  - Phrenic n.
- Brachial plexus
  - Suprascapular n.

VEINS
- Internal jugular v.
- External jugular v.
  - Anterior jugular v.
    - Jugular venous arch

ARTERIES
- Aorta
  - Subclavian a.
  - Thyrocervical trunk
    - Transverse cervical a.
    - Suprascapular a.
  - Common carotid a.
    - External carotid a.
      - Occipital a.

CERVICAL FASCIA
- Superficial cervical fascia
- Deep cervical fascia
  - Investing fascia
  - Pretracheal fascia
  - Prevertebral fascia
  - Carotid sheath

MISCELLANEOUS
- Subtriangles of the posterior triangle of the neck
  - Supraclavicular triangle
  - Suboccipital triangle
  - Interscalene triangle

Lab 19 Dissection Overview

The purpose of this laboratory session is to learn the anatomy of the posterior triangle of the neck through dissection. You will do so through the following suggested sequence:

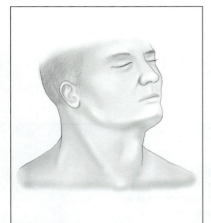

1. Identify surface anatomy and make skin incisions.

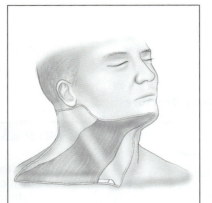

2. Identify and carefully reflect the platysma m.

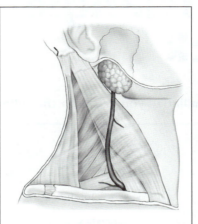

3. Identify cutaneous veins and nerves in the posterior triangle of the neck.

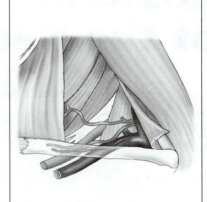

4. Identify the muscles, vessels, and nerves in the posterior triangle of the neck.

Table 19-1 Muscles of the Posterior Triangle of the Neck

Muscle	Attachments		Action	Innervation
Platysma	Inferior border of the mandible and subcutaneum	Fascia over the pectoralis major and deltoid mm.	Controls the grimace expression; tightens the skin of the neck	Cervical branch of the facial n. (CN VII)
Trapezius	Occipital bone, nuchal ligament, C7–T12 vertebrae	Lateral one third of the clavicle; acromion and spine of the scapula	Rotates, elevates, adducts, and depresses the scapula	Spinal accessory n. (CN XI) and cervical n. (C3–C4)
Sternocleidomastoid	Clavicle and manubrium	Mastoid process of the temporal bone	Individually, they tilt the head toward the shoulder on the same side, rotating the head to turn the face to the opposite side; acting together, they draw the head forward	Spinal accessory n. (CN XI)
Omohyoid	Superior border of the scapula medial to the scapular notch	Inferior border of the body of the hyoid bone	Depresses the hyoid bone	Ansa cervicalis; anterior rami of C1–C3
Scalene, anterior	Transverse processes of C3–C6 vertebrae	Rib 1	Elevate the ribs; laterally flex the neck; bilaterally stabilize the neck	Anterior rami of the cervical nn. C4–C7
Scalene, middle	Posterior tubercle of the transverse processes of C4–C6 vertebrae			Anterior rami of C3–C7
Scalene, posterior		Rib 2		Anterior rami of C5–C7
Levator scapulae	Transverse processes of C1–C4 vertebrae	Superior angle of the scapula	Elevates the scapula	C3, C4, and dorsal scapular n. (C4, C5)
Splenius capitis	Lower half of the nuchal ligament; spinous processes of C7–T4 vertebrae	Mastoid process, skull below the lateral one third of the superior nuchal line	Individually, they draw and rotate the head to the same side; acting together, they draw the head backward	Posterior rami of the middle cervical nn.

Table 19-2 Schematic of the Cervical Plexus

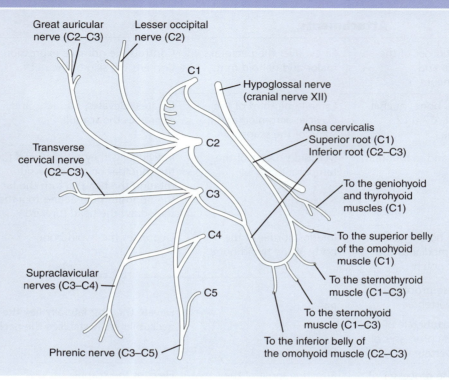

Fascial Planes — Overview

- Throughout the dissections of the neck, observe the following fascial planes in the neck as you dissect from superficial to deep **(Figure 19-1)**:

  - **Skin**

  - **Superficial cervical fascia (subcutaneum)** — encircles the neck and surrounds the structures in the neck; envelopes the platysma m.

  - **Deep cervical fascia**

    - **Investing fascia** — envelops the sternocleidomastoid and trapezius mm.

    - **Pretracheal fascia** — covers the anterior aspect of the neck; encloses the thyroid gland, trachea, and esophagus

    - **Prevertebral fascia** — covers the prevertebral muscles and is continuous with the deep fascia covering the muscular floor of the posterior triangle of the neck

    - **Carotid sheath** — contains the common carotid a., internal jugular v., and vagus n.; part of the ansa cervicalis courses within the connective tissue that comprises the carotid sheath

  - **Retropharyngeal space** — potential space between the pretracheal fascia and prevertebral fascia

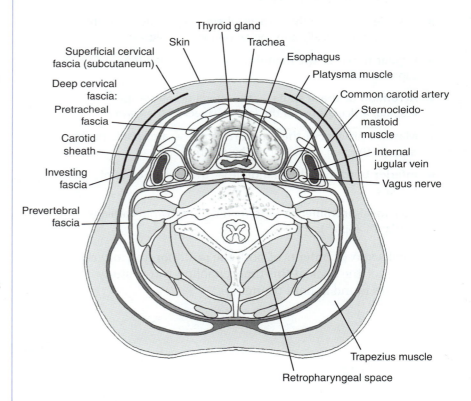

Figure 19-1 Overview of the fascial planes of the neck

Surface Anatomy of the Neck

- Use your fingers to palpate and identify the following surface landmarks **(Figure 19-2)**:

  - **Clavicle** — palpate the clavicle where it articulates with the manubrium medially and the acromion laterally
  - **Jugular notch of the manubrium** — also called the suprasternal notch
  - **Acromion of the scapula** — the lateral tip of the spine of the scapula; articulates with the lateral aspect of the clavicle
  - **Mastoid process of the temporal bone** — a palpable bump deep to the skin, posterior to the external ear
  - **Inferior border of the mandible** — the inferior edge of the jaw
  - **Laryngeal prominence** — formed by the thyroid cartilage ("Adam's apple")

- You will expose contents of both the posterior and anterior triangles of the neck at this time, enabling you to study structures found in both triangles

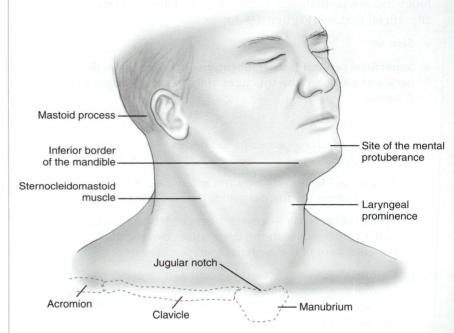

Figure 19-2 Surface anatomy of the neck

Superficial Aspect of the Neck

- Use a scalpel to make the following skin incisions on both sides of the neck; make the scalpel cuts shallow because the facial skin is thin **(Figure 19-3A)**:
  - Mandible *(A)* to the jugular notch *(B)*, bilaterally
  - Acromion *(C)* to the jugular notch *(B)* along the superior border of the clavicle, bilaterally
  - Mental protuberance *(A)* of the mandible along the inferior margin of the mandible; continue the cut far enough posteriorly (inferior to the ear) to expose the anterior 2 cm of the trapezius m. *(D)*, bilaterally

- Grasp an edge of the skin with forceps to cut the skin from the superficial fascia; *use a sharp scalpel!*

- *Note:* The platysma m. is attached to the skin; try not to remove the platysma m. or cutaneous branches of the cervical plexus of nerves as you remove the skin (stay superficial to the platysma m.)

- Identify the following (see Figure 19-3B):
  - **Platysma m.** — located in the superficial fascia and attached to the skin of the neck; covers superficial regions of both the posterior and anterior triangles of the neck
  - **Supraclavicular nn.** — cutaneous branches of the cervical plexus of nerves; medial, intermediate, and lateral branches; formed by the ventral rami of C3–C4 (cervical plexus); the nerves emerge through the platysma m. 1–2 cm above the clavicle
  - Use forceps to separate the supraclavicular nn. from the clavicular end of the platysma m.

- Carefully use a scalpel to dissect and reflect the platysma m. from the clavicle toward the face, leaving the supraclavicular nn. intact in the neck; do not cut the platysma m. from the mandible

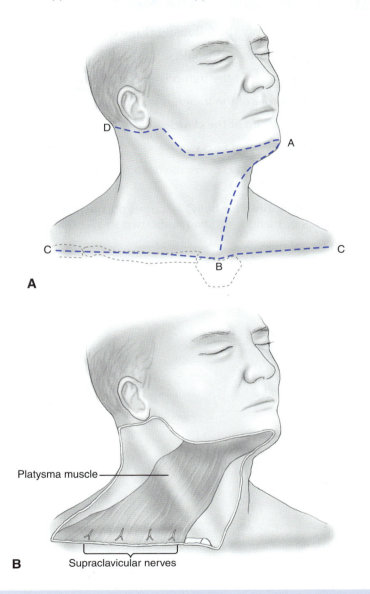

Figure 19-3 Superficial aspect of the neck. **A,** Skin incisions of the neck. **B,** Platysma muscle

Unit 4 • Lab 19   Posterior Triangle of the Neck

Posterior Triangle of the Neck

- Use forceps to identify the following **(Figure 19-4)**:
  - Borders of the posterior triangle:
    - Posterior border of the sternocleidomastoid m.
    - Anterior border of the trapezius m.
    - Middle one third of the clavicle
    - "Roof" — investing fascia
    - "Floor" — deep fascia over the deep muscles of the neck (prevertebral fascia)
  - **Omohyoid m. (inferior belly)** — passes obliquely through the posterior triangle, dividing it into two smaller triangles:
    - Occipital triangle
    - Supraclavicular triangle

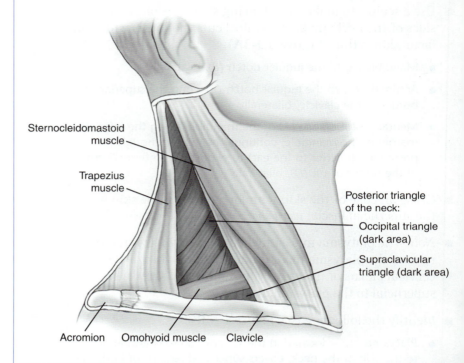

Figure 19-4 Borders of the right posterior triangle of the neck

Posterior Triangle of the Neck — Contents

- Use forceps to identify the following spaces and structures (**Figure 19-5**):

  - **Occipital triangle** — the larger, superior triangle bordered by the trapezius, sternocleidomastoid, and omohyoid mm.; the occipital a. appears at the apex of this triangle

  - **Supraclavicular triangle** — the smaller, inferior triangle bounded by the omohyoid m., sternocleidomastoid m., and clavicle

  - **External jugular v.** — emerges posterior to the ramus of the mandible and crosses superficial to the sternocleidomastoid m.; pierces the fascial "roof" of the posterior triangle

  - **Investing fascia** — forms the "roof" of the posterior triangle; spans from the sternocleidomastoid m. to the trapezius m.; this fascia is tough, so be patient as you dissect through it, and be prepared to use a sharp scalpel and forceps; you will likely have to remove it in a piecemeal fashion

- Use forceps to identify the following nerves:

  - **Spinal accessory n. (CN XI)** — emerges from the posterior border of the sternocleidomastoid m., approximately 5 cm above the clavicle, and courses obliquely to the deep surface of the trapezius m.

  - **Great auricular n.** — usually posterior and parallel to the external jugular v.; ascends on the superolateral surface of the sternocleidomastoid m. toward the ramus of the mandible

  - **Lesser occipital n.** — emerges from the posterior border of the sternocleidomastoid m.; trace the lesser occipital n. superiorly along the posterior border of the sternocleidomastoid m.

  - **Transverse cervical n.** — traverses anteriorly across the middle of the sternocleidomastoid m. toward the anterior triangle of the neck

GAFS pp 920–927   ACGA pp 147–157   NAHA Plates 24, 27–28

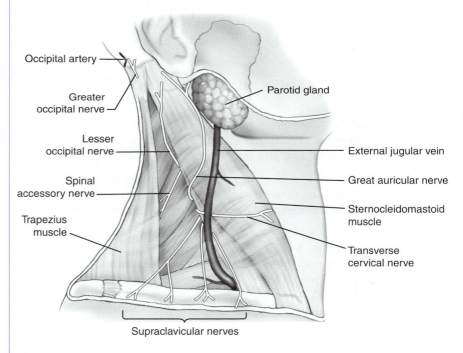

Figure 19-5 Contents of the superficial layer of the right posterior triangle of the neck

Posterior Triangle of the Neck — Contents Continued

Posterior Triangle of the Neck — Contents—cont'd

- Use forceps to trace the great auricular, lesser occipital, and transverse cervical nn. to a common trunk (C2–C3) immediately deep to the posterior border of the sternocleidomastoid m.; do *not* cut the sternocleidomastoid m. at this time

- Use forceps to reveal and identify the following structures **(Figure 19-6)**:
  - **Omohyoid m.** — the inferior belly passes through the posterior triangle, deep to the clavicular portion of the sternocleidomastoid m. and trapezius m.
  - **Transverse cervical a.** (expect variation) — branch of the **thyrocervical trunk** (branch of the subclavian a.) that is deep to the sternocleidomastoid m. and superficial to the anterior scalene m.
    - Courses laterally and posteriorly across to the posterior triangle to supply the trapezius m. **(superficial branch)** and the rhomboid mm. and levator scapulae m. **(deep branch)**
  - **Occipital a.** — branch of the external carotid a.; enters the posterior triangle at its apex

- Use forceps to peel or shred the prevertebral fascia from the "floor" of the posterior triangle; try not to damage previously dissected structures to identify the following muscles:
  - **Splenius capitis m.** — at the apex of the posterior triangle
  - **Levator scapulae m.** — inferior and parallel to the splenius capitis m.; usually has the spinal accessory n. on its superficial surface
  - **Scalene mm.** — inferior and parallel to the levator scapulae m.; there are three scalene muscles, named the **posterior, middle,** and **anterior scalenes,** from superior to inferior; all three muscles are crossed superficially by the transverse cervical a.

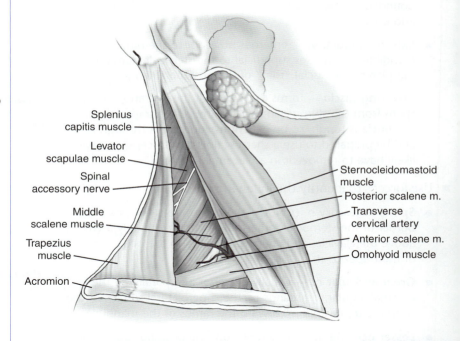

Figure 19-6 Contents of the intermediate layer of the right posterior triangle of the neck

Posterior Triangle of the Neck — Contents—cont'd

- Use forceps to lift up and free the inferior portion of the sternocleidomastoid m. and identify the following deeper structures **(Figure 19-7)**:

  - **Suprascapular a.** — branch of the thyrocervical trunk (not visible at this point); passes inferolaterally across the anterior scalene m., near the clavicle
    - Crosses the subclavian a. and the cords of the brachial plexus as it courses toward the scapula (do *not* dissect the scapular area at this time)
  - **Interscalene triangle**
    - Borders — lateral border of the anterior scalene m., superior border of the first rib, and medial border of the middle scalene m.
    - Contents — brachial plexus and subclavian a.
  - **Phrenic n.** — located on the anterior surface of the anterior scalene m.

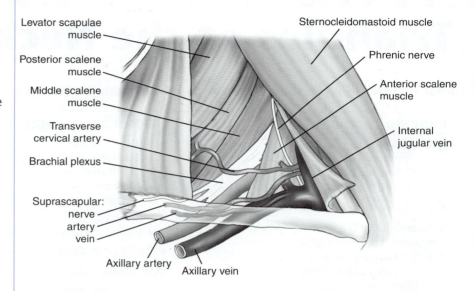

Figure 19-7 Contents of the deep layer of the right posterior triangle of the neck

Anterior and Visceral Triangles of the Neck

Lab 20

Prior to dissection, you should familiarize yourself with the following structures:

CAROTID TRIANGLE
- Carotid sheath
  - Common carotid a.
  - Internal jugular v.
  - Vagus n.
- Cervical sympathetic chain
- External carotid a.
  - Ascending pharyngeal a.
  - Superior thyroid a.
    - Superior laryngeal a.
  - Lingual a.
  - Facial a.
  - Occipital a.
  - Posterior auricular a.
- Internal carotid a.
- Carotid body and sinus
- Nerves
  - Hypoglossal n.
  - Ansa cervicalis
    - Superior root
    - Inferior root
  - Spinal accessory n.
  - Superior laryngeal n.
    - Internal laryngeal n.
    - External laryngeal n.
- Deep cervical lymph nodes

MUSCULAR TRIANGLE
- Infrahyoid mm.
  - Sternohyoid m.
  - Omohyoid m.
  - Sternothyroid m.
  - Thyrohyoid m.
- Thyroid gland
  - Right lobe, left lobe, and isthmus
- Parathyroid glands

SUBMANDIBULAR TRIANGLE
- Suprahyoid mm.
  - Digastric m.
    - Intermediate tendon
    - Fibrous sling
  - Mylohyoid m.
  - Stylohyoid m.
  - Geniohyoid m.
- Submandibular gland
- Submandibular lymph nodes
- Hypoglossal n.
- Mylohyoid n.
- Facial a. and v.
- Submental a. and v.

SUBMENTAL TRIANGLE
- Mylohyoid m. (fibrous raphe)
- Submental lymph nodes
- Small veins from the anterior jugular v.

MUSCLES
- Longus colli m.
- Anterior scalene m.
- Sternocleidomastoid m.

ARTERIES
- Subclavian a.
  - Vertebral aa.
  - Thyrocervical trunk
    - Inferior thyroid a.

VEINS
- Brachiocephalic v.
  - Inferior thyroid v.
- Internal jugular v.
  - Common facial v.
    - Facial v.
    - Retromandibular v.
  - Superior thyroid v.
  - Middle thyroid v.
- External jugular v.
  - Posterior auricular v.
  - Anterior jugular v.

LYMPHATICS
- Superficial cervical lymph nodes
- Deep cervical lymph nodes
- Submental lymph nodes
- Submandibular lymph nodes
- Thoracic (lymphatic) duct

MISCELLANEOUS
- Hyoid bone
- Thyrohyoid membrane
- Thyroid cartilage
- Cricothyroid membrane
- Cricoid cartilage
- First tracheal ring
- Laryngeal prominence
- Larynx
- Branches of the cervical plexus
- Phrenic n.

Lab 20 Dissection Overview

The purpose of this laboratory session is to learn the anatomy of the anterior and visceral triangles of the neck through dissection. You will do so through the following suggested sequence:

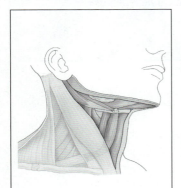

1. Identify the borders of the anterior triangle of the neck and the subtriangles (carotid, muscular, submental, and submandibular).

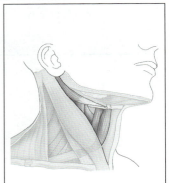

2. Identify the borders and contents of the carotid triangle, including the cervical plexus of nerves.

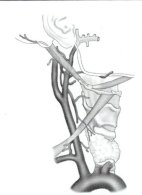

3. Dissect and identify branches of the external carotid artery.

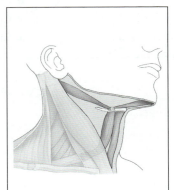

4. Identify the borders and contents of the muscular triangle.

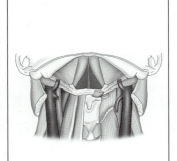

5. Identify the borders and contents of the submental triangle.

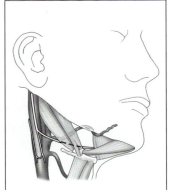

6. Identify the borders and contents of the submandibular triangle.

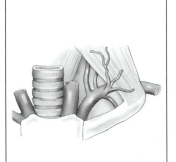

7. Identify the vertebral artery, thoracic duct, and costocervical trunk.

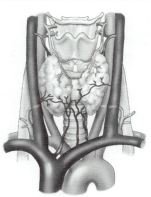

8. Dissect the thyroid gland and its associated vasculature and nerves. Identify the parathyroid glands.

Table 20-1 Muscles Associated with the Anterior Triangle of the Neck

Muscles	Attachments		Action	Innervation
Sternocleidomastoid	Manubrium and medial part of the clavicle	Occipital bone and mastoid process	Individually, they tilt the head toward the shoulder on the same side, rotating the head to turn the face to the opposite side; acting together, they draw the head forward	Spinal accessory n. (CN XI) and branches from anterior rami of C2–C3 (C4)
Suprahyoid muscles				
• Mylohyoid	Mylohyoid line of the mandible	Hyoid bone	Supports and elevates the floor of the mouth; elevates the hyoid	Mylohyoid n.: inferior alveolar n. (CN V-3)
• Geniohyoid	Inferior mental spine on the inner surface of the mandible	Body of the hyoid bone	Fixed mandible elevates and pulls the hyoid bone forward; fixed hyoid bone pulls the mandible downward and inward	Branch from the anterior ramus of C1 (carried along the hypoglossal n. CN XII)
• Stylohyoid	Styloid process (temporal bone)	Body of the hyoid bone	Elevates the hyoid bone	Facial n. (CN VII)
• Digastric	Anterior belly: digastric fossa of the mandible Posterior belly: mastoid notch on the mastoid process of the temporal bone	Attachment of the tendon between the two bellies to the body of the hyoid bone	Opens the mouth by lowering the mandible; raises the hyoid bone	Anterior belly: mylohyoid n. (inferior alveolar n., CN V-3) Posterior belly: facial n. (CN VII)
Infrahyoid muscles				
• Sternohyoid	Manubrium and medial part of the clavicle	Body of the hyoid bone	Depresses the hyoid bone	Anterior rami of C1–C3 (ansa cervicalis)
• Omohyoid	Superior border of the scapula medial to the scapular notch	Inferior border of the hyoid bone	Depresses and stabilizes the hyoid bone	Anterior rami of C1–C3 (ansa cervicalis)
• Sternothyroid	Dorsal region of the manubrium	Thyroid cartilage	Depresses the hyoid bone and larynx	Anterior rami of C2–C3 (ansa cervicalis)
• Thyrohyoid	Thyroid cartilage	Greater horn of the hyoid bone	Depresses the hyoid bone and elevates the thyroid cartilage	Anterior ramus of C1 (via hypoglossal n.)

Table 20-2 Schematic of the Cervical Plexus

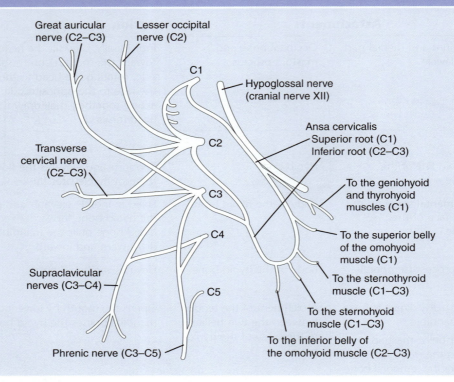

Anterior Triangle of the Neck

■ Raise the platysma m. onto the mandible to identify the following:

- Borders of the anterior triangle of the neck **(Figure 20-1A)**:
  - Midline of the neck
  - Anterior border of the sternocleidomastoid m.
  - Inferior border of the mandible
- The four smaller triangles into which the anterior triangle is subdivided include the following (see Figure 20-1B):
  1. **Carotid**
  2. **Muscular**
  3. **Submental**
  4. **Submandibular**

■ During this dissection, you will identify anatomic structures within each smaller triangle

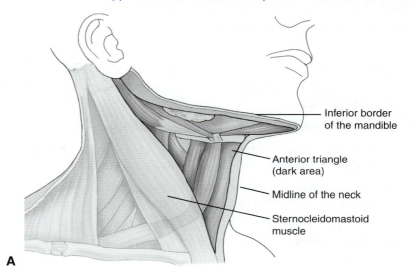

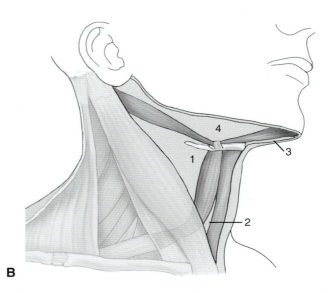

Figure 20-1 Anterior triangle of the neck. **A,** Lateral view of the borders. **B,** Lateral view of the subtriangles

Anterior Triangle of the Neck — Superficial Structures

- Identify and palpate the following surface landmarks, from superior to inferior, along the anterior midline of the anterior triangle of the neck on your cadaver **(Figure 20-2)**:

  - **Hyoid bone** — superior to the thyroid cartilage
  - **Thyroid cartilage** — referred to as the Adam's apple; inferior to the hyoid bone
  - **Cricoid cartilage** — signet-shaped cartilaginous ring located inferior to the thyroid cartilage; the only complete ring of cartilage in the respiratory tree of airways
  - **Thyroid gland** — endocrine gland located superficial to the trachea
  - **Trachea** — also known as the windpipe; inferior and continuous with the thyroid cartilage

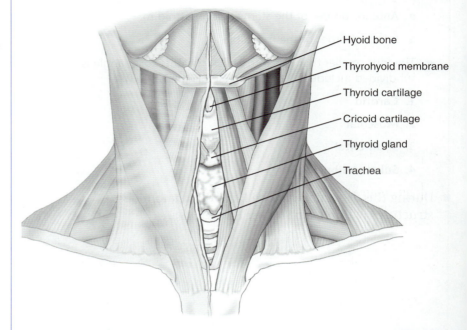

Figure 20-2 Superficial structures in the anterior triangle

Anterior Triangle of the Neck — Superficial Structures—cont'd

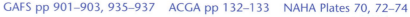

- This dissection may be easier if the neck is flexed to the side of the dissection to remove tension from the sternocleidomastoid m. so that it can be moved away from underlying structures

- Use forceps to reveal and identify the following (expect variation) **(Figure 20-3A** and **20-3B)**:

  - **External jugular v.** — located superficial to the sternocleidomastoid m.); dissect superiorly along this vein to reveal its course posterior to the mandible; dissect inferiorly along this vein to reveal that it pierces the investing fascia about 2–3 cm superior to the clavicle before joining the subclavian v.

  - **Superficial cervical lymph nodes** — pea-sized lymph nodes parallel to the external jugular v.

  - **Retromandibular v.** — formed by union of the superficial temporal and maxillary vv. (studied further in another laboratory session)
    - The posterior branch of the retromandibular v. unites with the posterior auricular v. (deep to the parotid gland) to form the external jugular v.

  - **Posterior auricular v.** — tributary to the external jugular v.; courses posterior to the ear

  - **Facial v.** — locate this vein where it crosses the inferior border of the mandible; joined by the anterior branch of the retromandibular v. to form the common facial v.

  - **Common facial v.** — connects the facial v. to the internal jugular v. deep to the sternocleidomastoid m.; lift the sternocleidomastoid m. to reveal the course of the common facial v.

  - **Anterior jugular v.** — located in the superficial fascia of the inferior part of the anterior triangle of the neck; occasionally, this vein joins the facial v. via a communicating branch (not shown)

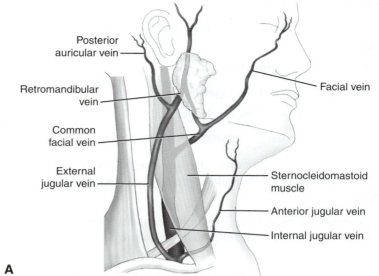

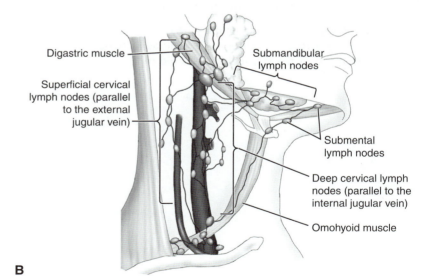

Figure 20-3 Superficial structures of the neck. **A,** Lateral view of veins. **B,** Lateral view of the superficial lymph nodes

Carotid Triangle

GAFS pp 762, 905   ACGA pp 136–139   NAHA Plates 28, 34

- Use forceps to reveal and identify the following **(Figure 20-4)**:
  - Borders of the carotid triangle
    - Posterior belly of the digastric m.
    - Superior belly of the omohyoid m.
    - Anterior border of the sternocleidomastoid m.

- On one side of the neck only, use a scalpel to make the following transections to allow access to deeper structures **(Figure 20-5)**:
  - **Sternocleidomastoid m.** — cut horizontally across the center of its belly; use forceps to free and clean the superior portion of this muscle
    - *Note:* Try not to damage the cervical plexus of nerves that radiate from the posterior border of this muscle
  - **External jugular v.** — may already be cut; if not, cut horizontally across the center of the vein as it crosses superficially over the sternocleidomastoid m.

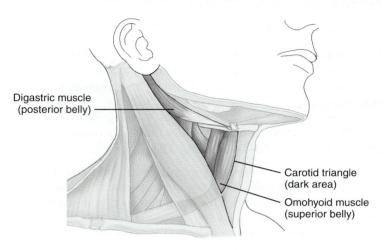

Figure 20-4   Boundaries of the carotid triangle

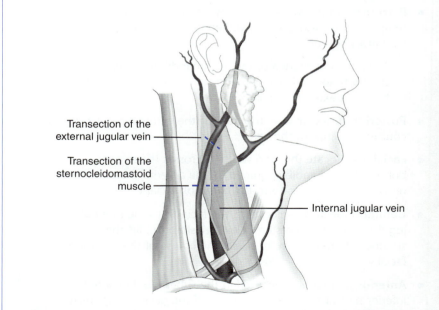

Figure 20-5   Transections

Carotid Triangle—cont'd

- Use forceps to reveal and identify the following structures:

  - **Spinal accessory n. (CN XI) (Figure 20-6)** — pull the superior part of the sternocleidomastoid m. away from the internal jugular v. to find the spinal accessory n. on the muscle's deep surface about 4 cm inferior to the mastoid process

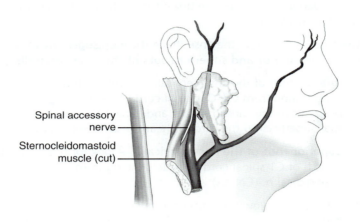

Figure 20-6 Spinal accessory nerve

Carotid Triangle Continued

Carotid Triangle—cont'd

- **Ansa cervicalis (C1–C3 spinal cord segments)** — embedded in the connective tissue that is the carotid sheath (*ansa* means loop)

- Use forceps to dissect the ansa; trace the loop superiorly to reveal the **inferior and superior roots of the ansa cervicalis**

  - **Inferior root** of the ansa cervicalis — look for this contribution from C2–C3 spinal cord levels originating posterior to the carotid sheath and joining the superior root superficial to the carotid sheath (expect variation)

  - **Superior root of the ansa cervicalis** — look for this branch of C1 spinal cord level descending from the hypoglossal n. (CN XII)

  - Attempt to follow the terminal branches of the ansa cervicalis peripherally to the infrahyoid muscles that they supply (see Table 20-2)

- **Hypoglossal n. (CN XII)** — courses parallel to the inferior border of the posterior digastric m.; use forceps to push that muscle superiorly to aid identification of the hypoglossal n.; the nerve emerges between the internal jugular v. and common carotid a. and crosses anterior to the common carotid a.; at the hyoid bone, the nerve courses immediately superior to the tip of the greater horn of the hyoid bone

  - Trace the hypoglossal n. posteriorly to locate where it passes deep to the posterior belly of the digastric m.

  - Retract the posterior belly of the digastric m. to reveal the course of the hypoglossal n. from the hypoglossal canal (base of the skull)

  - **Carotid sheath** — a tubular fascial investment that extends from the base of the skull to the root of the neck; surrounds the following **(Figure 20-7)**:

    ◆ **Common carotid a., internal carotid a., internal jugular v.,** and the **vagus n.**

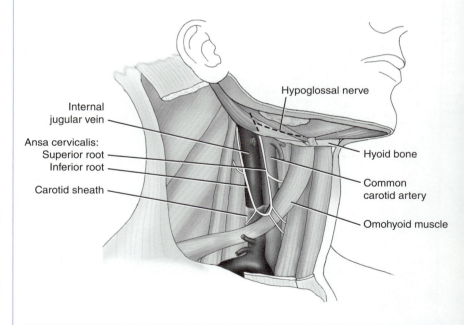

Figure 20-7 Carotid sheath contents

Carotid Triangle—cont'd

■ Use forceps to bluntly dissect through the remaining parts of the carotid sheath to reveal and identify the following:

- **Deep cervical lymph nodes** along the carotid sheath, near the internal jugular v. **(Figure 20-8A)**

- **Vagus n.** — deep, between the common carotid a. and the internal jugular v. (see Figure 20-8B); use forceps to separate the artery from the vein to reveal the vagus n.

- **Common carotid a.** — medial position within the carotid sheath

  - Bifurcates to become the **internal** and **external carotid aa.**; the proximal portion of the internal carotid a. is dilated and is called the **carotid sinus** (contains blood pressure receptors)

  - **Carotid body** — small, dark fibrous mass of tissue at the carotid bifurcation; contains chemoreceptors for oxygen; difficult to identify (not illustrated)

- **Internal carotid a.** — has no branches in the neck; the artery enters the skull via the carotid canal to supply the brain and orbital structures

- **External carotid a.** — anteromedial to the internal carotid a.; provides arterial branches to the neck and face

  - Terminates deep to the parotid gland, where it divides into the maxillary and superficial temporal aa.

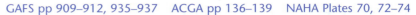

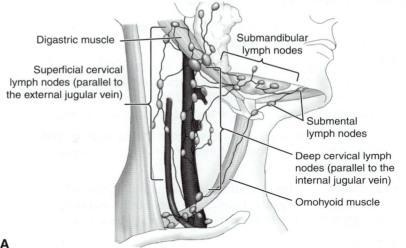

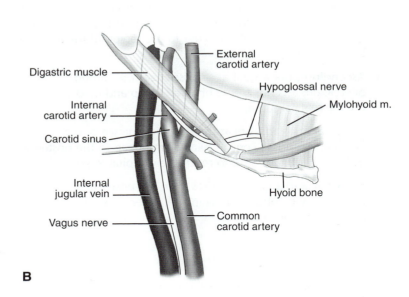

Figure 20-8 Carotid region. **A,** Lateral view of the deep lymph nodes. **B,** Lateral view

Carotid Triangle Continued

Carotid Triangle—cont'd

- Use forceps to reveal and identify the following branches of the external carotid a. **(Figure 20-9)**:

  - **Superior thyroid a.** — most inferior branch of the external carotid a.; inferior and posterior to the greater horn of the hyoid bone; descends anteriorly and inferiorly, deep to the infrahyoid mm., to reach the thyroid gland (superior pole)

    - **Superior laryngeal a.** — arises from the superior thyroid a.; pierces the thyrohyoid membrane with the **internal laryngeal n.**

  - **Lingual a.** — arises from the external carotid a., immediately posterior to the greater horn of the hyoid bone and deep to the posterior belly of the digastric m. and stylohyoid m.

  - **Facial a.** — arises superior to the lingual a. (sometimes the lingual and facial aa. branch from a common trunk); enters a groove under the mandible and emerges around the inferior border of the mandible, anterior to the region of the angle of the mandible (seen later)

  - **Ascending pharyngeal a.** — arises near the carotid bifurcation; ascends to the pharynx, deep and medial to the internal carotid a.

  - **Occipital a.** — arises near the posterior surface of the external carotid a.; courses parallel and deep to the posterior belly of the digastric m. to reach the occipital region

  - **Posterior auricular a.** — arises from the posterior surface of the external carotid a.; small in size; ascends between the ear and mastoid process

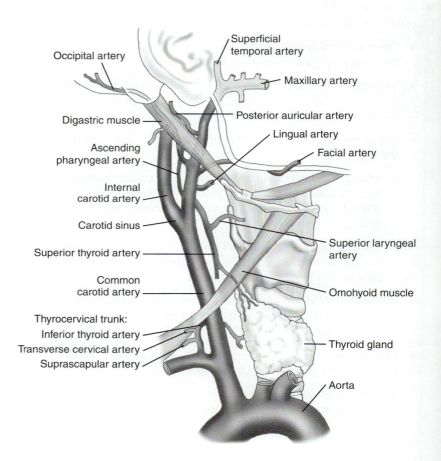

Figure 20-9 Branches of the external carotid artery

Carotid Triangle—cont'd

- On one side of the neck only, use a scalpel to cut the omohyoid and sternohyoid mm. from their attachments to the hyoid bone

- Reflect the two cut muscles superiorly to identify the following **(Figure 20-10)**:

  - **Thyrohyoid membrane** — connective tissue sheath that spans the space from the thyroid cartilage to the hyoid bone
  - **Superior laryngeal n.** — arises from the vagus n. (CN X) and passes deep to the carotid a.; divides into two branches:
    - **Internal laryngeal n.** — arises from the superior laryngeal n.; pierces the thyrohyoid membrane, inferior to the greater horn of the hyoid bone, to reach the larynx
      - Do *not* pursue this nerve into the larynx; this will be studied in another laboratory session
    - **External laryngeal n.** — also arises from the superior laryngeal n.; motor to the cricothyroid m.

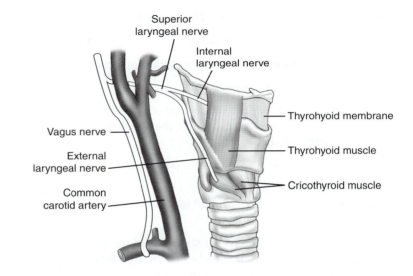

Figure 20-10 Branches of the superior laryngeal nerve

Muscular Triangle and Infrahyoid Muscles

- The muscular triangle contains the infrahyoid ("strap") mm. and thyroid and parathyroid glands

- Use forceps to reveal and identify the following:

  - Borders of the muscular triangle (**Figure 20-11**):

    - Superior belly of the omohyoid m.

    - Anteroinferior border of the sternocleidomastoid m.

    - Midsagittal plane in the neck

  - **Infrahyoid mm.** — named by their muscular attachments; the longest muscles are superficial and the shortest muscles are deep (**Figure 20-12**):

    - **Sternohyoid m.** — superficial and parallel to the midline of the neck

    - **Omohyoid m.** — superficial and lateral to the sternohyoid m.

    - **Thyrohyoid m.** — deep to the sternohyoid m.; as the name implies, the muscle attaches to the thyroid cartilage inferiorly and the hyoid bone superiorly

    - **Sternothyroid m.** — deep to the sternohyoid m.; as the name implies, the muscle attaches to the sternum inferiorly and the thyroid cartilage superiorly

GAFS pp 905–909 ACGA pp 136–139 NAHA Plates 27–29

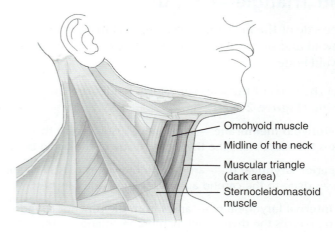

Figure 20-11 Borders of the muscular triangle

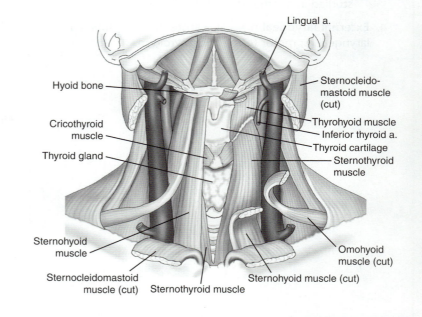

Figure 20-12 Chin tilted upward to show the infrahyoid muscles

Submental Triangle

- Hyperextend the neck, if possible, to improve the view of the neck superior to the hyoid bone

- Use forceps to reveal and identify the following **(Figure 20-13)**:

  - Borders of the submental triangle
    - Inferior: Hyoid bone
    - Lateral: Anterior bellies of both digastric mm.

  - **Mylohyoid m.** — paired muscle; the two muscles are fused along the median fibrous raphe and form the floor of both submental triangles

  - **Submental lymph nodes** — tiny; rest on the mylohyoid mm. (not illustrated)

  - **Submental v.** — drains blood to the anterior jugular v. and/or facial v. (not illustrated)

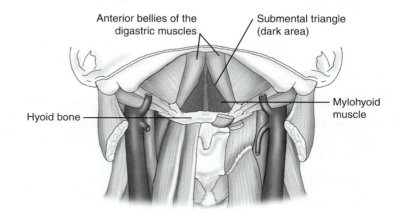

Figure 20-13 Submental triangle (chin lifted up)

Submandibular Triangle

- Hyperextend the neck, if possible, to improve the view of the neck superior to the hyoid bone

- Use forceps to reveal and identify the following **(Figure 20-14)**:
  - Borders of the submandibular triangle
    - Inferior border of the mandible
    - **Anterior belly of the digastric m.**
    - **Posterior belly of the same digastric m.**
  - **Submandibular gland** — almost fills the triangle; this gland has superficial and deep parts that form a U shape superficial and deep to the mylohyoid m.
  - Submandibular lymph nodes **(Figure 20-15)**:
    - These are tiny and may be difficult to identify
  - Facial a. and v. — identify these vessels as they exit the submandibular triangle en route to the face
    - **Facial a.** — usually takes a course *deep* to the submandibular gland
    - **Facial v.** — usually takes a course *superficial* to the submandibular gland

- On one side of the neck, remove the superficial part of the submandibular gland to locate the deep contents of the submandibular triangle

GAFS pp 905, 911–912, 935–936   ACGA pp 122–123   NAHA Plates 27, 72–73

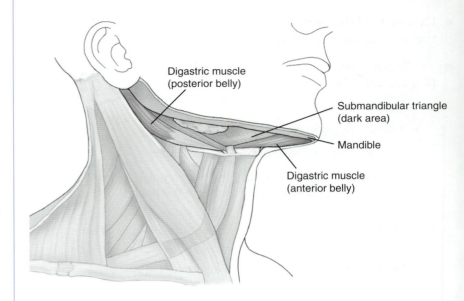

Figure 20-14 Borders of the submandibular triangle

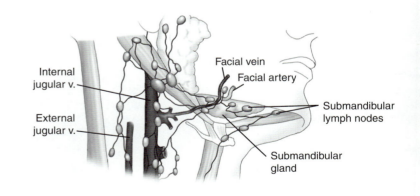

Figure 20-15 Contents of the submandibular triangle

Contents of the Submandibular Triangle

- Hyperextend the neck, if possible, to improve the view of the neck superior to the hyoid bone

- Use forceps to reveal and identify the following **(Figure 20-16)**:

  - **Digastric m.** (anterior and posterior bellies) — identify the **intermediate tendon** attached to the greater horn of the hyoid bone via a **fibrous sling**

  - **Stylohyoid m.** — anterior to the digastric m.; the intermediate tendon of the digastric m. splits the stylohyoid m. near the greater horn of the hyoid bone

  - **Mylohyoid n.** — pull the anterior belly of the digastric m. medially to expose the mylohyoid n. (branch of CN V-3)

  - **Facial a.** and **v.** — deep to the stylohyoid m. and posterior belly of the digastric m.

  - **Hypoglossal n. (CN XII)** — courses through the submandibular triangle; this nerve is posterior and deep to the intermediate tendon of the digastric mm. and disappears under the mylohyoid m.; reveal the course of this nerve, using forceps

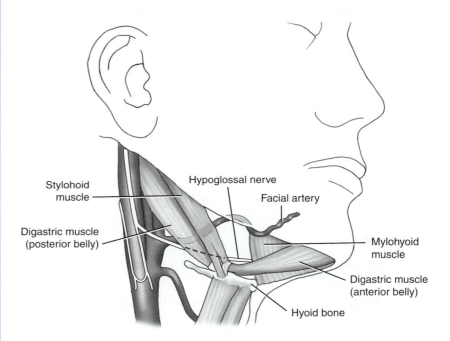

Figure 20-16 Contents of the submandibular triangle after removal of the submandibular gland

Root of the Neck

- Follow these dissection instructions on the left side of the neck only **(Figure 20-17A)**:

  - On the left side, if not already done, use scissors to cut the sternohyoid and sternothyroid mm. from the manubrium; use scissors to also cut and reflect the superior belly of the omohyoid m.

  - Use forceps to dissect the left subclavian a. and v. from the middle one third of the clavicle; use an electric or hand bone saw to cut the middle one third of the clavicle to expand the dissection field

- Use forceps to reveal and identify the following (see Figure 20-17B):

  - Borders of the root of the neck

    - Manubrium (anteriorly), rib 1 (laterally), and the body of T1 vertebra (posteriorly)

  - **Thoracic duct**

    - Find the junction of the left subclavian v. and the left internal jugular v.

    - The thoracic duct is usually located on the posterior surface of the venous junction; it often has a dilated segment (due to valves) at its junction with the veins

  - An alternative approach is to locate the thoracic duct in the posterior mediastinum, from where you may follow the thoracic duct superiorly into the root of the neck

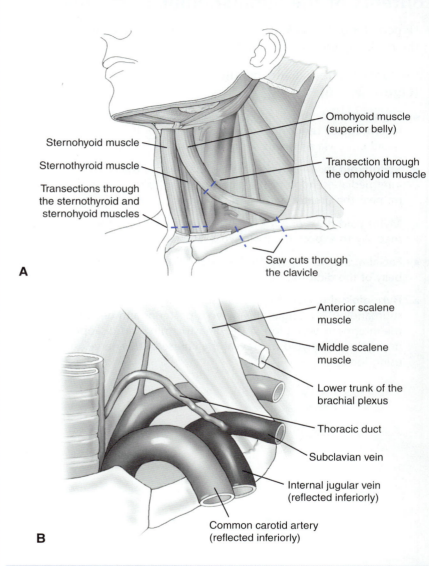

Figure 20-17 Thoracic duct at the left root of the neck. **A,** Lateral view. **B,** Anterior view

Root of the Neck—cont'd

- Continue the dissection on the left side of the neck only
- Use forceps to reveal and identify the following (Figure 20-18):

  - **Phrenic n.** — courses on the anterior surface of the anterior scalene m.
  - **Thyrocervical trunk** — arises from the subclavian a. near the medial border of the **anterior scalene m.**; divides into three branches:
    - **Inferior thyroid a.** — a branch of the thyrocervical trunk; supplies the inferior region of the thyroid gland; arising from the inferior thyroid artery is the ascending cervical a.
    - **Transverse cervical a.** — courses laterally over the superficial surface of the anterior scalene m. and phrenic n. toward the shoulder region
    - **Suprascapular a.** — also crosses superficial to the anterior scalene m. and phrenic n. toward the scapula
- **Triangle of the vertebral a.**
  - Borders — **longus colli m.** and **anterior scalene m.** form two sides; the apex of the triangle is the transverse process of C6 vertebra (the common carotid a. passes anterior to C6 vertebra)
  - **Vertebral a.** — enters the transverse foramen of C6 vertebra at the apex of this triangle
  - **Costocervical a.** — lateral to the vertebral a.; supplies the deep neck region around rib 1
  - **Internal thoracic a.** — arises from the inferior surface of the left subclavian a., deep to the clavicle

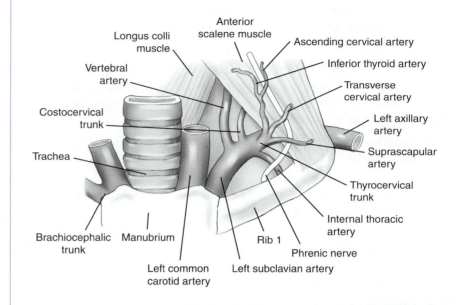

Figure 20-18 Triangle of the vertebral artery on the left side of the neck

Thyroid Gland and Associated Structures

■ Using forceps identify the following **(Figure 20-19)**:

- **Thyroid gland** — reflect the infrahyoid mm. (you may want to bisect one side of the infrahyoid mm. to increase the dissection field)
  - **Left** and **right lobes** of the thyroid gland
  - **Isthmus** — midline connection between the left and right lobes of the thyroid gland; inferior to the cricoid cartilage, on the anterior surface of the trachea
- **Superior thyroid a.** — branch of the external carotid a. that descends to the superior poles of the thyroid gland
- **Inferior thyroid a.** — use forceps to pull a lobe of the thyroid gland anteriorly; the inferior thyroid a. is deep to the inferior poles of the thyroid gland; arises from the thyrocervical trunk
- **Superior, middle,** and **inferior thyroid vv.** — drain blood from the thyroid gland to the internal jugular vv. and brachiocephalic vv.
- **Laryngeal prominence** — the anterior projection of thyroid cartilage ("Adam's apple")
- **Thyrohyoid membrane** — deep to the thyrohyoid m.; spans the space between the thyroid cartilage and hyoid bone; perforated by the superior laryngeal a., v., and internal laryngeal n.
- **Cricothyroid membrane** — use forceps to dissect and lift cricothyroid m. from the underlying cricothyroid membrane; spans the space between the cricoid and thyroid cartilages
- **Cricoid cartilage** — the only complete ring (shaped like a signet ring) of cartilage in the respiratory tract; inferior to the thyroid cartilage
- **First tracheal ring** — C-shaped plate of hyaline cartilage; inferior to the cricoid cartilage

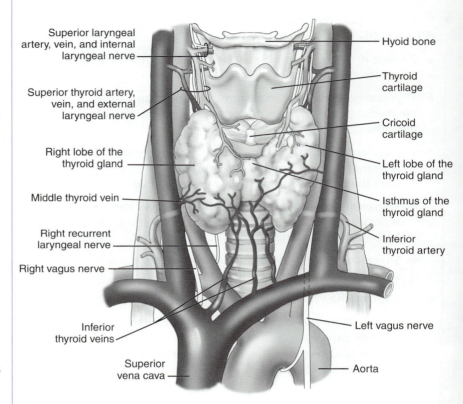

Figure 20-19 Thyroid gland and associated structures

Recurrent Laryngeal Nerves and the Parathyroid Glands

- Follow these dissection instructions:
  - Use scissors to cut through the isthmus of the thyroid gland
  - Reflect the lobes laterally; leave their blood vessels and nerves attached

- Use forceps to reveal and identify the following structures associated with the posterior surface of the lobes of the thyroid gland (**Figures 20-20** and **20-21**):
  - **Recurrent laryngeal nn.** — ascend bilaterally between the thyroid gland and trachea; locate these nerves near the root of the neck, in the groove between the esophagus and trachea, and follow the nerves superiorly to the thyroid gland and larynx
  - **Parathyroid glands** — usually located lateral to the recurrent laryngeal nn.; small, brownish bodies about 1–2 mm in diameter; two to five glands on each side
    - *Note:* You may not be able to locate the parathyroid glands because of their tiny size and because they are usually embedded in the fascia surrounding the thyroid gland

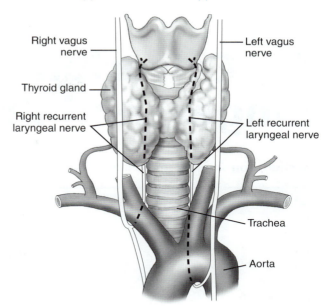

Figure 20-20   Anterior view of the thyroid gland

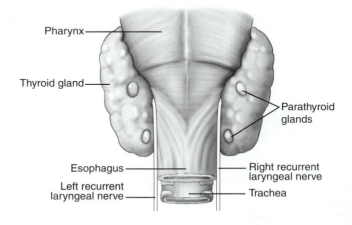

Figure 20-21   Posterior view of the thyroid gland

Lab 21

Scalp, Calvarium, Meninges, and Brain

Prior to dissection, you should familiarize yourself with the following structures:

OSTEOLOGY
- Calvarium
- Sutures
  - Sagittal suture
  - Coronal suture
  - Lambdoid suture
- Bregma and lambda (cranial landmarks)
- Frontal bone
- Parietal bones
- Occipital bone
  - External occipital protuberance
  - Internal occipital protuberance
  - Grooves for the transverse and occipital sinuses, and confluence of sinuses
- Temporal bone
  - Mastoid process
- Ethmoid bone
  - Cribriform plate and crista galli
- Sphenoid bone
- Cranial fossae
  - Anterior cranial fossa
  - Middle cranial fossa
  - Posterior cranial fossa
  - Foramen magnum

SCALP LAYERS
- Skin
- Superficial fascia
- Aponeurosis of the muscular layer (occipitofrontalis m.)
- Loose connective tissue
- Pericranium

ARTERIES
- Subclavian a.
  - Vertebral a.
    - Posterior inferior cerebellar a.
    - Basilar a.
      - Anterior inferior cerebellar a.
        - Labyrinthine a.
      - Pontine a.
      - Superior cerebellar a.
      - Posterior cerebral a.
      - Posterior communicating a.
- Common carotid a.
  - External carotid a.
    - Maxillary a.
      - Middle meningeal a.
  - Internal carotid a.
    - Ophthalmic a.
    - Anterior cerebral a.
      - Anterior communicating a.
    - Middle cerebral a.

VEINS
- Brachiocephalic v.
  - Internal jugular v.
    - Superior bulb of the jugular v.
    - Retromandibular v.
      - Pterygoid plexus of vv.
        - Middle meningeal v.
        - Deep temporal v.
  - Subclavian v.
    - External jugular v.
      - Posterior auricular v.
        - Occipital v.

DURAL VENOUS SINUSES
- Superior sagittal sinus
- Inferior sagittal sinus
- Straight sinus
- Transverse sinuses
- Occipital sinus
- Confluence of sinuses
- Sigmoid sinuses
- Inferior petrosal sinuses
- Superior petrosal sinuses
- Basilar plexus
- Cavernous sinuses
- Sphenoparietal sinus

MENINGES
- Dura mater
  - Falx cerebri
  - Tentorium cerebelli
  - Falx cerebelli
- Arachnoid mater
  - Arachnoid granulations
  - Subarachnoid space
- Pia mater

BRAIN
- Cerebral gyri (ridges)
- Cerebral sulci (valleys)
  - Lateral sulcus
  - Central sulcus
- Cerebrum
- Poles
  - Frontal pole
  - Temporal pole
  - Occipital pole
- Lobes
  - Frontal lobe
  - Temporal lobe
  - Parietal lobe
  - Occipital lobe
- Cerebellum

VENTRICULAR SYSTEM
- Lateral ventricles
  - Interventricular foramen
- Third ventricle
  - Cerebral aqueduct
- Fourth ventricle
  - Median aperture
  - Lateral apertures
  - Central canal of the spinal cord

NERVES
- Cranial nn.
  - Olfactory n. (CN I)
  - Optic n. (CN II)
  - Oculomotor n. (CN III)
  - Trochlear n. (CN IV)
  - Trigeminal n. (CN V)
  - Abducens n. (CN VI)
  - Facial n. (CN VII)
  - Vestibulocochlear n. (CN VIII)
  - Glossopharyngeal n. (CN IX)
  - Vagus n. (CN X)
    - Superior laryngeal n.
      - Internal laryngeal n.
      - External laryngeal n.
    - Recurrent laryngeal n.
  - Spinal accessory n. (CN XI)
  - Hypoglossal n. (CN XII)

MISCELLANEOUS
- Posterior atlanto-occipital membrane

Lab 21 Dissection Overview

The purpose of this laboratory session is to learn the anatomy of the scalp, calvarium, meninges, and brain through dissection. You will do so through the following suggested sequence:

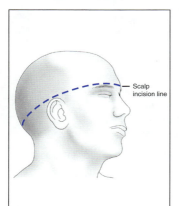

1. Using a scalpel, make a circumferential cut around the scalp.

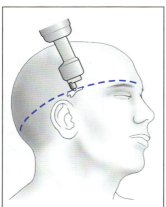

2. Using a bone saw, cut through the bone of the calvarium and remove the calvarium.

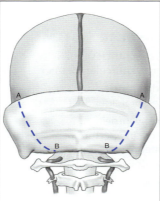

3. Using a bone saw, remove a wedge of the occipital bone.

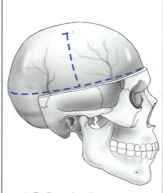

4. Reflect the dura mater.

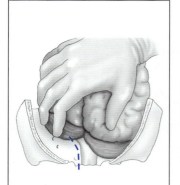

5. Transect the spinal cord, vertebral arteries, and superior spinal nerves in preparation for removal of the brain.

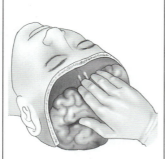

6. Reflect the frontal lobes of the brain to transect the anterior cranial nerves; remove the brain from the base of the skull.

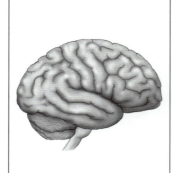

7. Identify the lobes and regions of the brain.

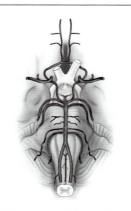

8. Dissect and identify the internal carotid and vertebral arteries and their associated branches.

Scalp

- Using a scalpel, make the following continuous incision through the scalp to the underlying bone **(Figure 21-1)**:
  - Around the circumference of the skull, approximately 2 cm above the supraorbital margin and 2 cm above the external occipital protuberance

- Use a scalpel and forceps to reveal and identify the following **(Figure 21-2)**:
  - **Scalp layers** — five layers, from superficial to deep:
    1. **(S) Skin** — external surface covered with hair
    2. **(C) Superficial Connective tissue (fascia)** — deep to the skin; consists of dense connective tissue; many nerves and vessels are contained within it
    3. **(A) Aponeurosis** — deep to the superficial connective tissue; of the **frontalis m.** anteriorly and the **occipitalis m.** posteriorly, connected by a broad aponeurosis called the **galea aponeurotica**
    4. **(L) Loose connective tissue** — deep to the aponeurosis; provides a plane for gliding of the more superficial layers of the scalp
    5. **(P) Pericranium** — the deepest layer is the periosteum that ensheaths the cranial bones

- The bones of the skull are flat bones that have an external lamina, a central spongy bone (diploë), and an internal lamina

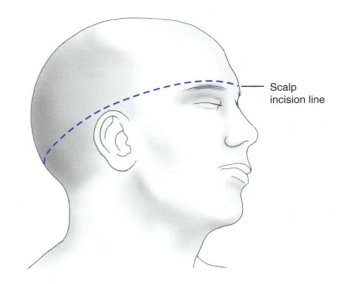

Figure 21-1 Scalp skin incision

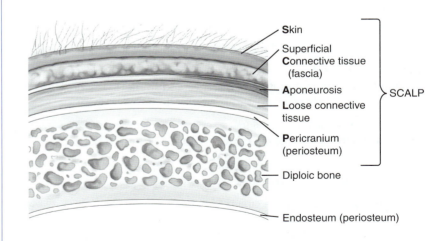

Figure 21-2 Scalp layers

Removal of the Calvarium

- You will use a bone saw, chisel, mallet, and finally your fingers to remove the calvarium from the rest of the skull

- *Note:* Make sure that the bone saw is turned off before plugging it in

- Follow these instructions to remove the calvarium **(Figure 21-3)**:

  - **Bone saw *(A)*** — cut through the skull where the skin incision was made with the scalpel

    - The key to sawing through the skull *(B)* is to only saw into the diploë region and leave the internal lamina intact; this approach minimizes damage (cuts) to the underlying dura mater and brain; if the saw cuts through the full thickness of the skull bone, you will feel the saw drop because of less resistance

  - **Chisel and mallet *(C)*** — once you have completed sawing the circumference, break through the internal lamina of the skull by repeatedly inserting a chisel along the saw cut and striking the chisel with a mallet; hit the mallet with sufficient force to break the internal layer of compact bone but not too much force, which will push the chisel into the underlying brain

    - Continue this procedure until the calvarium is loose

  - **Separate the calvarium from the dura mater *(D)*** — this step sounds easier than it is; it takes patience and strength; the goal is to remove the calvarium and leave the dura mater intact

    - Using a probe and your fingers, separate the dura mater from the internal surface of the calvarium; they are strongly bonded

    - *Be careful* of sharp edges of the bone; they will pierce rubber gloves and puncture your skin

    - Keep prying along the circumference to separate the dura mater from the calvarium; place a chisel in the saw cut and twist the chisel to increase the separation between the dura mater and calvarium

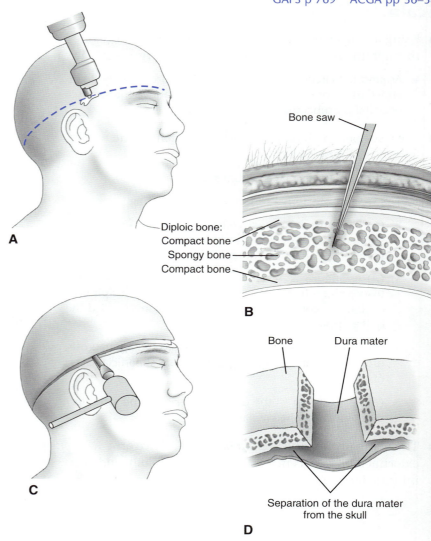

Figure 21-3 Cutting the skull with a bone saw. **A,** Saw along the scalpel incision line. **B,** Desired depth of penetration of the saw blade. **C,** Hammer and chisel use along the saw-cut line. **D,** Separation of the dura mater from the inside of the skull

Calvarium — Internal Surface

- Once the calvarium is removed, examine its internal surface
- Identify the following **(Figure 21-4)**:
  - Grooves of the middle meningeal a.
  - Groove for the superior sagittal sinus
    - Indentations (impressions) of the arachnoid villi (granulations)
  - Frontal bone
  - Parietal bones
  - Occipital bone
  - Coronal suture
  - Sagittal suture
  - Lambdoid suture
  - **Sutural bones** — extra bones within a suture; sutural bones are commonly found in the lambdoid region (not shown)

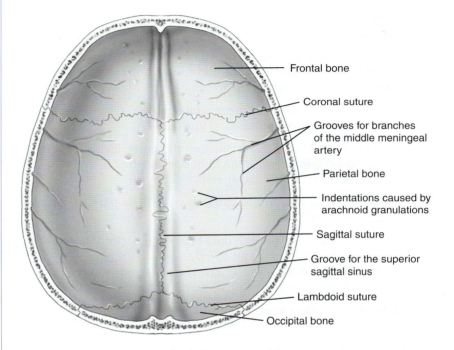

Figure 21-4 Internal view of the calvarium

Removal of a Wedge of the Occipital Bone to Better Expose the Brain

- Place the cadaver prone, place a wooden block under the sternum to allow the neck to flex, and follow these instructions:

  - Use a scalpel to scrape away skin, muscles, and soft tissue that attach to the occipital bone and surround the posterior half of the **foramen magnum**

  - Locate the space between the occipital bone and C1 vertebra (atlas); preserve the vertebral aa. **(Figure 21-5A)**:

    - With a scalpel, carefully cut through the **posterior atlanto-occipital membrane** from one vertebral a. to the other, without cutting the arteries

    - Ensure that all muscle and connective tissue have been removed from the area

    - Insert a probe between the dura mater and occipital bone; sweep the probe from right to left to peel the dura mater from the occipital bone; continue the sweeping motion inferiorly and laterally

- **Make the following bone saw cuts** (see Figure 21-5A and 21-5B):

  - Along the lines indicated, from point A to point B, on both external sides of the occipital bone; as when you sawed through the calvarium, saw only into the spongy bone and use a chisel and mallet to finish the job

  - Pull away the occipital bone wedge from the underlying dura mater, using blunt dissection to remove dural connections

- Examine the removed bony wedge to identify the following (see Figure 21-5B):

  - **Grooves for the transverse dural sinuses**
  - **Groove for the confluence of dural venous sinuses**
  - **Groove for the occipital dural sinus**

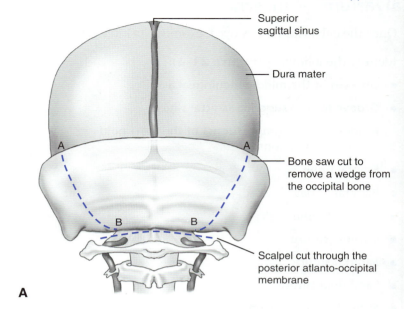

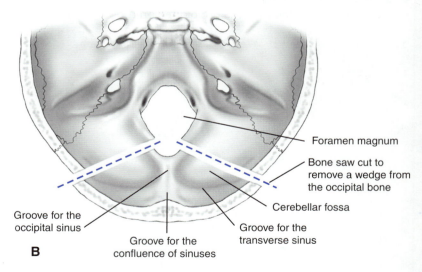

Figure 21-5 Occipital wedge removal. **A,** Posterior view. **B,** Superior view.

Examination of the Cranial Dura Mater and Dural Venous Sinuses

■ Identify the following structures **(Figure 21-6)**:

- **Dura mater** — surrounds the cerebrum and cerebellum

- **Branches of the middle meningeal a. and v.** — observe the anterior and posterior branches along the dura mater; observe the corresponding grooves on the internal surface of the calvarium

- **Dural venous sinuses** — venous sinuses are not true veins but are endothelial-lined venous structures that drain venous blood from the brain; the dural venous sinuses are formed by separation of the two layers of the dura mater (endosteal and meningeal layers)

  - **Superior sagittal sinus** — extends from anterior to posterior in the midline, deep to the calvarium

  - **Arachnoid granulations** — visible as outward bulges of the dura mater, lateral to the superior sagittal sinus; internally, formed by capillary tufts that provide absorption of cerebrospinal fluid into the dural venous sinuses (see Figure 21-6B):

    ◆ Use scissors or a scalpel to cut open the superior sagittal sinus to observe these numerous cauliflower-like masses; you can usually see their outline through the dura mater

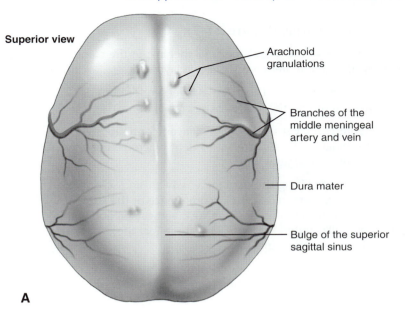

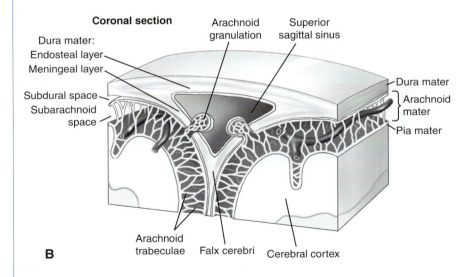

Figure 21-6 Dura mater. **A,** Superior view. **B,** Coronal section

Unit 4 • **Lab 21** Scalp, Calvarium, Meninges, and Brain

Cranial Meninges

- Identify the following **(Figure 21-7)**:

  - **Dura mater** — the most superficial meninx; in the cranial cavity, the dura mater consists of two layers:

    - **Endosteal layer** — the external layer; endosteum (periosteum on the inside of the cranial bones)

    - **Meningeal layer** — the internal layer; continuous with the spinal cord's dura mater; evident where you opened the superior sagittal sinus

  - Use forceps to lift up the dura mater while using scissors to cut the dura mater along the circumference of the edge of the saw cut through the skull; make a vertical incision with a scalpel, as illustrated in Figure 21-7, to reflect the dura mater to help expose the brain

  - **Arachnoid mater** — the second meninx; smoothly drapes over the surface of the brain; does not drop into the sulci (valleys)

    - **Subarachnoid space** — space deep to the arachnoid mater in which cerebrospinal fluid is located

  - **Pia mater** — probe through the arachnoid mater and note that the third, and deepest, meninx cannot be distinguished from the surface of the brain; intimately applied to every **gyrus** (ridge) and sulcus

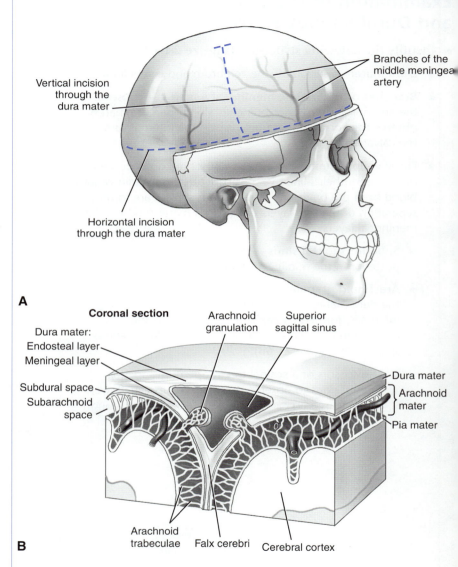

Figure 21-7 Dura mater dissection. **A,** Lateral view of the skull to demonstrate removal of the dura mater. **B,** Coronal section

Cranial Dural Folds

■ Lift up (invert) the cut dura mater to fully expose both hemispheres of the brain to identify the following (**Figure 21-8**):

- **Dural folds** — perpendicular projections of the dura mater that compartmentalize the cranial cavity and thereby stabilize the brain; contain the dural venous sinuses
  - **Falx cerebri** — biggest dural projection; sickle-shaped septum between the two cerebral hemispheres; attached from the crista galli (ethmoid bone) anteriorly to the tentorium cerebelli posteriorly
  - **Tentorium cerebelli** — transverse projection between the cerebellum inferiorly and occipital lobes of the cerebrum superiorly; attached to the superior border of the petrous portion of the temporal bones
  - **Falx cerebelli** — short dural projection that separates the cerebellar hemispheres; attached to the internal occipital crest and tentorium cerebelli

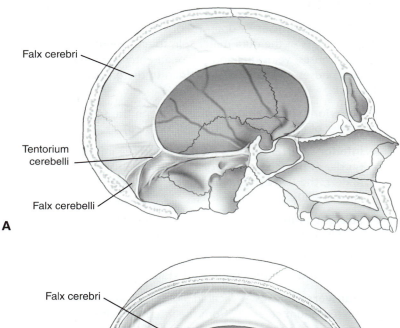

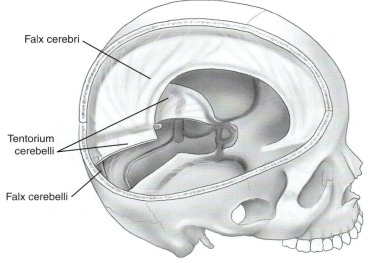

Figure 21-8 Brain removed to demonstrate the dural folds. **A**, Medial view. **B**, Superior and oblique view

Cranial Dural Venous Sinuses

- Use forceps and scissors to reveal and identify the following (**Figure 21-9**):

  - **Dural venous sinuses** — drain venous blood from the brain; the two layers of the dura mater split to enclose the dural venous sinuses; veins draining the brain enter the dural venous sinuses, which ultimately drain to the great veins of the neck

    - **Superior sagittal sinus** — located along the superior border of the falx cerebri (already opened)

    - **Inferior sagittal sinus** — located along the inferior "free" border of the falx cerebri; gently separate, using your fingers, the two cerebral hemispheres to observe this dural venous sinus

    - **Straight sinus** — located along the line of fusion between the falx cerebri and tentorium cerebelli

    - **Great cerebral v.** — drains into the junction of the inferior sagittal and straight sinuses; not visible at this point

    - **Transverse sinuses** — located along the lateral edges of the tentorium cerebelli, from the internal occipital protuberance to the petrous portion of the temporal bones; gently raise the occipital lobes to observe these dural venous sinuses

    - **Sigmoid sinuses** — S-shaped dural venous sinuses that end bilaterally at the jugular foramen where the jugular bulb (dilation) is located (beginning of the internal jugular v.)

    - **Superior and inferior petrosal sinuses** — located along the petrous portion of the temporal bone; not visible at this point

    - **Cavernous sinuses** — located on the sides of the sella turcica; not visible at this point

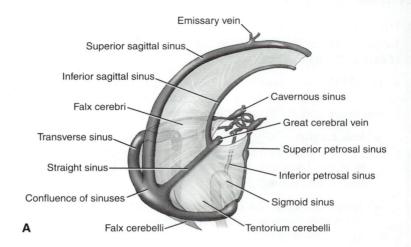

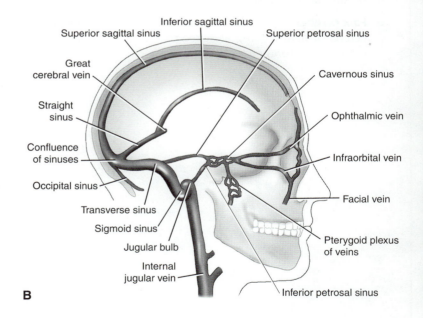

Figure 21-9 Dural venous sinuses. **A,** Superior and oblique view. **B,** Medial view

Removal of the Brain

- To remove the brain, cut all of its attachments bilaterally
  - Attachments include nerves, vessels, and dura mater at the base of the brain and skull
- To remove the brain, place the cadaver prone and complete the following instructions:
  - Use a scalpel to transect the spinal cord and both vertebral aa. inferior to the foramen magnum of the occipital bone **(Figure 21-10A)**
  - Cut the dura mater along the edge of the occipital bone (where the occipital wedge was removed) from A to B on both sides; extend the dural cuts to the foramen magnum
  - Reflect the dural flap superiorly to expose the brain
  - Use your fingers to gently lift up the occipital lobes (see Figure 21-10B)
  - Use a scalpel to cut the tentorium cerebelli from its internal cranial attachments along the occipital bones and the rim of the petrous portion of the temporal bones to expose the cerebellum

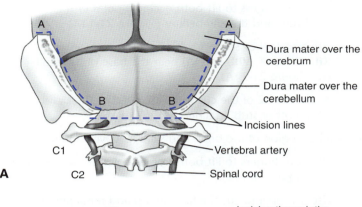

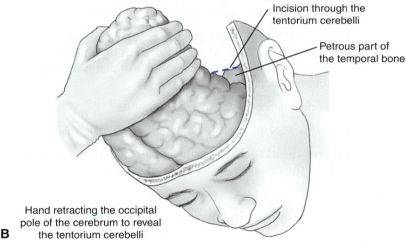

Figure 21-10 Removal of the brain. **A,** Posterior view of the skull. **B,** Superior and oblique view

Removal of the Brain Continued

Removal of the Brain—cont'd

- To finish removal of the brain, complete the following instructions, bilaterally:
  - Posterior region of the brain and skull (cadaver prone)
    - Use your fingers to lift both occipital poles of the cerebrum and the cerebellum (**Figure 21-11A**)
    - Use a scalpel or scissors to transect **cranial nerves XII, XI, X, IX, VIII,** and **VII** near the base of the skull (see Figure 21-11A)
      - Leave one of the cut stubs attached to the brain and the other stub attached to the skull
  - Anterior region of the brain and skull (cadaver supine)
    - Use your fingers to lift both frontal poles of the cerebrum (see Figure 21-11B)
    - Use a scalpel to cut the falx cerebri and remaining dura mater from the crista galli of the ethmoid bone
    - Identify the **olfactory bulbs** and **tracts** (CN I) on the **cribriform plates of the ethmoid bone**; using a probe, pry the bulbs and tracts from the cribriform plates to keep the bulbs and tracts attached to the brain
    - Identify and transect the following structures:
      - **Optic nn.** (CN II) — cut just anterior to the optic chiasma
      - **Internal carotid aa.** — cut the arteries close to the bone to keep the cerebral arterial circle intact on the brain
    - **Cut the following nerves sequentially:**
      - **Oculomotor nn. (CN III), abducens nn. (CN IV), trochlear nn. (CN VI),** and **trigeminal nn. (CN V)**

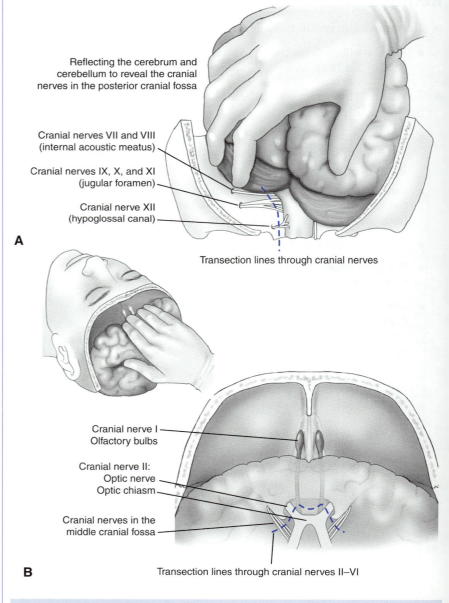

Figure 21-11 Removal of the brain. **A,** Posterior view. **B,** Superior view.

Examination of the Removed Brain

- Gently pull the brain out of the cranial vault and use a scalpel to cut remaining attachments, if necessary

- Identify the following **(Figure 21-12)**:
  - *Poles* of the cerebrum
    - **Frontal**
    - **Temporal**
    - **Occipital**
  - *Lobes* of the cerebrum
    - **Frontal** — anterior cranial fossae
    - **Temporal** — middle cranial fossae
    - **Parietal** — superior to the temporal lobes
    - **Occipital** — posterior cranial fossae
  - **Main sulci**
    - **Lateral sulcus** — separates the temporal lobe from the parietal and frontal lobes
    - **Central sulcus** — separates the primary motor cortex (located in the precentral gyrus of the frontal lobes) from the primary sensory cortex (located in the postcentral gyrus of the parietal lobes)

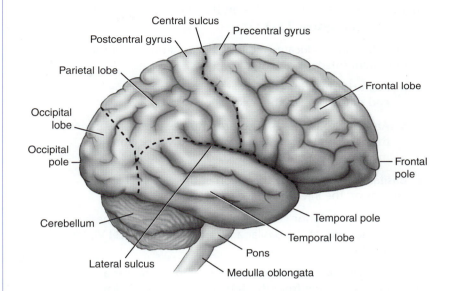

Figure 21-12 Lateral view of the brain

Arterial Supply of the Brain

- Probe and peel away the arachnoid mater to reveal arteries at the brain's base

- Identify the following arteries on the inferior surface (base) of the brain **(Figure 21-13)**:

  - **Vertebral aa.** — located along the ventral surface of the brainstem (medulla oblongata)

    - **Posterior inferior cerebellar aa.** — arise near the inferior end of the olive of the medulla oblongata

    - **Anterior spinal a.** — arises from the vertebral aa., prior to their union at the basal a.; courses down the anterior median fissure of the spinal cord

  - **Basilar a.** — formed by the union of the vertebral aa.; courses on the inferior surface of the pons

    - **Anterior inferior cerebellar aa.** — branch from the inferior part of the basilar a.; course ventral to CN VI, VII, and VIII

    - **Labyrinthine aa.** — may branch from the basilar a. but more often from the anterior inferior cerebellar a.; accompany the facial (CN VII) and vestibulocochlear nn. (CN VIII) into the internal acoustic meatus; separated from the anterior inferior cerebellar aa. by the abducens n. (CN VI)

    - **Pontine aa.** — branch from the basilar a. to supply the pons

    - **Superior cerebellar aa.** — arise near the superior end of the basilar a.

    - **Posterior cerebral aa.** — also arise from the superior end of the basilar a.; separated from the superior cerebral a. by the oculomotor n. (CN III); supply the occipital and parietal lobes

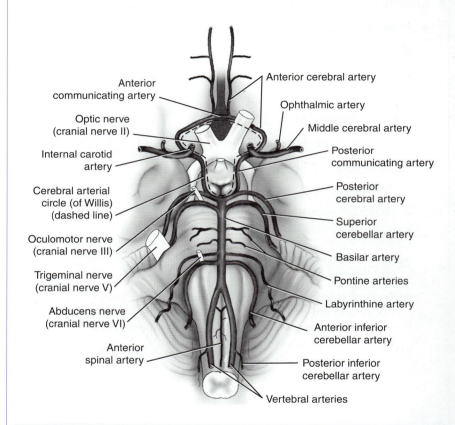

Figure 21-13 Arteries on the inferior surface of the brain

Arterial Supply of the Brain—cont'd

- **Internal carotid aa.** — enter the cranial base via the carotid canals and turn to travel anteriorly through the cavernous sinuses (on the side of the sphenoid bone); each internal carotid a. divides into the following branches **(Figure 21-14)**:

  - **Ophthalmic aa.** — leave the cavernous sinus medial to the anterior clinoid process of the sphenoid bone; enter the orbit via the optic canal, inferolateral to the optic n.

  - **Middle cerebral aa.** — course laterally to the temporal lobe in the lateral sulcus; largest of the branches of the internal carotid a.

  - **Anterior cerebral aa.** — course anteromedially superior to the optic n. to reach the longitudinal cerebral fissure and thence the frontal lobe

    - **Anterior communicating a.** — connects the right and left anterior cerebral aa.; about 4 mm long

  - **Posterior communicating aa.** — connect the right and left middle cerebral aa. to the right and left posterior cerebral aa., respectively

- **Cerebral arterial circle (of Willis)** — a hexagonal vascular ring that is formed by union of the internal carotid and vertebral aa. via the anterior and posterior communicating aa.; surrounds the optic chiasma and stalk of the pituitary gland

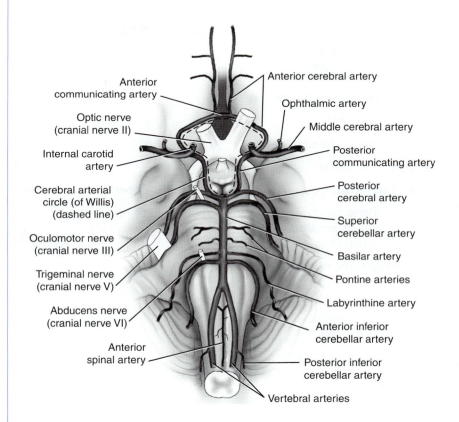

Figure 21-14 Arteries on the inferior surface of the brain

Ventricles of the Brain

- Unless the brain is sliced in the gross anatomy course, you will not identify the ventricular system of the brain, other than radiographically

- The following ventricular structures are identifiable on radiographs **(Figure 21-15)**:
  - **Lateral ventricles (paired)**
    - **Interventricular foramen**
  - **Third ventricle**
    - **Cerebral aqueduct**
  - **Fourth ventricle**
    - **Lateral apertures (paired) and the median aperture**
      - These apertures allow cerebrospinal fluid to flow into the **cisterna magna**, which communicates with the subarachnoid space
  - **Central canal of the spinal cord**

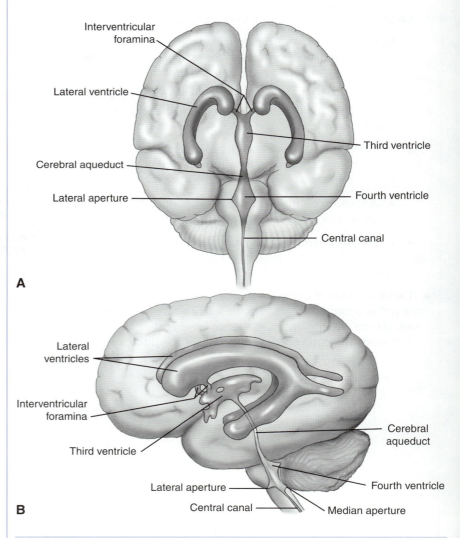

Figure 21-15 Ventricular system of the brain. **A,** Anterior view. **B,** Lateral view

Base of the Skull and Cranial Nerves

Lab 22

Prior to dissection, you should familiarize yourself with the following structures:

ANTERIOR CRANIAL FOSSA

Frontal Bone
- Orbital plates
- Foramen cecum
  - Emissary vv. to the superior sagittal sinus

Ethmoid Bone
- Crista galli
- Cribriform plate (bulbs of CN I)

Sphenoid Bone
- Lesser wings
- Anterior clinoid processes

MIDDLE CRANIAL FOSSA

Sphenoid Bone
- Greater wings
  - Grooves for the middle meningeal a.
- Chiasmatic groove (optic chiasma for CN II)
- Sella turcica and pituitary gland
  - Dorsum sellae
  - Posterior clinoid processes
- Groove for the internal carotid a.
- Foramen spinosum
  - Middle meningeal a. and v., meningeal branch of the mandibular n.
- Foramen ovale
  - Mandibular division of the trigeminal nerve (CN V-3)
- Foramen rotundum
  - Maxillary division of the trigeminal nerve (CN V-2)
- Superior orbital fissures
  - Oculomotor n. (CN III), trochlear n. (CN IV), ophthalmic division of the trigeminal nerve (CN V-1), abducens n. (VI), and superior ophthalmic v.
- Optic canal
  - Optic n. (CN II) and ophthalmic a.

Temporal Bone
- Greater petrosal canal with accompanying nerves
- Foramen lacerum

POSTERIOR CRANIAL FOSSA

Temporal Bone
- Internal acoustic meatus
  - Facial n. (CN VII), vestibulocochlear n. (CN VIII), and labyrinthine a.
- Groove for the superior petrosal sinus
- Groove for the sigmoid sinus

Parietal Bone
- Groove for the middle meningeal a.

Occipital Bone
- Clivus
- Groove for the inferior petrosal sinus
- Groove for the transverse and occipital sinuses
- Internal occipital crest and protuberance
- Groove for the superior sagittal sinus
- Foramen magnum
  - Medulla oblongata
  - Spinal cord
- Hypoglossal canal
  - Hypoglossal n. (CN XII)
- Jugular foramen
  - Inferior petrosal sinus, glossopharyngeal n. (CN IX), vagus n. (CN X), spinal accessory n. (CN XI), sigmoid sinus, and posterior meningeal a.

Continued

DURAL VENOUS SINUSES
- Superior sagittal sinus
- Inferior sagittal sinus
- Straight sinus
- Transverse sinus
- Sigmoid sinus
- Confluence of sinuses
- Occipital sinus
- Basilar plexus
- Cavernous sinus
- Inferior petrosal sinus
- Superior petrosal sinus
- Sphenoparietal sinus

CRANIAL NERVES (CN)
- Olfactory n. (I)
- Optic n. (II)
- Oculomotor n. (III)
- Trochlear n. (IV)
- Trigeminal n. (V)
  - Trigeminal ganglion
  - V-1 — ophthalmic division
  - V-2 — maxillary division
  - V-3 — mandibular division
- Abducens n. (VI)
- Facial n. (VII)
  - Nerve to the pterygoid canal
- Vestibulocochlear n. (VIII)
- Glossopharyngeal n. (IX)
- Vagus n. (X)
- Spinal accessory n. (XI)
- Hypoglossal n. (XII)

Lab 22 Dissection Overview

The purpose of this laboratory session is to learn the anatomy of the base of the skull and identify vessels, nerves, and associated structures located therein through dissection. You will do so through the following suggested sequence:

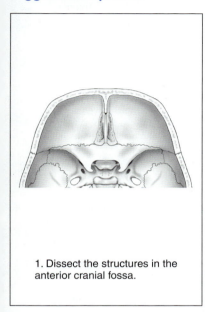

1. Dissect the structures in the anterior cranial fossa.

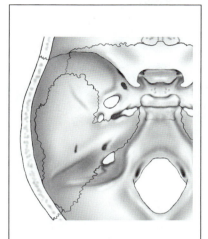

2. Dissect the structures in the middle cranial fossa.

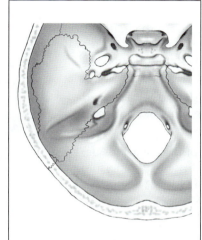

3. Dissect the structures in the posterior cranial fossa.

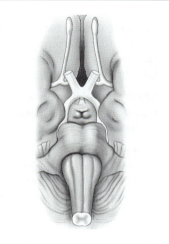

4. Identify the cranial nerves on the base of the skull as well as the base of the brain.

Cranial Fossae

- The base of the skull (internal surface of the cranium) is divided into three depressions (fossae) **(Figure 22-1A)**

- Use a dry skull to identify the three cranial fossae (see Figure 22-1B):

  - **Anterior cranial fossa** — separated from the middle cranial fossa by the sharp posterior crests of the lesser wings of the sphenoid bone and the anterior margin of the optic (chiasmatic) groove

  - **Middle cranial fossa** — butterfly-shaped fossa formed mainly by the greater wings of the sphenoid bone and the temporal bones

  - **Posterior cranial fossa** — largest of the cranial fossae; separated from the middle cranial fossa by the dorsum sellae and the posterior superior margins of the **petrous parts of the right and left temporal bones**

- Also identify the three cranial fossae on the cadaver's skull

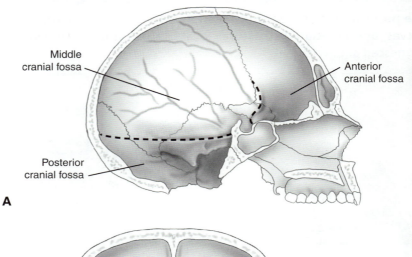

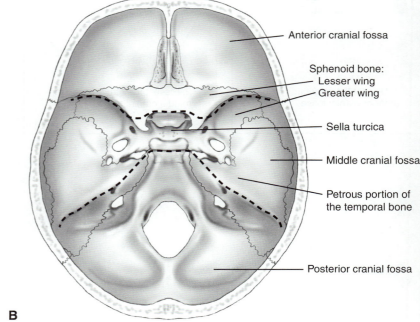

Figure 22-1 Cranial fossae of a dry skull. **A,** Medial view in sagittal section. **B,** Superior view; the *black dashed lines* identify boundaries for the cranial fossae

Anterior Cranial Fossa

- Identify the following in a dry skull and the cadaver's skull (**Figure 22-2**):

  - **Frontal bone**
    - **Orbital plates** — form the roof of the orbits
    - **Foramen cecum** — transmits an emissary v. en route to the superior sagittal sinus
  - **Ethmoid bone**
    - **Crista galli** — attachment for the dura mater (falx cerebri)
    - **Cribriform plate** — location of the olfactory bulbs of CN I
  - **Sphenoid bone**
    - **Lesser wings** — their posterior edge contributes to the boundary between the anterior cranial fossa and the middle cranial fossa
    - **Anterior clinoid processes** — form the anterior boundary around the pituitary gland

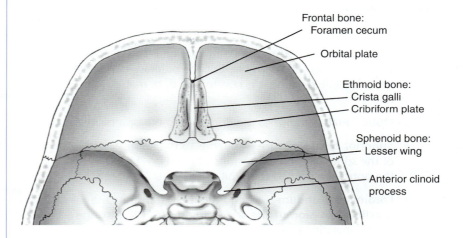

Figure 22-2 Internal view of the anterior cranial fossa of a dry skull

Middle Cranial Fossa

■ Identify the following in a dry skull and the cadaver's skull **(Figure 22-3)**:

- **Sphenoid bone**
  - **Sella turcica** — houses the pituitary gland; the stalk of the pituitary gland will be visible, but the pituitary gland will not be visible because it is covered by dura mater (diaphragm sellae)
  - **Optic canal** — transmits the optic n. and the ophthalmic a.
  - **Superior orbital fissure** — inferior to the lesser wings of the sphenoid bone; transmits CN III, IV, V-1, and VI and the ophthalmic vv. to the orbit
  - **Foramen rotundum** — round foramen; transmits the **maxillary division of the trigeminal n. (CN V-2)** to the pterygopalatine fossa
  - **Foramen ovale** — oval foramen; posterolateral to the foramen rotundum; transmits the **mandibular division of the trigeminal n. (CN V-3)** to the infratemporal fossa
  - **Foramen lacerum** — jagged gap superior to the carotid canal; filled with cartilage
  - **Foramen spinosum** — small round foramen posterolateral to the foramen ovale; transmits the **middle meningeal vessels** and the **accessory meningeal branch of the mandibular division of the trigeminal n. (CN V-3)**

- **Temporal bone**
  - **Hiatus for the greater petrosal n.**
  - **Petrous portion** — the densest bone in the skull, which is necessary for sound conduction

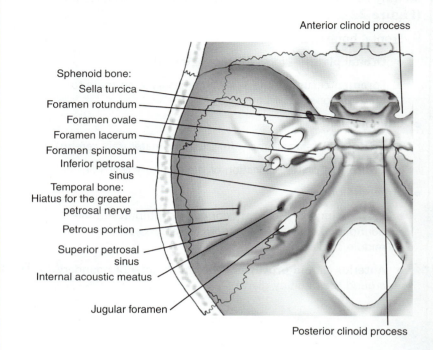

Figure 22-3 Internal view of the middle cranial fossa of a dry skull

Middle Cranial Fossa and Dural Venous Sinuses

GAFS pp 775–777, 794–796   ACGA p 18   NAHA Plates 9–11, 103–104

- Identify the following structures in the cadaver's skull **(Figure 22-4A)**:

  - **Superior petrosal sinuses** — paired dural venous sinuses located along the superior border of the petrous portions of the temporal bones; located at the lateral attachment of the tentorium cerebelli

  - **Inferior petrosal sinuses** — paired dural venous sinuses located inferior to the superior petrosal sinuses; course from the cavernous sinuses along the petro-occipital sutures to the anterior compartment of the jugular foramen to terminate at the bulb of the internal jugular vv.

  - **Basilar venous plexus** — located in the posterior cranial fossa

    - The superior petrosal sinuses, inferior petrosal sinuses, and basilar venous plexus are located in the posterior cranial fossa but are associated with the cavernous sinus

  - **Cavernous sinuses** — paired, irregularly shaped dural venous sinuses located on the lateral walls of the sella turcica; the dura mater that forms the lateral wall of the cavernous sinus contains the following, from superior to inferior (see Figure 22-4B); use a scalpel to make a coronal cut completely through the cavernous sinus:

    - Oculomotor n. (CN III)
    - Trochlear n. (CN IV)
    - Trigeminal n. (CN V) branches V-1 and V-2

  - **Lumen of the cavernous sinus** — the following course through the lumen of the cavernous sinus, surrounded by venous blood:

    - Internal carotid a.
    - Abducens n. (CN VI)

  - **Sphenoparietal sinuses** — drain to the cavernous sinuses

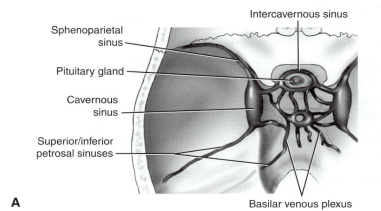

Figure 22-4 Cavernous sinuses. **A,** Internal view. **B,** Coronal section through the sphenoid bone

Middle Cranial Fossa and Dural Venous Sinuses Continued

Middle Cranial Fossa and Dural Venous Sinuses—cont'd

■ Identify the following in the cadaver's skull **(Figure 22-5)**:

- On one side of the petrous portion of the temporal bone, peel away the dura mater to reveal the divisions of the trigeminal n. and the trigeminal ganglion:
  - **Trace V-1 (ophthalmic division)** — exits through the superior orbital fissure
  - **Trace V-2 (maxillary division)** — exits through the foramen rotundum
  - **Trace V-3 (mandibular division)** — exits through the foramen ovale
- Study a dry skull to see the foramina of the middle cranial fossa

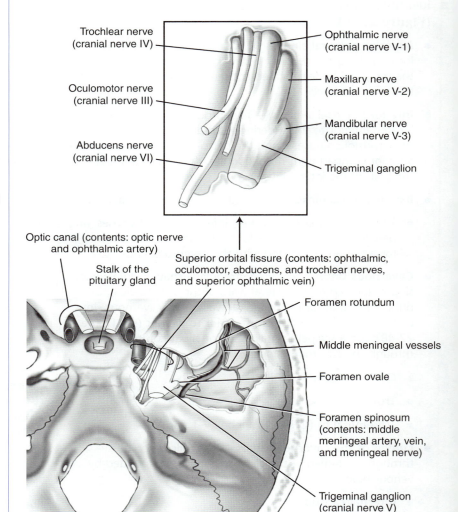

Figure 22-5 Internal view of the middle cranial fossa

Middle Cranial Fossa and Dural Venous Sinuses—cont'd

- Use forceps to reveal and identify the following in the cadaver's skull **(Figure 22-6)**:

  - **Middle meningeal aa.** — branches of the maxillary aa. (infratemporal fossa; to be dissected in a future laboratory session); embedded in the outer layer of the dura mater in the middle cranial fossa

    - Follow the middle meningeal aa. to the foramen spinosum on each side of the skull's base

  - **Greater petrosal n. (branch of CN VII)** — courses from the greater petrosal hiatus on the superior surface of the temporal bone; passes deep to the trigeminal ganglion before it reaches the foramen lacerum; the greater petrosal n. (parasympathetic) joins the deep petrosal n. (sympathetic) to form the nerve of the pterygoid canal (to be dissected in a future laboratory session)

GAFS pp 784, 804–805   ACGA p 18   NAHA Plates 9–11, 103–104

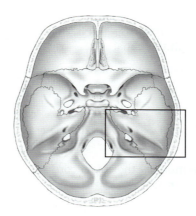

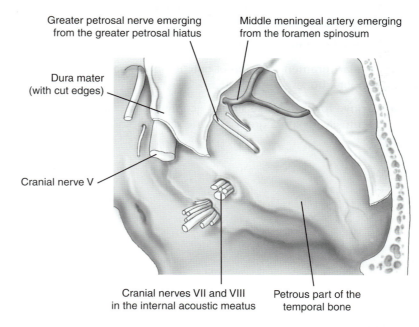

Figure 22-6 Internal view of the petrous part of the temporal bone

Unit 4 • Lab 22   Base of the Skull and Cranial Nerves

Posterior Cranial Fossa

■ Identify the following structures **(Figure 22-7)**:

- **Temporal bone**
  - **Internal acoustic meatus** — CNs VII and VIII exit the cranium through this canal
  - **Jugular foramen** — union of notches in the temporal and occipital bones

- **Occipital bone**
  - **Hypoglossal canal** — CN XII exits the cranium through this canal
  - **Foramen magnum** — the spinal cord exits the cranium through this foramen
  - **Clivus** — the inclined surface from the dorsum sellae to the foramen magnum; supports the pons and medulla oblongata
  - **Internal occipital protuberance**
  - **Jugular foramen** — union of notches in the occipital and temporal bones
  - **Groove for transverse sinus** — continues laterally eventually joining a groove for the sigmoid sinus

GAFS pp 777–778   ACGA p 18   NAHA Plates 9–11

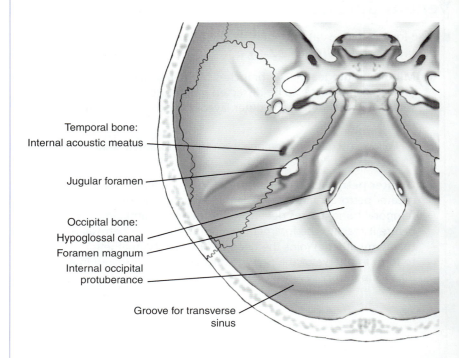

Figure 22-7   Internal view of the posterior cranial fossa

Posterior Cranial Fossa—cont'd

- Use forceps to reveal and identify the following in the cadaver's skull **(Figure 22-8)**:

  - **Foramen magnum** — largest foramen in the skull; transmits the following:
    - **Medulla oblongata** — at the level of the foramen magnum, the medulla oblongata becomes continuous with the spinal cord
    - **Vertebral aa.**
    - **Spinal roots of the spinal accessory nn. (CN XI)**
    - **Venous plexus of the spinal cord and cranial cavity** — these veins have no valves

  - **Hypoglossal canal** — located along the anterolateral margin of the foramen magnum; the **hypoglossal n. (CN XII)** exits the base of the skull through the hypoglossal canal

  - **Jugular foramen** — between the petrous portion of the temporal bone and occipital bone; transmits the following:
    - **Jugular bulb** — origin of the internal jugular v.
    - **Cranial nerves IX, X, and XI**
    - **Posterior meningeal a.**

  - **Internal acoustic meatus** — superior to the jugular foramen; transmits CN VII and VIII and the labyrinthine a.

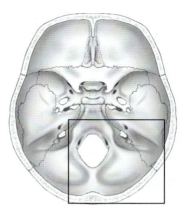

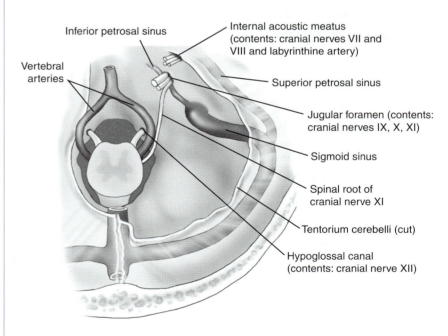

Figure 22-8   Internal view of the posterior cranial fossa

Review of the Cranial Nerves

- **Cranial nerves** (12 pairs):
  - Receive their name because they arise from the brain; emerge through foramina/fissures in the base of the skull
  - Numbered I through XII, from anterior to posterior, according to their attachment on the brain

- View the inferior surface of the brain to identify the following cranial nerves **(Figure 22-9)**:
  - Olfactory n. (CN I)
  - Optic n. (CN II)
  - Oculomotor n. (CN III)
  - Trochlear n. (CN IV)
  - Trigeminal n. (CN V)
  - Abducens n. (CN VI)
  - Facial n. (CN VII)
  - Vestibulocochlear n. (CN VIII)
  - Glossopharyngeal n. (CN IX)
  - Vagus n. (CN X)
  - Spinal accessory n. (CN XI)
  - Hypoglossal n. (CN XII)

- Review the same cranial nerves by locating their stubs on the base of the skull of the cadaver

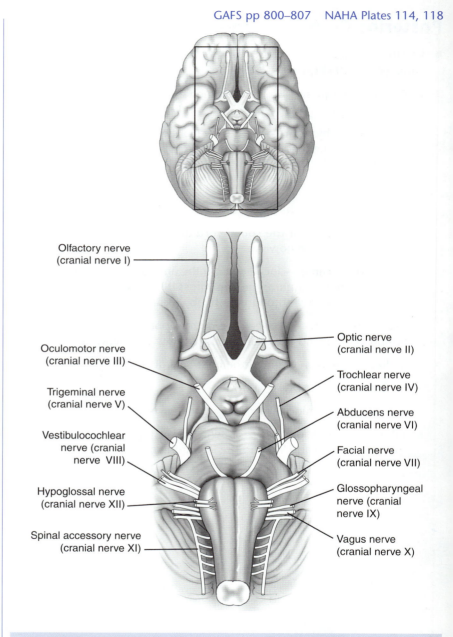

Figure 22-9 Cranial nerves on the inferior surface of the brain

Orbit

Lab 23

Prior to dissection, you should familiarize yourself with the following structures:

OSTEOLOGY
- Frontal bone
  - Superior orbital margin
  - Frontal sinus
- Lacrimal bone
- Ethmoid bone
  - Ethmoid labyrinth of air cells
  - Anterior and posterior ethmoid foramina
- Sphenoid bone
  - Anterior clinoid process
  - Optic canal
    - Contents: optic n. and ophthalmic a.
  - Superior orbital fissure
    - Contents: superior ophthalmic v., oculomotor n. (CN III), trochlear n. (CN IV), ophthalmic division of the trigeminal n. (lacrimal, frontal, and nasociliary branches of the CN V-1), and abducens n. (CN VI)
  - Inferior orbital fissure
  - Infraorbital groove
- Zygomatic bone

NERVES
- Optic n. (CN II)
- External nasal n. (CN V-1)
- Frontal n. (CN V-1)
  - Supraorbital n.
  - Supratrochlear n.
- Lacrimal n. (CN V-1)
- Infratrochlear n. (CN V-1)
- Nasociliary n. (CN V-1)
  - Long ciliary n.
  - Anterior and posterior ethmoid nn.
- Trochlear n. (CN IV)
- Abducens n. (CN VI)
- Oculomotor n. (CN III)
  - Superior and inferior divisions
  - Ciliary ganglion
  - Short ciliary nn.

VESSELS
- Ophthalmic a.
  - Branches are named the same as nerves in the orbit
  - Central a. of the retina

GLANDS
- Lacrimal gland
- Tarsal glands

MUSCLES
- Orbicularis oculi m.
- Levator palpebrae superioris m.
- Superior oblique m. (trochlea)
- Inferior oblique m.
- Medial rectus m.
- Lateral rectus m.
- Superior rectus m.
- Inferior rectus m.

EYEBALL (GLOBE)
- Sclera
- Cornea
- Choroid
  - Ciliary body
  - Zonular fibers
- Iris
- Lens
- Chambers
  - Anterior chamber
  - Posterior chamber
  - Vitreous body
- Retina

MISCELLANEOUS
- Periorbita
- Annulus tendineus

Lab 23 Dissection Overview

The purpose of this laboratory session is to learn the anatomy of the right orbit from a superior approach followed by an anterior (surgical) approach through dissection. You will do so through the following suggested sequence:

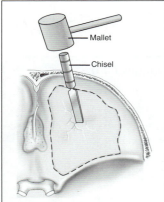

1. Using a mallet and chisel, remove the orbital plate covering the right orbit.

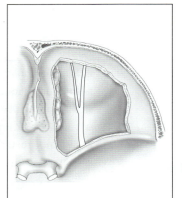

2. Identify the periorbita as well as the frontal nerve.

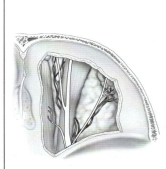

3. Dissect the periorbita away to reveal nerves, arteries, veins, and muscles associated with the orbit.

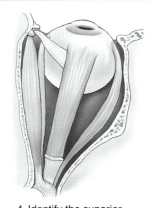

4. Identify the superior extraocular eye muscles.

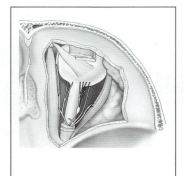

5. Dissect and identify branches of the oculomotor nerve (CN III).

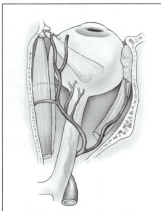

6. Identify branches of the ophthalmic artery.

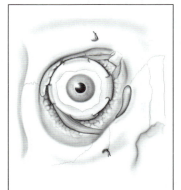

7. Dissect the eyelids away to identify the extraocular eye muscles from an anterior (surgical) approach.

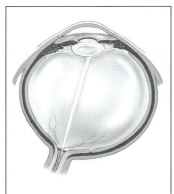

8. You may want to cut the eyeball in half to identify its structural anatomy.

APPROACHES TO DISSECT THE ORBIT

- During this dissection, the right orbit will be dissected via
  1. Superior approach — removal of the orbital roof
  2. Anterior (surgical) approach — removal of the eyelids

Superior Approach

- Follow these instructions to remove the orbital plate over the right eye:
  - With hemostats or forceps, peel the dura mater from the orbital plate of the right frontal bone
  - With a chisel and mallet, gently break the center of the roof of the orbit **(Figure 23-1A)**
  - Remove bone pieces with forceps (see Figure 23-1B)
  - Expand the exposure of the orbit as far anteriorly as possible, but leave the superior orbital margin intact; expand the exposure medially and laterally as well
  - Push a probe through the superior orbital fissure; remove the lesser wing of the sphenoid bone that is superior to the probe
  - Carefully break away the roof of the optic canal
  - Also remove the anterior clinoid process (sphenoid bone)

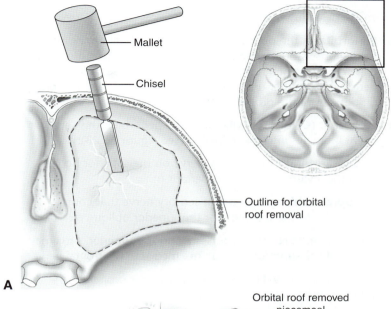

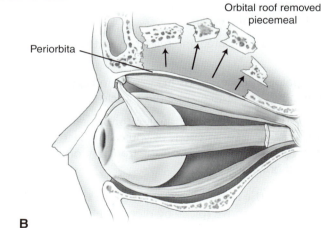

Figure 23-1 Removal of the right orbital plate. **A,** Superior view. **B,** Lateral view of a sagittal section

Superior Approach Continued

Superior Approach—cont'd

■ Identify the following:

- **Periorbita** — the periosteal lining of the orbital bones; use a scalpel or scissors to open the exposed periorbita but do *not* damage the frontal n. (usually seen through the translucent periorbita) or other underlying structures; use forceps to pick out lobules of the orbital fat **(Figure 23-2A)**

- **Frontal n. (CN V-1)** — inferior to the periorbita; this sensory nerve branches into the following (see Figure 23-2B):
  - **Supraorbital n.** — sensory nerve on the superior border of the levator palpebrae superioris m.
  - **Supratrochlear n.** — a thin sensory nerve that courses superior to the **trochlea** for the superior oblique m.

- **Trochlear n. (CN IV)** — courses along the superior, proximal border of the **superior oblique m.**, medial to the frontal nerve

- **Lacrimal n. (CN V-1)** — enters the superior orbital fissure lateral to the frontal n.; trace the lacrimal n. anteriorly to the lacrimal region of the eyelid

- **Lacrimal gland** — located anterolaterally in the superior part of the orbit

- **Levator palpebrae superioris m.** — with forceps, carefully pick out lobules of fat to expose this muscle
  - With scalpel or scissors, cut the levator palpebrae superioris m. as far anteriorly as you can; reflect the muscle posteriorly; do not cut the frontal n. or its terminal branches

■ *Note:* To identify the remaining structures in this laboratory session, carefully remove (piece by piece) fat lobules within the orbit. Motor nerves to the ocular mm. will enter the muscles at the orbit's apex, on the surface of the muscle closest to the optic n. Other nerves and main trunk arteries and veins will course through the orbital fat. Use caution when removing fat to avoid destroying these structures

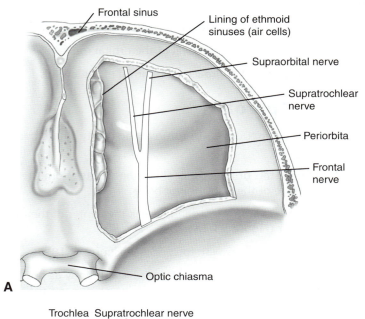
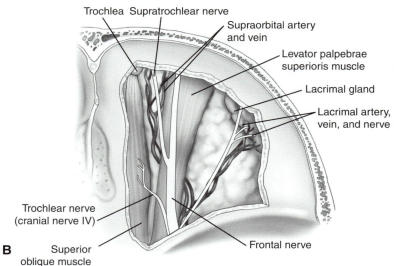

Figure 23-2 Superficial view of the right orbital contents. **A**, Periorbita. **B**, Periorbita removed

Superior Approach—cont'd

GAFS pp 842–843, 846–850   ACGA pp 65–68   NAHA Plates 83–87

- Use forceps to continue removing orbital fat to reveal and identify the following **(Figure 23-3A)**:

  - **Superior rectus m.** — directly inferior to the levator palpebrae superioris m.; attacks superiorly on the sclera
    - With a scalpel or scissors, cut the superior rectus m. close to the eyeball; reflect the cut muscle posteriorly
  - **Superior oblique m.** — medial to the superior rectus m.; trace anteriorly to the **trochlea**, where the tendon bends at a sharp angle around the trochlea to attach to the lateral, posterior surface of the sclera
  - **Medial rectus m.** — between the superior oblique and superior rectus mm.; also slightly inferior to the superior oblique m.; attaches medially on the sclera
  - **Lateral rectus m.** — lateral to the superior rectus m.; attaches laterally on the sclera

- Identify the following nerves around the optic n. (see Figure 23-3B):

  - **Abducens n. (CN V-1)** — enters the deep surface of the lateral rectus m.
  - **Superior division of the oculomotor n. (CN III)** — enters the deep surface of the levator palpebrae and superior rectus mm.
  - **Inferior division of the oculomotor n. (CN III)** — supplies the medial rectus, inferior rectus, and inferior oblique mm.
    - **Ciliary ganglion** — a parasympathetic ganglion (preganglionic fibers from CN V-3) approximately 1–2 mm in diameter; located posteriorly in the orbit, between the optic n. and the lateral rectus m.; may be difficult to find
    - **Short ciliary n., a., and v.** — postganglionic parasympathetic nerves that arise (synapse) in the ciliary ganglion and course to the posterior region of the eyeball
  - **Optic n. (CN II)** — deep to the superior rectus m.; the central a. of the retina is located within the optic n.; you may cut the optic n. in cross section to reveal this artery

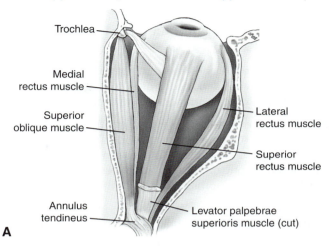
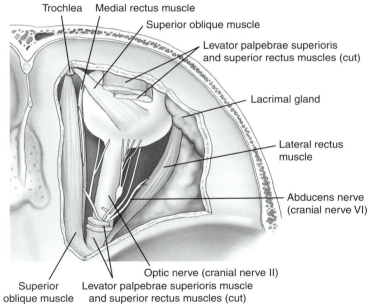

Figure 23-3 Intermediate view of the right orbital contents. **A,** Superior view (superficial). **B,** Superior view (deep)

Superior Approach Continued

Superior Approach—cont'd

■ Use forceps to reveal and identify the following (**Figures 23-4** and **23-5**):

- **Nasociliary n.** — courses between the optic n. and superior rectus m. in an anterior and medial direction; at the trochlea, the nasociliary n. exits the orbit as the infratrochlear n.

- **Ophthalmic a.** — enters the orbit via the optic canal, inferolateral to the optic n.; crosses the optic n. (accompanied by the nasociliary n.) between the superior rectus m. and the optic n.; terminal branches are the supratrochlear and supraorbital aa. and central artery of the retina

- **Ophthalmic v.** — the superior branch crosses over and the inferior branch crosses under the optic n., and both terminate in the cavernous sinus

■ Identify the following branches of the nasociliary n. and ophthalmic a. and v.:

- **Anterior ethmoidal n.** — traverses the anterior ethmoidal foramen; exits the nasal cavity as the external nasal n.

- **Posterior ethmoidal n., a.,** and **v.** — exit the orbit by the posterior ethmoidal foramen

- **Long ciliary n., a.,** and **v.** — two or three long ciliary nn. branch from the nasociliary n. as it crosses the optic n., accompanied by branches of the ophthalmic a. and v.

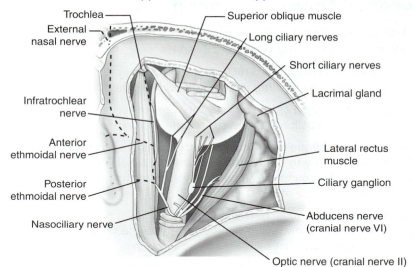

Figure 23-4 Deeper view of the right orbital contents

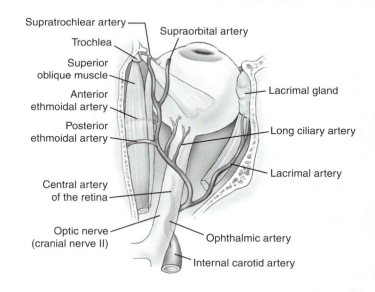

Figure 23-5 Superior view of the right ophthalmic artery

Anterior (Surgical) Approach

- To facilitate this dissection, use a scalpel to remove the upper and lower eyelids and the orbital septum (alternatively, you may use a scalpel to cut horizontally through the upper and lower eyelids)

- Identify the following structures in the anterior approach on the right orbit **(Figure 23-6)**:
  - **Lacrimal gland** — superior and lateral to the eyeball
  - **Trochlea** — superior and medial to the eyeball; attached to the internal surface of the bony orbit; the tendon of the superior oblique m. passes through the trochlea
  - **Inferior oblique m.** — inferior and medial to the eyeball; attaches inferiorly on the sclera

- Observe (do not cut) the insertions of the four recti mm. and two oblique mm. on the sclera of the eyeball
  - **Superior rectus m.**
  - **Superior oblique m.**
  - **Medial rectus m.**
  - **Lateral rectus m.**
  - **Inferior rectus m.**
  - **Inferior oblique m.**

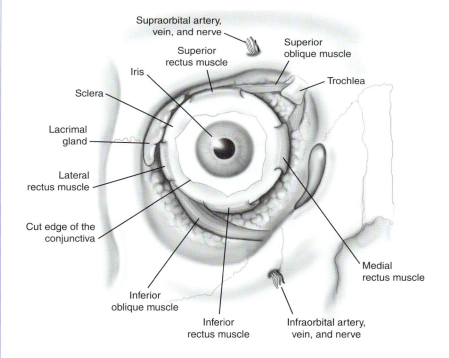

Figure 23-6 Facial/surgical approach to the right orbit

Dissection of the Eyeball In Situ (Right Eye Only)

- If you would like to examine the interior of the eyeball, use a scalpel to make a horizontal incision through the eyeball, along its anterior surface **(Figure 23-7)**

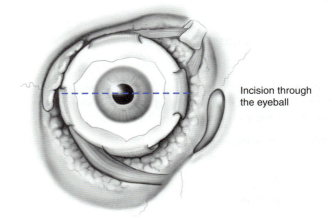

Figure 23-7 Horizontal incision across the right eyeball

Dissection of the Eyeball In Situ (Right Eye Only)—cont'd

■ Identify the following **(Figure 23-8)**:

- **Sclera** — the white, external tunic; continuous with the cornea
- **Iris** — pigmented drape superficial to the lens
- **Lens** — a transparent, flexible, biconvex, refractive structure located posterior to the iris and anterior to the vitreous humor
- **Choroid** — the dark-colored, middle tunic of the eyeball; blood vessels and ciliary nn. are contained in this layer
  - **Ciliary body** — the anterior termination of the choroid; has protrusions on its internal surface called ciliary processes
  - **Zonular fibers** — attach the lens to the ciliary processes
- **Retina** — internal tunic of the eyeball; in a hydrated eye, this layer is wispy and pinkish in color
  - When you cut open the eye, loss of vitreous pressure may result in detachment of the retina
- **Chambers**
  - **Anterior chamber** — anterior to the lens; located between the cornea and iris; contains aqueous humor; continuous with the posterior chamber at the pupil
  - **Posterior chamber** — anterior to the lens; located between the iris and the lens; contains aqueous humor
- **Vitreous body** — posterior to the lens; contains vitreous humor

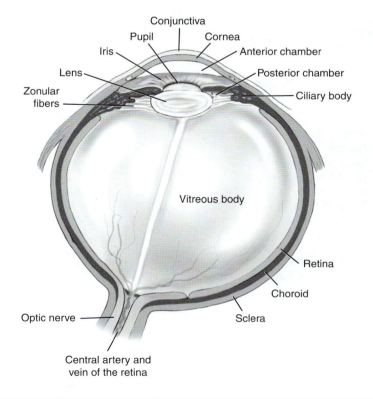

Figure 23-8 Cross-section of the right eyeball

Lab 24

Superficial Face

Prior to dissection, you should familiarize yourself with the following structures:

MUSCLES
- Muscles of facial expression
  - Frontalis m.
  - Orbicularis oculi m.
  - Corrugator supercilii m.
  - Nasalis m.
  - Procerus m.
  - Levator labii superioris alaeque nasi m.
  - Levator labii superioris m.
  - Levator anguli oris m.
  - Zygomaticus major and minor mm.
  - Orbicularis oris m.
  - Risorius m.
  - Depressor anguli oris m.
  - Depressor labii inferioris m.
  - Mentalis m.
  - Buccinator m.
  - Platysma m.
- Muscles of mastication
  - Temporalis m.
  - Masseter m.
  - Medial and lateral pterygoid mm.
- Prevertebral muscles
  - Scalene mm. (anterior, middle, and posterior)
  - Longus capitis and colli mm.
  - Rectus capitis anterior m.
  - Rectus capitis lateralis m.

LIGAMENTS
- Cruciate ligament
  - Superior longitudinal ligament
  - Inferior longitudinal ligament
  - Transverse ligament of the atlas
- Alar ligaments

NERVES
- Sympathetic trunk
  - Superior, middle, and inferior cervical ganglia
- Trigeminal n. (CN V)
  - V-1 — ophthalmic division
    - Supraorbital n.
    - Supratrochlear n.
    - Infratrochlear n.
    - Lacrimal n.
    - External nasal n.
  - V-2 — maxillary division
    - Infraorbital n.
    - Zygomaticofacial n.
    - Zygomaticotemporal n.
  - V-3 — mandibular division
    - Auriculotemporal n.
    - Buccal n.
    - Mental n.
- Facial n. (CN VII)
  - Posterior auricular n.
  - Temporal branch
  - Zygomatic branch
  - Buccal branch
  - Mandibular branch
  - Cervical branch

FASCIA
- Prevertebral fascia
  - Anterior layer (alar part)
    - Retropharyngeal space (danger space)
  - Posterior layer
- Buccopharyngeal fascia

OSTEOLOGY
- Atlas (C1)
- Axis (C2)
  - Odontoid process (dens)
- Pharyngeal tubercle
- Stylomastoid foramen
- Frontal bone
  - Supraorbital margin
  - Supraorbital foramen (notch)
- Maxilla
  - Infraorbital foramen
- Nasal bone
- Lacrimal bone
- Mandible
  - Ramus, neck, and body
  - Mental and mandibular foramina
  - Coronoid and condyloid processes

ARTERIES
- External carotid a.
  - Facial a.
    - Inferior and superior labial aa.
  - Superficial temporal a.
- Transverse facial a.

VEINS
- Internal jugular v.
  - Facial v.
    - Superior and inferior labial vv.
  - Retromandibular v.
    - Superficial temporal v.
    - Transverse facial v.

PAROTID REGION
- Parotid gland, duct, and fascia
- Buccal fat pad

Lab 24 Dissection Overview

The purpose of this laboratory session is to remove the skull from the vertebral column in order to bisect the head. This will improve the field of dissection for the face and internal structures, as well as the superficial aspect of the face. You will perform this laboratory through the following suggested sequence:

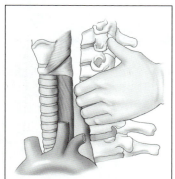

1. To remove the skull from the vertebral column, use your fingers to separate the vertebrae from the visceral compartment of the neck.

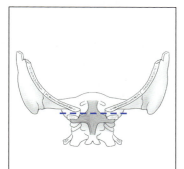

2. Cut all attachments from the vertebral area to the base of the skull using a scalpel.

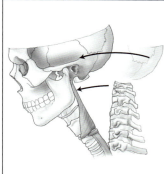

3. Reflect the skull anteriorly from the vertebral column.

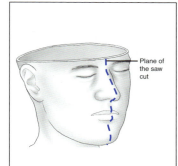

4. Bisect the head midsagittally, from the base of the skull through the mandible, but sparing the larynx.

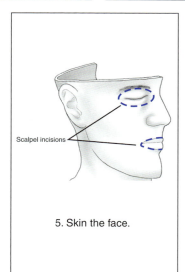

5. Skin the face.

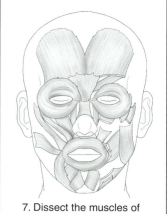

6. Dissect and identify the parotid gland, branches of the facial artery and vein, as well as the cranial nerves (CN V general sensory and CN VII muscles of facial expression).

7. Dissect the muscles of facial expression.

Table 24-1 Muscles of Facial Expression

Muscle	Attachments		Action	Innervation
Frontal belly of the occipitofrontalis	Epicranial aponeurosis	Skin of the forehead and eyebrows	Elevates the eyebrows and the skin of the forehead	Facial n. (CN VII)
Procerus	Nasal bone and nasal cartilage	Skin between the eyebrows	Wrinkles the skin over the bridge of the nose	
Corrugator supercilii	Medial region of the supraorbital margin	Skin of the medial half of the eyebrow	Draws the eyebrows downward and medial	
Orbicularis oculi	Frontal and maxillary bones around the orbit	Superficial fascia of the eyelid	Closes the eyelid; acts as sphincter of the eyelids	
Zygomaticus major and minor	Zygomatic arch	Angle of the mouth	Elevate lateral corners of the mouth	
Risorius	Superficial fascia overlying the masseter m.	Angle of the mouth	Draws the corners of the lip laterally	
Levator labii superioris	Frontal process of the maxilla, infraorbital region, and zygomatic bone	Skin of the upper lip	Elevates the lip, dilates the nostril, and elevates the angle of the mouth	
Levator labii superioris alaeque nasi	Maxilla inferior to the infraorbital foramen	Alar cartilage of the nose and upper lip	Elevates the nostrils and lip	
Depressor labii inferioris	Mandible between the symphysis and the mental foramen	Into the orbicularis oris and skin of the lower lip	Depresses the lower lip	
Depressor anguli oris	Oblique line of the mandible	Angle of the mouth	Turns the corner of the mouth downward	
Orbicularis oris	Surrounds the oral orifice, forming intrinsic muscles of the lips; interlaces with other muscles associated with the lips		Closes and protrudes the lips (pursing action)	
Mentalis	Incisive fossa of the mandible	Skin of the chin	Protrudes the inferior lip; wrinkles the chin	
Buccinator	Pterygomandibular raphe, alveolar processes of the jaw	Angle of the mouth	Compresses the cheek (whistling, blowing, and sucking)	
Platysma	Superficial fascia of the pectoral and deltoid regions	Mandible, skin of the neck and cheek, angle of the mouth, and orbicularis oris	Depresses the mandible; tenses the skin of the neck	

Table 24-2 Muscles of Mastication

Muscle	Attachments		Action	Innervation
Masseter	Inferior border and deep surface of the zygomatic arch	Lateral surface of the ramus of the mandible	Elevates the mandible	Trigeminal n. (CN V-3)
Temporalis	Temporal fossa and temporal fascia	Coronoid process and anterior border of the ramus of the mandible via a tendon that passes deep to the zygomatic arch	Elevates and retracts the mandible; maintains the position of the mandible at rest	
Medial pterygoid	Medial surface of the lateral pterygoid plate of the sphenoid bone	Medial surface of the ramus of the mandible between the mandibular foramen and the angle	Elevates and protracts the mandible; draws the mandible toward the opposite side	
Lateral pterygoid	Lateral surface of the lateral pterygoid plate of the sphenoid bone	Neck of the mandible and capsule of the temporomandibular joint	Protracts and depresses the mandible; draws the mandible toward the opposite side	

Table 24-3 Muscles of Prevertebral Region

Muscle	Attachments		Action	Innervation
Scalene muscle group				
• Anterior scalene	Transverse processes of C4–C6 vertebrae	Rib 1	Bilaterally: stabilize the neck Unilaterally: flex the neck laterally	Cervical plexus and ventral rami of C4–C6 spinal nerves
• Middle scalene	Posterior tubercles of the transverse processes of C4–C6 vertebrae	Superior surface of rib 1		Ventral rami of cervical spinal nerves
• Posterior scalene		External border of rib 2		Ventral rami of C7–C8 spinal nerves
Longus capitis	Transverse processes of C3–C6 vertebrae	Basilar portion of the occipital bone	Flexes and rotates the head	Ventral rami of C1–C3 spinal nerves
Longus colli	Transverse processes and bodies of C3–T3 vertebrae	Anterior tubercle of C1 (atlas), vertebral bodies of C2–C4, and transverse processes of C5–C6 vertebrae	Flexes the neck and rotates to the opposite side if acting unilaterally	Ventral rami of C2–C6 spinal nerves
Rectus capitis lateralis	Transverse processes of C1 vertebra (atlas)	Jugular process of the occipital bone	Flexes and stabilizes the head	Ventral rami of C1–C2 spinal nerves
Rectus capitis anterior	Lateral mass of C1 vertebra (atlas)	Basilar portion of the occipital bone anterior to the occipital condyles	Flexes and rotates the head	

Special Dissection Instructions — Bisection of the Head and Neck

- To preserve the triangles of the cervical region for study and review, the instructions on this page are recommended to be followed by every fourth or fifth dissection group; ask for instructions from your laboratory staff

- This dissection is performed to save the cervical triangles and maintain structural continuity among the thorax, neck, and head

- Laboratory staff will help select which cadaver heads will be bisected based on the integrity of the previous dissections

- If you are not instructed to bisect the head and neck, proceed to the next page

- Follow these instructions to bisect the head **(Figure 24-1)**:
  - A member of the laboratory staff will bisect the head, neck, and thorax in a sagittal plane, using a band saw or the equivalent
    - *Note:* If your laboratory is not equipped with a band saw, follow directions from your laboratory staff
    - The intention is to bisect the head, midsagittally, from the base of the skull through the mandible, but sparing the larynx

- Proceed to the page entitled **Superficial Face** to continue your dissection

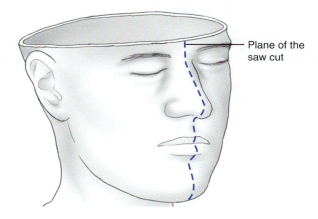

Figure 24-1 Special dissection instructions

Dissection of the Craniovertebral Joints

- Place the cadaver prone and peel the dura mater from the basioccipital region and underlying tectorial membrane; reflect the flap of dura to reveal the tectorial membrane

- Identify the following structures deep to the dura mater:

  - **Tectorial membrane** — this strong, longitudinally oriented band within the vertebral canal is the superior continuation of the posterior longitudinal ligament **(Figure 24-2A)**

    - The dura mater and tectorial membrane may be fused, in which case both may have been peeled away

    - Use a scalpel to cut the tectorial membrane transversely above the anterior border of the foramen magnum; reflect the membrane inferiorly

- At this point, the major ligaments of the craniovertebral region are exposed (these ligaments may manifest as thickenings of a continuous sheath):

  - **Cruciate ligament** — receives its name because the cruciate ligament looks like a cross; composed of the following (see Figure 24-2B):

    - **Transverse ligament of C1 (atlas)** — attaches to the medial surface of C1 vertebra on both sides

      - The ligament has a superior longitudinal band that extends to the basilar part of the occipital bone and an inferior longitudinal band that extends to the body of C2 vertebra

    - **Alar ligaments** — extend from the sides of the dens to the occipital condyles; immediately superior to the transverse ligament

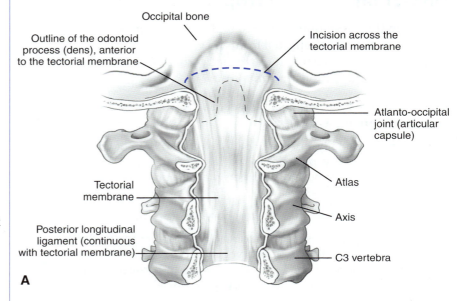

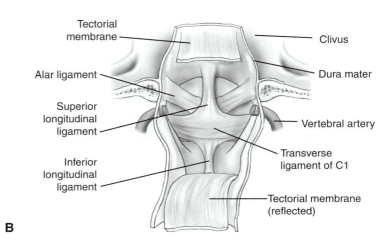

Figure 24-2 Craniovertebral joints. **A,** Internal view of the skull base: tectorial membrane incision. **B,** Internal view of the skull base: tectorial membrane reflected

Dissection of the Retropharyngeal Space

- During this dissection, the head and visceral compartment of the neck will be reflected from the vertebral column; the visceral compartment of the neck will remain attached to the superior mediastinum

- Follow these instructions to dissect the retropharyngeal space **(Figure 24-3)**:

  - Starting inferiorly, insert a finger or two from both of your hands bilaterally, posterior to the carotid sheaths, trachea, and esophagus; push your fingers medially until they meet posterior to the cervical viscera
    - Your fingers are in the **retropharyngeal space**

  - Work your fingers superiorly to reach the base of the skull (superior limit of the retropharyngeal space) and inferiorly to about the level of the T3 vertebra (where the **prevertebral fascia** fuses with the **buccopharyngeal fascia**)

  - Do not damage branches of the subclavian a. at the root of the neck

  - Attempt to leave the cervical sympathetic chains on the prevertebral muscular compartment; look for the cervical sympathetic chain in this compartment
    - If you do not find the cervical sympathetic chains, examine the posterior surface of the reflected cervical viscera
    - If the cervical sympathetic chains are attached to the posterior surface of the reflected cervical viscera, use forceps to dissect the chains from the cervical viscera

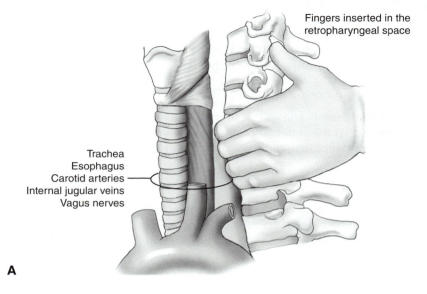

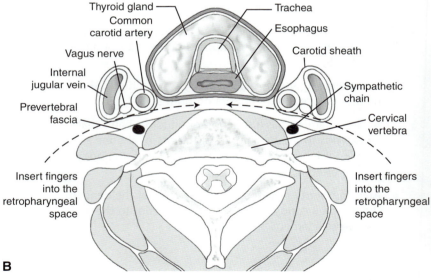

Figure 24-3 Fingers in the retropharyngeal space. **A,** Lateral view. **B,** Cross-section through the thyroid gland

Removal of the Head and Neck Viscera from the Vertebral Column

- *Note:* Do *not* decapitate the cadaver; your goal is to reflect the head and cervical viscera *together* from the vertebral column; in other words, the head will remain attached to the trachea and esophagus (cervical viscera)

- Reflect the head and neck in two steps:

  - **Transection of the tissue between C1 vertebra and the occipital bone**

    - Use a scalpel to circumscribe inferior to the foramen magnum, between C1 vertebra and the occipital bone; cut all tissue attachments; *use caution* to avoid cutting CN IX–XII and the internal jugular vv. as you do so (**Figure 24-4A** and **24-4B**)

    - Continue pulling the cervical viscera anteriorly to cut between the transverse processes of C1 vertebra and the occipital bone, severing the **rectus capitis lateralis mm.** bilaterally (see Figure 24-4A)

    - Carry the scalpel incision medially, cutting the **rectus capitis anterior** and **longus capitis mm.** (see Figure 24-4B)

    - Use a hammer and chisel to pry the base of the skull away from the C1 vertebra; cut remaining attachments with a scalpel (see Figure 24-4C); proceed with caution; you may need to approach your scalpel cuts from many angles

  - **Reflection of the head and cervical viscera from the vertebral column**

    - Place your fingers superiorly into the already defined retropharyngeal space

    - Pull the head and cervical viscera, vessels, and nerves anterior; use blunt dissection and a scalpel to cut the remaining attachments (prevertebral and erector spinae mm.) (see Figure 24-4D)

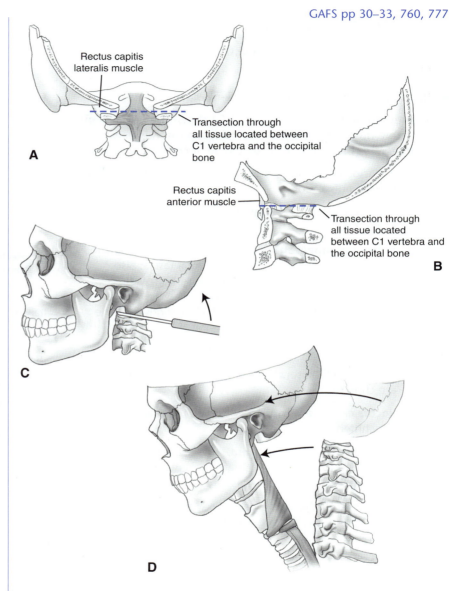

Figure 24-4 Removal of the head from the vertebral column. **A,** Posterior view. **B,** Lateral view. **C,** Reflection of the skull from C1. **D,** Reflection of the head and neck viscera from the vertebral column

Prevertebral Region

- Examine the prevertebral fascia that covers the prevertebral muscles

- Identify the following **(Figure 24-5A)**:

  - **Prevertebral fascia** — Figure 24-5A shows the fascial planes before dissection; the prevertebral fascia extends between transverse processes of the vertebrae; it consists of two layers

    - **Anterior layer (alar part)** — destroyed during previous dissection

    - **Posterior layer** — contiguous with the prevertebral fascia, bilaterally

    - **Retropharyngeal space** — space between the anterior and posterior layers of the prevertebral fascia; also known as the "danger space" because it provides a potential passageway for infection in the cervical region to spread from the base of the skull inferiorly into the posterior mediastinum

  - **Prevertebral muscles** (see Figure 24-5B):

    - **Rectus capitis lateralis m.** — locate the severed distal attachment

    - **Rectus capitis anterior m.** — locate the severed distal attachment

    - **Longus colli and capitis mm.** — attach along the cervical and superior thoracic vertebrae; the superior attachment of the longus capitis m. is severed

    - **Anterior, middle, and posterior scalene mm.** — attach to the transverse processes of the cervical vertebrae

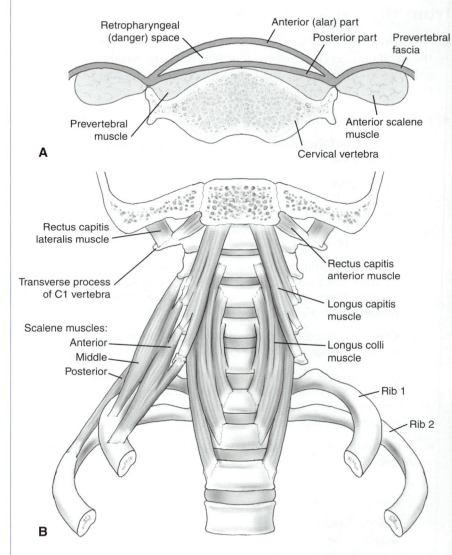

Figure 24-5 Prevertebral structures. **A**, Cross-section. **B**, Coronal section through the temporal bone with the cervical viscera removed

Superficial Face

- Those who did not bisect the head and neck of their cadaver will bisect the head only to facilitate the following:
  - Dissection of both sides of the superficial face (this laboratory session)
  - Dissection of both sides of the deep face (another laboratory session)

- Bisection allows both sides of the face to be dissected simultaneously

- Follow these instructions to bisect the head **(Figure 24-6)**:
  - Laboratory staff will bisect the head from the base of the skull through the mandible (*not* through the neck)
    - If your laboratory is not equipped with a band saw, follow the instructions of your laboratory staff
    - The intention is to bisect the head, midsagittally, from the base of the skull through the mandible, but spare the larynx
  - This approach preserves the pharyngeal constrictor muscles and larynx

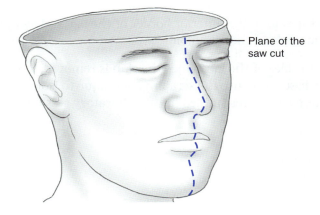

Figure 24-6   Saw cut through the face

Skin Removal from the Face

- Use a new scalpel blade to make the skin incisions shown in **Figure 24-7** to remove the skin of the face
  - Leave the mucous membrane on the lips and the skin attached to the eyelids and nostrils

- Remove *only* the skin because the muscles of the face (muscles of facial expression) attach to the skin, and the nerves and vessels are immediately deep to the skin

- View the cut edge of the skin along the saw line to gauge the skin's thickness

- Reflect the skin to the anterior border of the ear and away from the angle of the mandible

- Skin both sides of the face; once the skin is removed, bluntly dissect and use the scraping technique to isolate the remaining structures studied in this laboratory session

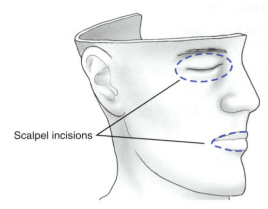

Figure 24-7 Incisions of the facial skin

Trigeminal Nerve (CN V)

- Identify the three foramina on a dry skull (aligned vertically) through which peripheral branches of CN V emerge:
  - **Supraorbital, infraorbital, and mental foramina**

- Use forceps to reveal and identify the cutaneous divisions of **CN V-1**; locate the nerves shown in **Figure 24-8**; trace the nerves back to the skull to locate their foramina:
  - **Supraorbital n.** — originates from the frontal n.; exits the skull through the supraorbital foramen (use a dry skull to orientate); locate the supraorbital foramen on the cadaver's skull by separating the fibers of the corrugator supercilii m. and orbicularis oculi m.
  - **Supratrochlear n.** — also originates from the frontal n.; emerges deep to the corrugator supercilii and frontalis mm. and usually pierces the orbicularis oculi m. to supply the skin of the inferior part of the forehead, near the midline
  - **Infratrochlear n.** — originates from the nasociliary n.; exits the orbit inferior to the trochlea and pierces the orbicularis oculi m. to supply the skin of the eyelids and side of the nose
  - **Lacrimal and external nasal nn.** — usually too small to identify

- Vessels that share the same name as the nerve (i.e., supraorbital n., a., and v.) accompany each of these nerves

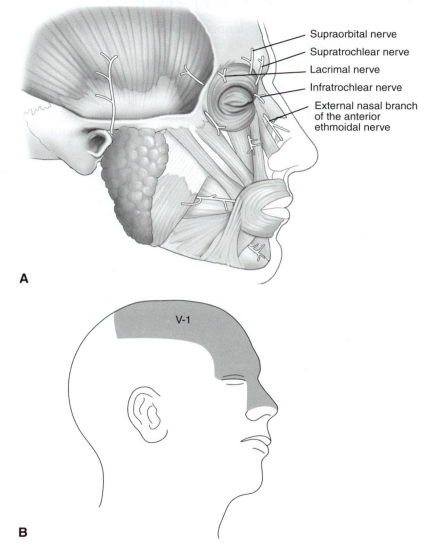

Figure 24-8 Lateral view of the cutaneous distribution of CN V-1. **A,** Cutaneous nerves of V-1. **B,** Cutaneous field for CN V-1

Trigeminal Nerve (CN V) Continued

Trigeminal Nerve (CN V)—cont'd

- Use forceps to reveal and identify the cutaneous divisions of **CN V-2**; locate the nerves shown in **Figure 24-9**; trace the nerves back to the skull to locate their foramina:

  - **Infraorbital n.** — locate the nerve by separating the levator labii superioris m. (superficial) from the levator anguli oris m. (deep); exits the skull through the infraorbital foramen (use a dry skull to orientate); locate the infraorbital foramen on the cadaver's skull by separating muscle fibers

  - **Zygomaticofacial n.** — originates from the zygomatico-orbital n.; exits the skull through the zygomaticofacial foramen (use a dry skull to orientate); pierces the orbicularis oculi m. to supply the skin over the cheek (may be hard to find)

  - **Zygomaticotemporal n.** — also originates from the zygomatico-orbital n.; exits the skull through the zygomaticotemporal foramen (use a dry skull to orientate); pierces the temporal fascia less than 3 cm above the zygomatic arch to supply the skin of the temple (may be hard to find)

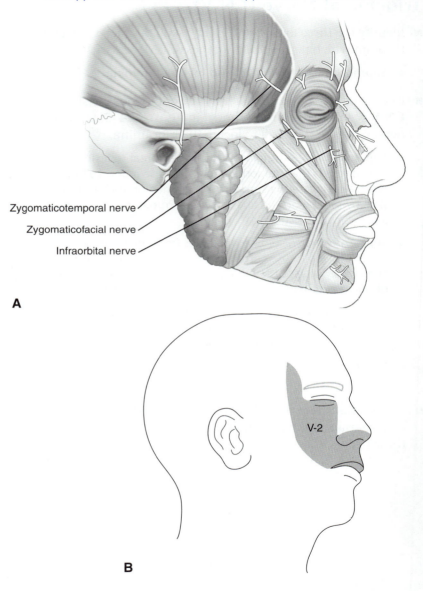

Figure 24-9 Lateral view of the cutaneous distribution of CN V-2. **A,** Cutaneous nerves of V-2. **B,** Cutaneous field for CN V-2

Trigeminal Nerve (CN V)—cont'd

- Use forceps to reveal and identify the cutaneous divisions of **CN V-3**; locate the nerves shown in **Figure 24-10**; trace the nerves back to the skull to locate their foramina:

  - **Auriculotemporal n.** — emerges posterior and inferior to the temporomandibular joint and ascends posterior to the superficial temporal vessels

  - **Buccal n.** — emerges anterior to the masseter m. to supply the skin superficial, and the mucous membrane deep, to the buccinator m.; courses between the two bellies of the lateral pterygoid m. and descends deep to the temporalis tendon; passes deep to the masseter m.

  - **Mental n.** — originates from the inferior alveolar n.; exits the mandible via the mental foramen (use a dry skull to orientate); locate by separating the fibers of the mentalis m. from the depressor anguli oris m.

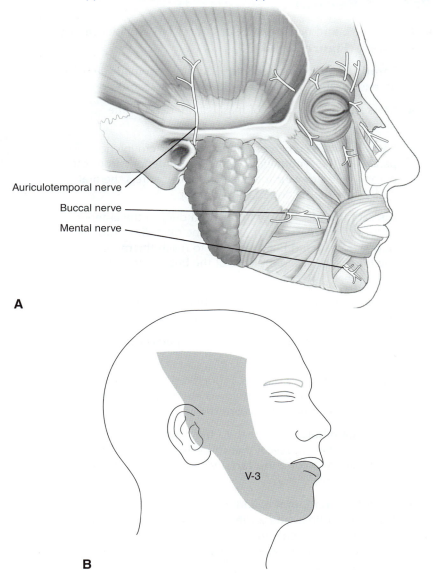

Figure 24-10 Lateral view of the cutaneous distribution of CN V-3. **A,** Cutaneous nerves of V-3. **B,** Cutaneous field for CN V-3

Parotid Region

- Use forceps, and perhaps scissors, to reveal and identify the following **(Figure 24-11)**:

  - **Parotid gland** — located inferior to the zygomatic arch and anterior to the ear; invested within a dense capsule

  - **Masseter m.** — muscle of mastication; deep to the parotid gland

  - **Parotid duct** — emerges approximately 3 cm inferior and parallel to the zygomatic arch; courses anteriorly from the parotid gland toward the cheek (mouth); enters the oral cavity near the second maxillary molar

  - **Buccal fat pad** — follow the parotid duct to the anterior border of the masseter m., where the duct dives into the buccal fat pad and buccinator m. to reach the mouth; use forceps to pick out pieces of the buccal fat pad until it is gone

  - **Buccinator m.** — removal of the buccal fat pad exposes the buccinator m., which is pierced by the parotid duct

  - **Transverse facial a. and v.** — located parallel and superior to the parotid duct

  - **Facial a. and v.** — both cross superficial to the mandible (at the anterior border of the masseter m.) and course medially and superiorly toward the angle of the eye

  - **Retromandibular v.** — deep to the parotid gland and inferior to the ear; reveal that this vein unites with the **facial v.**, forming the **common facial v.** (a tributary to the internal jugular v.); not shown

  - **Superficial temporal a. and v.** — a terminal branch of the external carotid a. and a tributary to the retromandibular v., respectively; located anterior to the ear; they course superficially over the temporalis m.

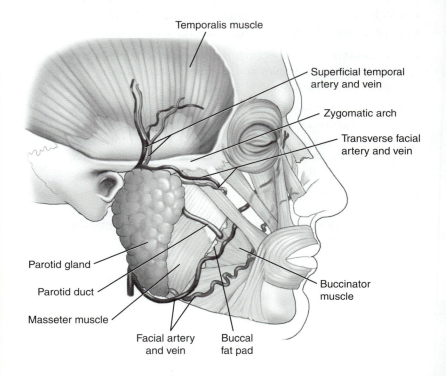

Figure 24-11 Parotid region and facial vasculature

Facial Nerve in the Parotid Region

- To identify the branches of the facial n., follow these instructions; use forceps, and perhaps scissors, to dissect parallel to the course of the nerves shown in **Figure 24-12**:

  - Look for white, flattened branches of the facial n. that emerge through the substance of (or deep to) the parotid gland; follow the branches through the parotid gland toward the stylomastoid foramen

  - To reveal the nerves, you will have to remove the parotid gland, piece by piece, especially to reveal the course of the facial n. (CN VII) from the stylomastoid foramen

  - The branches of the **facial n.** are named for the region that they innervate (may be several branches to each region):
    - **Temporal branches**
    - **Zygomatic branches**
    - **Buccal branches**
    - **Mandibular branches**
    - **Cervical branches**

  - **Posterior auricular n.** — attempt to identify this nerve where it courses along the posterior border of the ear

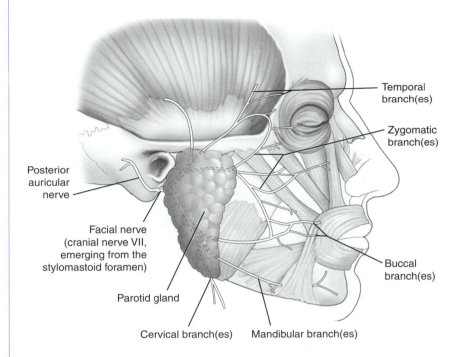

Figure 24-12 Branches of the facial nerve

Muscles of Facial Expression

- Identify the muscles of facial expression **(Figure 24-13)**:
  - **Frontal belly of the occipitofrontalis m. (1)**
  - **Auricular mm.** — anterior, superior, and posterior bellies (not illustrated)
  - **Corrugator supercilii m. (2)**
  - **Orbicularis oculi m. (3)**
  - **Nasalis m. (4)**
  - **Procerus m. (5)**
  - **Risorius m. (6)**
  - **Zygomaticus major m. (7)**
  - **Zygomaticus minor m. (8)**
  - **Levator labii superioris alaeque nasi m. (9)**
  - **Orbicularis oris m. (10)**
  - **Levator labii superioris m. (11)**
  - **Levator anguli oris m. (12)**
  - **Depressor anguli oris m. (13)**
  - **Depressor labii inferioris m. (14)**
  - **Mentalis m. (15)**
  - **Buccinator m. (16)** — deep to the buccal fat pad
  - **Platysma m.** — extends from the inferior border of the mandible inferiorly over the clavicles (not illustrated)

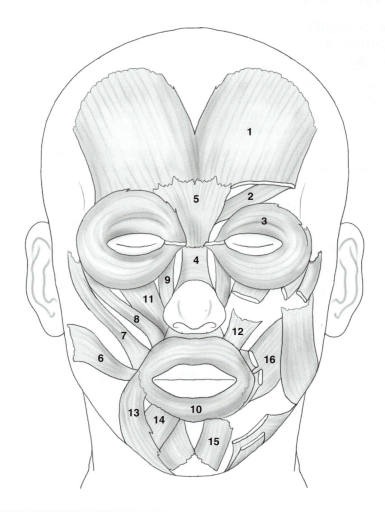

Figure 24-13 Muscles of facial expression

Muscles of Mastication

- Identify two of the four muscles of mastication **(Figure 24-14)**:

  - **Masseter m.** — attached to the zygomatic arch and external surface of the ramus of the mandible

  - **Temporalis m.** — attached within the temporal fossa; courses deep to the zygomatic arch; inserts on the coronoid process of the mandible

  - **Medial pterygoid m.** — deep to the mandible; will be dissected in another laboratory session

  - **Lateral pterygoid m.** — deep to the mandible; will be dissected in another laboratory session

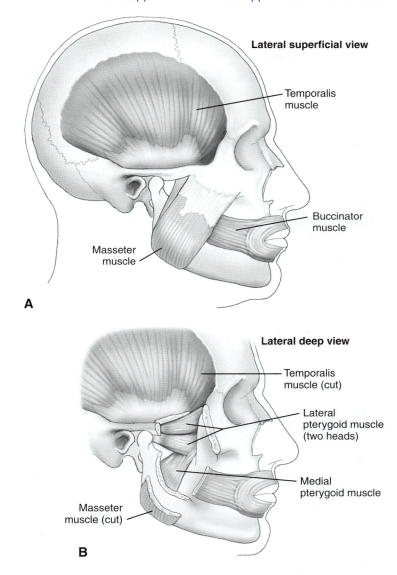

Figure 24-14 Muscles of mastication. **A,** Lateral superficial view. **B,** Lateral deep view for reference only (do not dissect these muscles at this time)

Lab 25

Deep Face and Pharynx

Prior to dissection, you should familiarize yourself with the following structures:

OSTEOLOGY
- Hyoid bone
  - Greater horns
  - Lesser horns
- Zygomatic bone and arch
- Temporal bone
  - Mastoid process
  - Styloid process
- Mandible
  - Ramus, body, and neck
  - Lingula
  - Coronoid and condylar processes
  - Mandibular notch
  - Mandibular foramen
  - Mylohyoid line
- Sphenoid bone
  - Lateral and medial pterygoid plates
    - Pterygoid hamulus
    - Pterygoid canal
- Maxilla
  - Palatine process
- Palatine bone
  - Perpendicular plate
  - Horizontal plate
- Occipital bone
  - Pharyngeal tubercle

INFRATEMPORAL FOSSA CONTENTS
- Muscles of mastication
  - Temporalis m.
  - Masseter m.
  - Medial pterygoid m.
  - Lateral pterygoid m.
- Pterygoid plexus of vv.
- Maxillary artery and branches
  - Maxillary a.
    - Middle meningeal a.
    - Deep temporal a.
    - Inferior alveolar a.
    - Posterior superior alveolar a.
    - Infraorbital a.
    - Muscular branches
    - Buccal a.
- Nerves
  - Trigeminal n.
    - CN V-2
      - Posterior superior alveolar n.
    - CN V-3
      - Inferior alveolar n.
      - Mylohyoid n.
      - Lingual n.
      - Buccal n.
      - Auriculotemporal n.
  - Facial n. (CN VII)
    - Chorda tympani n.
  - Glossopharyngeal n. (CN IX)
    - Otic ganglion
  - Vagus n. (CN X)
    - Superior laryngeal n.
      - Internal laryngeal n.
      - External laryngeal n.
    - Recurrent laryngeal n.
  - Cervical ganglia (superior, middle, and inferior)

PHARYNX
- Pharyngeal mm.
  - Superior pharyngeal constrictor m.
  - Middle pharyngeal constrictor m.
  - Inferior pharyngeal constrictor m.
  - Stylopharyngeus m.
  - Salpingopharyngeus m.
  - Palatopharyngeus m.

NASOPHARYNX
- Auditory (Eustachian) tube
- Torus tubarius
- Salpingopharyngeal fold
- (Naso)pharyngeal tonsils (adenoids)

MISCELLANEOUS
- Pterygomaxillary fissure
  - Pterygoid fossa
- Thyroid cartilage
  - Oblique line
- Cricoid cartilage
- Pterygomandibular raphe
- Temporomandibular joint
  - Joint capsule
- Sphenomandibular ligament
- Petrotympanic fissure
- Stylohyoid ligament

Lab 25 Dissection Overview

The purpose of this laboratory session is to learn the anatomy of the infratemporal fossa, pharynx, and associated structures through dissection. You will do so through the following suggested sequence:

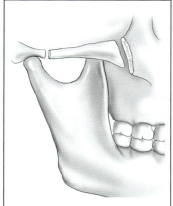

1. Using a bone saw, cut away the zygomatic arch.

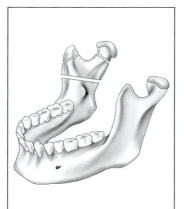

2. Using a bone saw, cut away the ramus of the mandible.

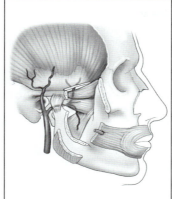

3. Dissect the superficial contents of the infratemporal fossa.

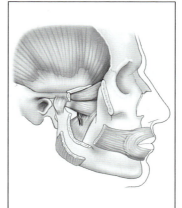

4. Remove the lateral pterygoid muscle in a piecemeal fashion.

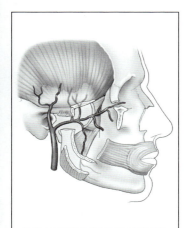

5. Dissect the deeper contents of the infratemporal fossa.

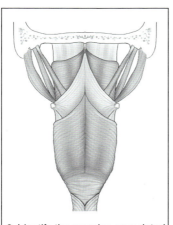

6. Identify the muscles associated with the pharynx from a posterior view.

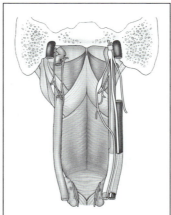

7. Dissect the nerves, arteries, and veins associated with the pharynx.

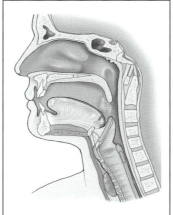

8. Dissect the structures associated with the nasopharynx and oropharynx.

Table 25-1 Muscles of Mastication

Muscle	Attachments		Action	Innervation
Masseter	Zygomatic arch and maxillary process of the zygomatic bone	Lateral surface of the ramus of the mandible	Elevates the mandible	Trigeminal n. (CN V-3)
Temporalis	Temporal fossa and temporal fascia	Coronoid process and anterior border of the ramus of the mandible via a tendon that passes deep to the zygomatic arch	Elevates and retracts the mandible	
Medial pterygoid	Deep head: medial surface of the lateral plate of the pterygoid process and pyramidal process of the palatine bone Superficial head: tuberosity and pyramidal process of the maxilla	Medial surface of the mandible near angle	Elevates the mandible and moves the mandible from side to side	
Lateral pterygoid	Upper head: roof of the infratemporal fossa Lower head: lateral surface of the lateral plate of the pterygoid process	Capsule of temporomandibular joint in the region of attachment to the articular disc and to the pterygoid fovea on the neck of the mandible	Protrudes and moves the mandible from side to side	

Table 25-2 Muscles of the Pharynx

Muscle	Attachments		Action	Innervation
Pharyngeal constrictor muscles				
• Superior constrictor	Pterygomandibular raphe and adjacent bone on the mandible and pterygoid hamulus	Pharyngeal tubercle and pharyngeal raphe	Constrict the pharynx	Vagus n. (CN X)
• Middle constrictor	Upper margin of the greater horn of the hyoid bone and adjacent margins of the lesser horn and stylohyoid ligament	Pharyngeal raphe		
• Inferior constrictor	Cricoid cartilage, oblique line of the thyroid cartilage, and a ligament that spans between these attachments and crosses the cricothyroid m.			
Palatopharyngeus	Upper surface of the palatine aponeurosis	Pharyngeal wall	Elevates the pharynx; closes the oropharyngeal isthmus	
Salpingopharyngeus	Inferior aspect of the pharyngeal end of the auditory tube		Elevates the pharynx	
Stylopharyngeus	Medial side of the base of the styloid process		Elevates the pharynx	Glossopharyngeal n. (CN IX)

Infratemporal Fossa — Overview

- Identify the following on a dry skull (**Figure 25-1A**):

  - **Infratemporal fossa** — an irregularly shaped space deep and inferior to the zygomatic arch and continuous with the temporal fossa; the fossa is located between these structures:

    - Lateral — deep surface of the **ramus of the mandible**
    - Medial — **lateral pterygoid plate of the sphenoid bone**
    - Anterior — posterior surface of the **maxilla**
    - Posterior — **temporomandibular joint (TMJ), carotid sheath,** and **styloid process**

- During this dissection, you will identify the following contents of the infratemporal fossa:

  - **Muscles of mastication**
    - Temporalis and medial and lateral pterygoid mm. (and the masseter m., which is superficial to the infratemporal fossa)

  - **Branches of the maxillary a.** (see Figure 25-4)
    - Middle meningeal, masseteric, inferior alveolar, deep temporal, posterior superior alveolar, sphenopalatine, infraorbital, buccal, and descending palatine aa.

  - **Nerves** (see Figure 25-1B)
    - Mandibular, inferior alveolar, lingual, buccal, deep temporal, masseteric, posterior superior alveolar, and chorda tympani nn.

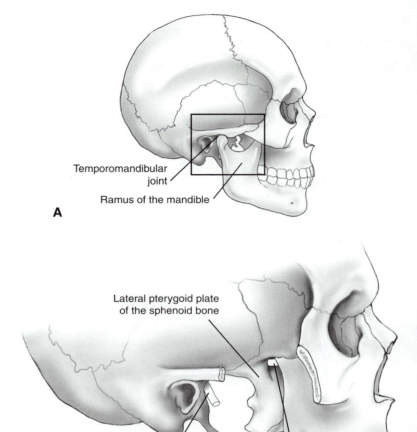

Figure 25-1 Infratemporal fossa. **A,** Lateral view. **B,** Lateral view close-up

Dissection of the Parotid Gland and Masseter Muscle

- Perform this dissection on the half of the head displaying the fewest muscles of facial expression and branches of the facial n.

- To access the infratemporal fossa, you must first remove the following:
  - Parotid gland
  - Masseter m.
  - Zygomatic arch
  - Ramus of the mandible

- To begin this dissection, follow these instructions:
  - **Remove the parotid gland** — use scissors to cut the parotid duct where it crosses the anterior border of the masseter m. and remove the gland (take care to preserve branches of the facial n. [CN VII]) **(Figure 25-2A)**
  - **Cut the masseter m.** — use a scalpel to cut along the inferior border of the zygomatic arch; use forceps to reflect the muscle inferiorly; preserve branches of the facial n. (CN VII)

- Identify the following (see Figure 25-2B):
  - **Masseteric n., a., and v.** — as you reflect the masseter m. inferiorly from the ramus of the mandible, look for the masseteric neurovascular bundle in the mandibular notch

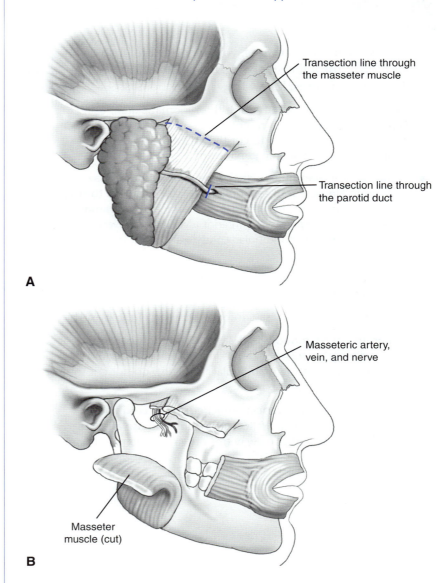

Figure 25-2 Dissection of the parotid gland and masseter muscle. **A,** Incisions. **B,** Reflection of the masseter muscle

Zygomatic Arch and Ramus of the Mandible

- *Before* you make any saw cuts, you may want to push a probe deep to the following bones to avoid cutting underlying structures; follow these instructions:

  - **Zygomatic arch** — saw through the zygomatic arch, using **Figure 25-3A** as a guide; remove the cut section of the arch; if necessary, use a scalpel to cut the attachments of the temporalis m. from the zygomatic arch

  - **Ramus of the mandible** — make the following three saw cuts, using Figure 25-3B as a guide; use sharp forceps to strip the periosteum from the inner (deep) surface of the ramus of the mandible to separate the inferior alveolar neurovascular structures from the mandibular condyle and neck to the mandibular foramen

    - **Neck of the mandibular condyle** — saw through this part of the mandible

    - **Coronoid process** — saw through this part of the mandible

    - **Ramus of the mandible** — saw through this part of the mandible; stay superior to the **lingula** of the mandible (a bony spike at the mandibular foramen); do not cut the inferior alveolar n., a., and v.

  - **Temporalis m.** — can remain attached to the coronoid process of the mandible; reflect superiorly and use a pin to hold the reflected muscle away from the dissection field

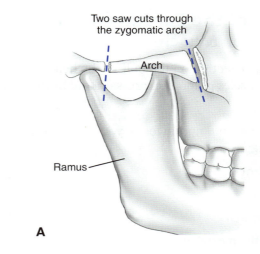

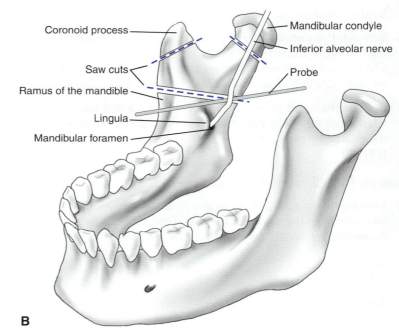

Figure 25-3 Instructions to reveal the infratemporal fossa. **A**, Removal of the zygomatic arch. **B**, Removal of the mandibular ramus

Infratemporal Fossa — Superficial Contents

- Use forceps to pick apart and remove the fat from the infratemporal fossa; this fat is continuous with the buccal fat pad; as you pick away the fat, note the **pterygoid plexus of vv.**, which will be broken

- Use forceps to reveal and identify the following (Figure 25-4):

  - **Lateral pterygoid m.** — oriented horizontally from the neck of the mandible to the lateral pterygoid plate; has two heads

  - **Medial pterygoid m.** — muscle fibers course parallel to the masseter m. on the internal surface of the ramus of the mandible; deep to the lateral pterygoid m. and oriented obliquely upward from the angle of the mandible to the lateral pterygoid plate

  - **Inferior alveolar n. (CN V-3), a., and v.** — emerge between the lateral and medial pterygoid mm.; use forceps to trace the neurovascular structures distally, where they enter the mandibular foramen

    - Trace the inferior alveolar n. proximally to the inferior border of the lateral pterygoid m.

  - **Sphenomandibular ligament** — courses from the spine of the sphenoid bone to the lingula of the mandible

  - **Lingual n. (CN V-3)** — courses anterior to the inferior alveolar n., then enters the oral cavity between the medial pterygoid m. and the ramus of the mandible

  - **Maxillary a.** — arises from the external carotid a., posterior to the neck of the mandible; crosses superficial or deep to the lateral pterygoid m. en route to the pterygopalatine fossa

    - **Deep temporal nn.** and **aa.** — branches of the maxillary a. that course deep to the temporalis m.

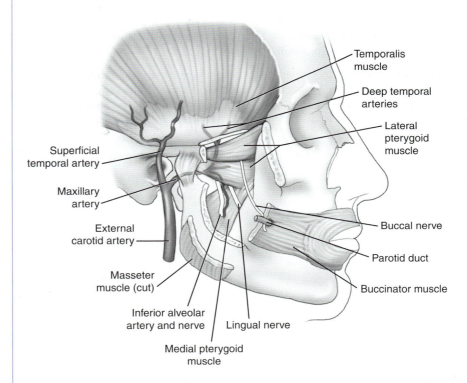

Figure 25-4 Lateral view of the infratemporal fossa for superficial dissection (only part of the mandibular ramus is shown removed)

Removal of the Lateral Pterygoid Muscle

- To obtain a complete view of the infratemporal region, the lateral pterygoid m. must be removed

- Follow these directions **(Figure 25-5)**:

  • Use forceps to separate the lateral pterygoid m. completely from the medial pterygoid m.; insert a probe between the lateral and medial pterygoid mm.

    • *Note:* The inferior alveolar and lingual nn. and vessels mark the plane of separation between the lateral and medial pterygoid mm.

  • Use forceps to pick apart and completely remove the lateral pterygoid m. in a piecemeal fashion; preserve the nerves, arteries, and veins that course around or through the lateral pterygoid m.

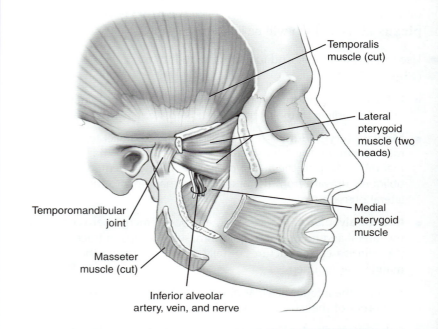

Figure 25-5 Lateral view of the removal of the lateral pterygoid muscle (only part of the mandibular ramus is shown removed)

Infratemporal Fossa — Deep Contents

- Use forceps to reveal and identify the following nerves and arteries **(Figure 25-6)**:

  - **Lingual n., a., and v.** — course to the tongue
  - **Inferior alveolar n., a., and v.** — course to the mandibular teeth
  - **Mylohyoid n.** — branch of the inferior alveolar n. to the mylohyoid m.; originates from the posterior surface of the inferior alveolar n.

- Trace the lingual and inferior alveolar nn. to the base of the skull; remove remaining remnants of the lateral pterygoid m. to reveal and identify the following:

  - **Chorda tympani n.** — a branch of CN VII; emerges from the petrotympanic fissure (medial to the temporomandibular joint); joins the lingual n. posteriorly
  - **Buccal n. (CN V-3)** and **buccal a.** — course anteriorly to pierce the buccinator m. to supply skin of the cheek (the buccal n. and a. may have been destroyed while removing the buccal fat pad)
  - **Auriculotemporal n. (CN V-3)** — characteristically splits and rejoins (forms a loop) around the middle meningeal a., at the base of the skull
  - **Middle meningeal a.** — branch of the maxillary a.; courses superiorly through the foramen spinosum; supplies the cranial dura mater
  - **Posterior superior alveolar n. (CN V-2)** and **a.** — enter the posterior surface of the maxilla
  - **Sphenopalatine** and **infraorbital aa.** — terminal branches of the maxillary a. (dissected in a future laboratory session)

- Branches of CN V-3 and the maxillary a. that may be destroyed or are too small to identify include **the anterior tympanic, deep auricular, muscular branches to the pterygoids,** and **accessory meningeal a.**

GAFS pp 882–886   ACGA pp 46–51   NAHA Plates 46, 54–55, 69–71

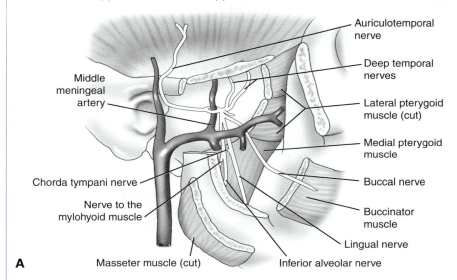

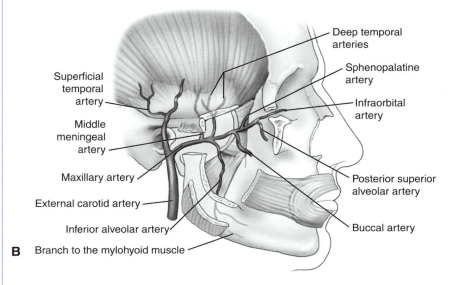

Figure 25-6 Lateral view of the infratemporal fossa deep dissection. **A,** Nerves. **B,** Arteries (mandibular condyle removed to provide a better view of infratemporal fossa contents)

Temporomandibular Joint

- Use a scalpel and forceps to reveal and identify the following:

  - **Joint capsule** — use a scalpel to cut away muscle remnants to reveal the fibrous capsule surrounding the temporomandibular joint; attaches to the articular area of the temporal bone and around the neck of the mandible **(Figure 25-7A)**

    - Use a scalpel to make a horizontal incision through the lateral surface of the joint capsule to reveal the internal structures

  - **Articular disc** — a fibrocartilaginous disc that divides the joint cavity into superior and inferior compartments; fused with the articular capsule surrounding the joint (see Figure 25-7B); use forceps to delineate the articular disc

- Review the following ligaments (see Figure 25-7A):

  - **Sphenomandibular ligament** — spans from the spine of the sphenoid bone to the lingula of the mandible (you may not see this)

  - **Stylomandibular ligament** — spans from the styloid process of the temporal bone to the internal surface of the mandible

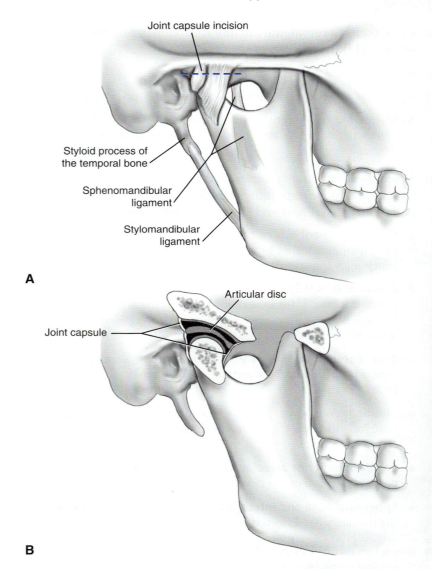

Figure 25-7 Lateral views of the temporomandibular joint. **A,** Superficial view. **B,** Deep view (mandible is shown intact)

Pharynx (Posterior Approach)

- Place the cadaver supine and pull the head and attached visceral compartment away from the vertebral column to straighten the visceral compartment; you will dissect the posterior surface of the visceral compartment, which is the location of the posterior pharyngeal wall

- Use forceps to reveal the pharyngobasilar fascia and pharyngeal constrictor mm.; the three pharyngeal constrictor mm. meet in a median raphe on the posterior surface of the pharynx and receive support superiorly from the pharyngobasilar fascia

- Identify the following **(Figure 25-8)**:

  - **Superior pharyngeal constrictor m.** — superiorly arises from the medial pterygoid plates and attaches to the posterior median raphe; inferiorly, the fibers disappear deep to the middle pharyngeal constrictor m.

  - **Middle pharyngeal constrictor m.** — easiest to identify because its fibers arise superiorly from the greater horns of the hyoid bone and attach to the posterior median raphe; inferiorly, the fibers disappear deep to the inferior pharyngeal constrictor m.

  - **Inferior pharyngeal constrictor m.** — superiorly arises from the thyroid and cricoid cartilages; attaches to the posterior median raphe and esophagus; inferiorly, the fibers disappear deep to the musculature of the esophagus

  - **Stylopharyngeus m.** — arises superiorly from the medial side of the styloid process and inserts inferiorly in the pharyngeal wall; courses between the superior and middle pharyngeal constrictor mm.

  - **Stylohyoid m.** — arises superiorly from the posterior surface of the styloid process and inserts inferiorly on the hyoid bone; also courses between the superior and middle pharyngeal constrictor mm.

  - **Posterior belly of the digastric m.** — arises superiorly from the medial surface of the mastoid process (mastoid notch) and courses inferiorly to the hyoid bone, where the anterior belly arises

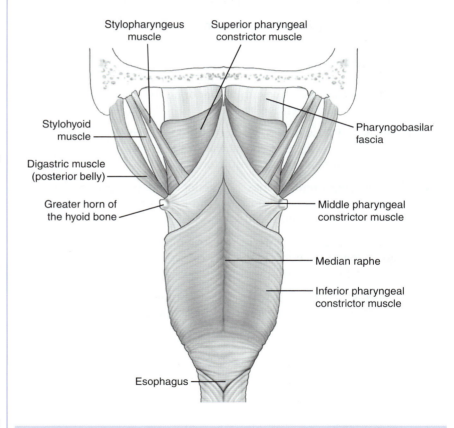

Figure 25-8 Posterior view of the pharyngeal constrictor muscles

Pharynx — Posterior and Lateral Aspects

■ Use forceps to probe the area near the base of the skull and styloid process to locate and identify the following (**Figure 25-9A** and **25-9B**):

- **Stylopharyngeus m. and glossopharyngeal n. (CN IX)** — pass between the internal and external carotid aa. and enter the pharynx by passing between the superior and middle pharyngeal constrictor mm.

- **Vagus n.** — trace the vagus n. inferiorly from the jugular foramen, between the internal jugular v. and internal carotid a.

  - **Inferior ganglion of the vagus n.** — a 2-cm-long swelling on the vagus n., inferior to the jugular foramen

  - **Internal laryngeal n.** and the **superior laryngeal vessels** — course along the middle and inferior pharyngeal constrictor mm. to perforate the thyrohyoid membrane to reach the larynx

  - **Recurrent laryngeal n.** — ascends from the thorax to the larynx; enters the pharyngeal wall at the inferior border of the inferior pharyngeal constrictor m.

- **Cervical sympathetic trunks** — anterior to the prevertebral fascia or on the dissected posterior surface of the pharynx; posterior to the carotid sheaths

- **Superior, middle,** and **inferior cervical ganglia** — expanded regions along the course of the cervical sympathetic trunks; the superior cervical ganglion is usually the largest

  - When the inferior cervical ganglion is fused with the superior thoracic ganglion, the fused structure is called the **stellate ganglion**

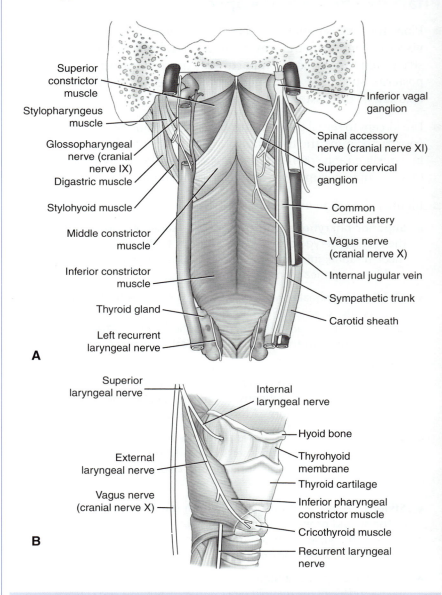

Figure 25-9 Pharyngeal wall structures. **A**, Posterior view. **B**, Lateral view.

Nasopharynx

- To study the nasopharynx, choose the side of the bisected head without the nasal septum

- The borders of the nasopharynx **(Figure 25-10A)**:
  - Anterior — choana
  - Roof — mucous membrane attached to the basilar portions of the sphenoid and occipital bones
  - Lateral and posterior walls — superior pharyngeal constrictors
  - Inferior — soft palate

- Identify the following (see Figure 25-10B):
  - **Torus tubarius**
  - **Opening of the auditory tube**
  - **Salpingopharyngeal fold**
  - **Nasopharyngeal tonsils (adenoids)** — probably difficult to identify because they atrophy later in life

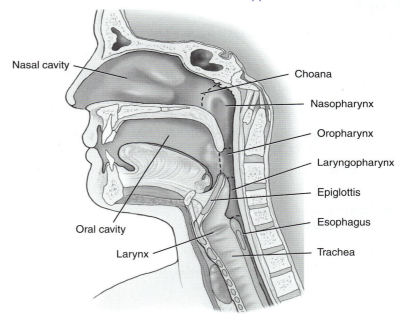

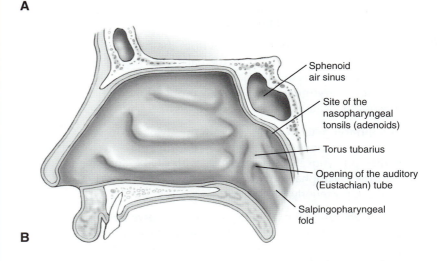

Figure 25-10 Medial views of the nasopharynx. **A,** Midsagittal view. **B,** Sagittal view of the lateral nasal wall

Oropharynx

- Identify the following **(Figure 25-11)**:

  - **Soft palate** — located along the posterior border of the hard palate; mobile muscular partition projecting between the nasopharynx and oropharynx

    - **Uvula** — a conical midline projection of the soft palate
    - **Palatoglossal arch** — the anterior fold from the soft palate to the tongue; covers the palatoglossal m.
    - **Palatopharyngeal arch** — the posterior fold from the soft palate to the pharynx; covers the palatopharyngeus m.

  - **Palatine tonsil** — a lymphoid aggregate located between the palatoglossal and palatopharyngeal arches

- Use forceps to peel away the mucous membrane from the palatoglossal and palatopharyngeal arches; the underlying muscle fibers are thin and delicate

  - **Palatopharyngeus m.** — arises from the hard palate and attaches to the thyroid cartilage; blends with the other vertical muscles of the pharynx

  - **Salpingopharyngeus m.** — arises from the cartilage of the auditory tube and blends with the palatopharyngeus m.; the muscle and its overlying mucosa form a ridge called the **salpingopharyngeal fold**; you may probe through the mucosa to locate this thin muscle

  - **Stylopharyngeus m.** — arises from the styloid process of the temporal bone, passes between the superior and middle pharyngeal constrictor mm. with CN IX, and blends with the palatopharyngeus m.; attaches to the thyroid cartilage posteriorly

  - **Glossopharyngeal n. (CN IX)** — find the nerve by stripping the mucous membrane from the posterior wall of the pharynx, immediately posterior to the base of the tongue and inferior to the styloglossus m.

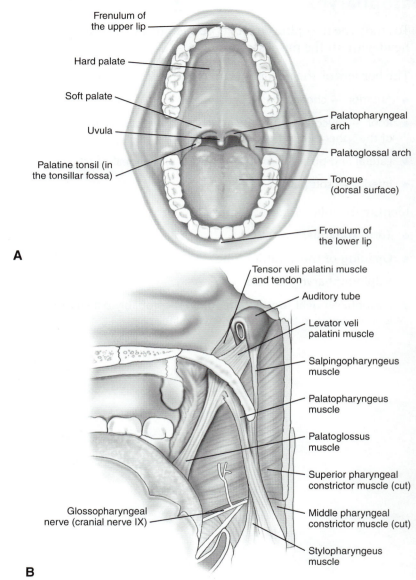

Figure 25-11 Pharyngeal arches. **A**, Anterior view. **B**, Medial view.

Nasal Cavity, Palate, and Oral Cavity

Lab 26

Prior to dissection, you should familiarize yourself with the following structures:

OSTEOLOGY
- Ethmoid bone
  - Ethmoid labyrinth of air cells
  - Perpendicular plate
  - Superior nasal concha (superior meatus)
  - Middle nasal concha (middle meatus)
  - Ethmoidal bulla
- Inferior nasal concha (inferior meatus)
- Palatine bone
  - Greater and lesser palatine foramina
  - Palatine canal
- Maxilla
  - Palatine process of the maxilla
  - Incisive canal
  - Maxillary sinus
  - Infraorbital foramen and canal
  - Posterior superior alveolar foramen
- Sphenoid bone
  - Sphenoid sinus
  - Sphenoethmoidal recess
  - Pterygomaxillary fissure
  - Sphenopalatine foramen
  - Pterygoid canal
  - Pterygoid hamulus
- Zygomatic bone
  - Zygomaticofacial foramen
  - Zygomaticotemporal foramen
- Mandible
  - Mylohyoid line
  - Sublingual fossa
- Temporal bone
  - Greater and lesser petrosal foramina/grooves

STRUCTURES ASSOCIATED WITH THE NASAL CAVITY
- Nasal septum
  - Perpendicular plate of the ethmoid bone
  - Vomer bone
  - Septal cartilage
- Vestibule
- Atrium
- Nasolacrimal duct opening
- Hiatus semilunaris

NERVES
- Trigeminal n. (CN V)
  - V-2 — maxillary division
    - Zygomatic n.
      - Zygomaticotemporal n.
      - Zygomaticofacial n.
    - Pterygopalatine ganglion
    - Greater and lesser palatine nn.
    - Nasopalatine n.
    - Infraorbital n.
    - Anterior, middle, and posterior superior alveolar nn.
  - V-3 — mandibular division
    - Lingual n.
    - Nerve to the mylohyoid m.
- Facial n. (CN VII)
  - Greater petrosal n. (contributes to the nerve of the pterygoid canal [Vidian n.])
- Glossopharyngeal n. (CN IX)
- Hypoglossal n. (CN XII)

ARTERIES
- Ophthalmic a.
  - Posterior ethmoid a.
  - Anterior ethmoid a.
- Maxillary a.
  - Sphenopalatine a.
    - Posterior lateral nasal aa.
    - Posterior septal aa.
  - Greater and lesser palatine aa.
- Facial a.
  - Superior labial a.
  - Lateral nasal a.
  - Ascending palatine a.
- Lingual a.

Continued

PALATE
- Levator veli palatini m.
- Tensor veli palatini m.
- Uvula
- Palatine aponeurosis
- Soft palate
- Palatoglossal and palatopharyngeal arches
- Palatine tonsil

TONGUE
- Genioglossus m.
- Styloglossus m.
- Hyoglossus m.
- Vallate (circumvallate) papillae (taste buds)
- Filiform/fungiform papillae (taste buds)
- Sulcus terminalis
- Median and lateral glossoepiglottic folds
- Vallecula
- Foramen cecum
- Lingual tonsils

MISCELLANEOUS
- Pterygomandibular raphe
- Auditory tube
- Pharyngobasilar fascia
- Plica sublingualis
- Sublingual gland
- Submandibular salivary gland and duct
- Submandibular ganglion
- Geniohyoid m.
- Mylohyoid m.
- Digastric m.
- Superior, middle, and inferior pharyngeal constrictor mm.
- Stylopharyngeal m.

Lab 26 Dissection Overview

The purpose of this laboratory session is to learn the anatomy of the nasal cavity, palate, and oral cavity through dissection. You will do so through the following suggested sequence:

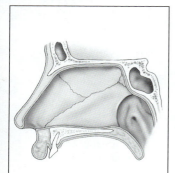

1. Strip the mucosa from the nasal septum on the side of the bisected head possessing the nasal septum; identify the nerves and vessels in the nasal septum.

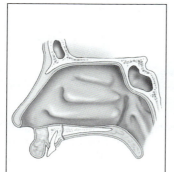

2. Strip the mucosa from the nasal septum on the other side of the bisected head; identify the nerves and vessels associated with the lateral wall of the nasal cavity and palatine canal.

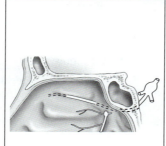

3. Remove the lateral wall of the nasal cavity to follow the infraorbital canal through the roof of the maxillary sinus.

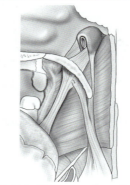

4. Strip the mucosa from the palate and identify structures associated with the palate.

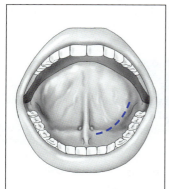

5. Make an incision along the floor of the oral cavity.

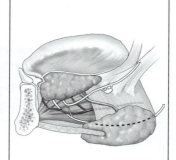

6. Identify the nerves, vessels, and salivary glands associated with the tongue.

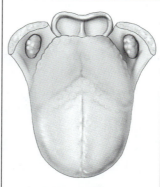

7. Study the superior surface of the tongue.

Table 26-1 Muscles of the Tongue

Muscle	Attachments		Action	Innervation
Genioglossus	Superior mental tubercles	Body of the hyoid bone; entire length of the tongue	Protrudes the tongue; depresses the center of the tongue	Hypoglossal n. (CN XII)
Hyoglossus	Greater horn and adjacent part of the body of the hyoid bone	Lateral surface of the tongue	Depresses and retracts the tongue	
Styloglossus	Styloid process		Elevates and retracts the lateral aspect of the tongue	
Palatoglossus	Inferior surface of the palatine aponeurosis	Lateral side of the tongue	Depresses the palate; moves the palatoglossal fold toward the midline; elevates the back of the tongue	Vagus n. (CN X) (via the pharyngeal branch of the pharyngeal plexus)

Table 26-2 Muscles of the Soft Palate

Muscle	Attachments		Action	Innervation
Tensor veli palatini	Scaphoid fossa of the medial pterygoid plate, spine of the sphenoid bone and cartilage of the auditory tube	Palatine aponeurosis	Tenses the soft palate; opens the pharyngotympanic tubes	Mandibular n. (CN V-3) via the branch to the medial pterygoid m.
Levator veli palatini	Cartilage of the auditory tube and the petrous part of the temporal bone		Elevates the soft palate during swallowing and yawning	Vagus n. (CN X) via the pharyngeal branch to the pharyngeal plexus
Palatoglossus	Inferior surface of the palatine aponeurosis	Lateral margin of the tongue	Depresses the palate; moves the palatoglossal arch toward the midline; elevates the back of the tongue	
Palatopharyngeus	Superior surface of the palatine aponeurosis	Pharyngeal wall	Depresses the soft palate; moves the palatopharyngeal arch toward the midline; elevates the pharynx	

Table 26-3 Branches of the Mandibular Division of the Trigeminal Nerve (CN V-2)

Pterygopalatine Fossa and CN V-2

- During this dissection, you will find the following branches of CN V-2 (and the associated vessels) in the nasal and oral cavities:

A. Schematic of the pterygopalatine fossa

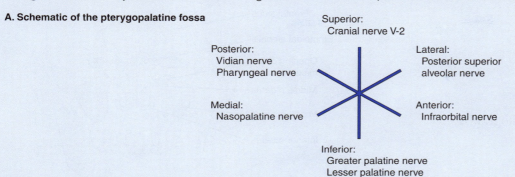

B. Schematic of CN V-2

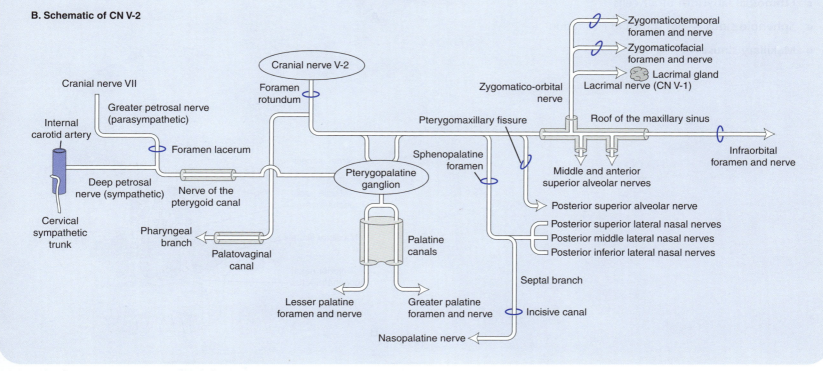

Paranasal Sinuses — Overview

- The paranasal sinuses are air-filled extensions of the nasal cavity and are located in the following bones **(Figure 26-1A)**:
  - Frontal
  - Ethmoid
  - Sphenoid
  - Maxilla

- Paranasal sinuses are easily identified on radiographs (see Figure 26-1B):
  - **Frontal sinuses**
  - **Ethmoidal labyrinth of air cells**
  - **Sphenoid sinus** — not shown in illustration
  - **Maxillary sinuses**

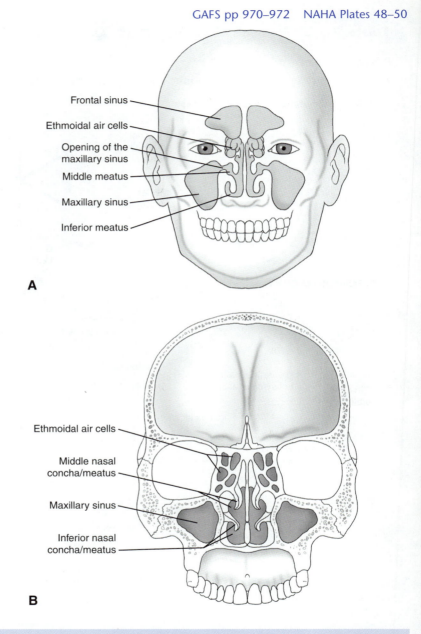

Figure 26-1 Paranasal sinuses. **A,** Anterior view. **B,** Coronal sectional view

Nasal Cavity

- The two sides of the nasal cavity are separated by the nasal septum; examine the half of the bisected head containing the nasal septum to identify the following **(Figure 26-2)**:

  - **Choana** — posterior opening into the nasopharynx; each nasal cavity begins at each nostril and ends posteriorly at the choana

  - **Nasal septum** — composed of three structures:
    - **Perpendicular plate of the ethmoid bone**
    - **Vomer bone**
    - **Septal cartilage**

- Use forceps to gently peel away the mucous membrane from the nasal septum; be gentle because vessels and nerves are located between the mucous membrane and nasal septum (see next page)

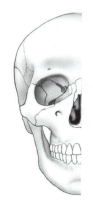

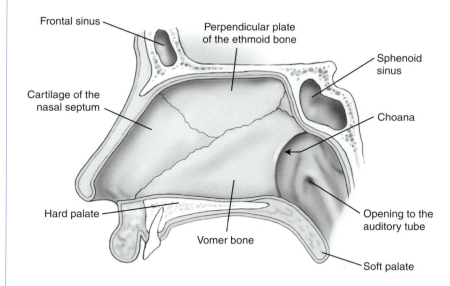

Figure 26-2 Medial view of the nasal septum

Nasal Septum

- Use a scalpel and/or forceps to cut the mucous membrane from the inferior portion of the nasal septum to reveal and identify the following **(Figure 26-3)**:

  - **Nasopalatine n.** — accompanied by vessels that have a different name (**sphenopalatine a.** and **v.**)
    - Look for septal branches on the deep surface of the mucous membrane peeled from the nasal septum

  - **Incisive canal** — anterior portion of the hard palate, just posterior to the incisors; follow the nasopalatine n. and sphenopalatine a. and v. across the nasal septum and through the incisive canal, where they reach the hard palate

  - **Palatine branches of the nasopalatine n. and sphenopalatine a.** — use hemostats and a scalpel to peel the mucous membrane from the anterior portion of the hard palate to locate these structures

GAFS pp 894–898, 978–980   ACGA pp 87–90, 99–100   NAHA Plates 36–44

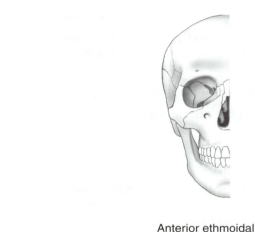

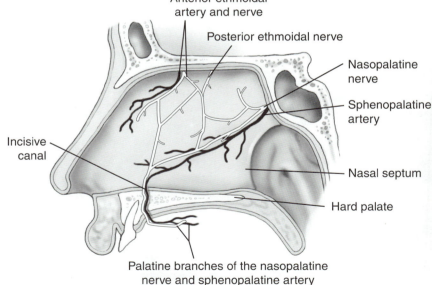

Figure 26-3 Medial view of the nerves and vessels of the nasal septum

Lateral Nasal Wall

- Identify the following on the lateral wall of the nasal cavity (**Figure 26-4**):

  - **Inferior concha** — a separate bone (*not* part of the ethmoid bone); ends 1 cm anterior to the auditory tube
    - **Inferior meatus** — the space inferior to the inferior concha
  - **Middle concha** — part of the ethmoid bone
    - **Middle meatus** — the space inferior to the middle concha
  - **Superior concha** — also part of the ethmoid bone; anterior to the sphenoid sinus
    - **Superior meatus** — the space inferior to the superior concha
  - **Sphenoethmoidal recess** — space posterosuperior to the superior concha
  - **Vestibule** — located superior to the nostril and anterior to the inferior meatus; note the presence of hairs (vibrissae)
  - **Atrium** — located superior to the vestibule and anterior to the middle meatus
  - **Opening of the nasolacrimal duct** (tear duct) — use scissors to cut away the inferior concha to identify the duct in the inferior meatus (**Figure 26-5**)

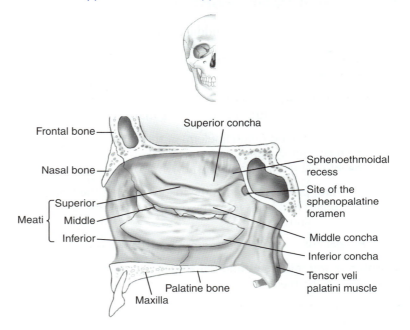

Figure 26-4 View of the lateral nasal wall

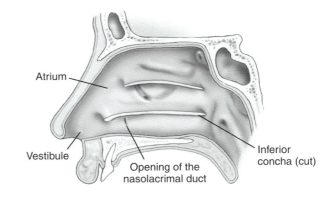

Figure 26-5 Opening of the nasolacrimal duct in the lateral nasal wall

Lateral Nasal Wall Continued

Lateral Nasal Wall—cont'd

- Use scissors to cut away the middle concha
- Use forceps to reveal and identify the following **(Figure 26-6)**:
  - **Hiatus semilunaris** — a curved slit inferior to the middle concha (middle meatus) that drains the maxillary air sinus
    - Note an opening (infundibulum) at the anterior margin of the hiatus semilunaris; the frontal air sinus drains through the infundibulum (middle meatus)
    - **Uncinate process** — forms the medial edge of the hiatus semilunaris and helps form the medial wall of the maxillary sinus
  - **Ethmoidal bulla** — an elevation superior to the hiatus semilunaris
  - **Anterior** and **middle ethmoidal air cells** — openings are located on the medial aspect of the ethmoid bulla
  - **Posterior ethmoidal air cells** — communicate with the superior meatus
  - **Sphenoid air sinus** — look for its opening into the **sphenoethmoidal recess** (space superior to the superior concha)

GAFS pp 968–975   ACGA pp 87–90, 99–100   NAHA Plates 36–44

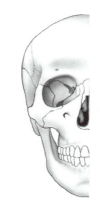

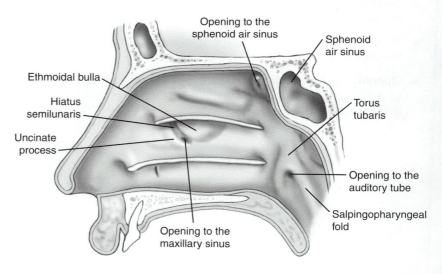

Figure 26-6 View of the lateral nasal wall

Vasculature of the Lateral Nasal Cavity

- Use forceps to gently peel away the mucous membrane from the lateral wall of the nasal cavity to identify the following arteries (be gentle because the vessels and nerves are located between the mucous membrane and bones of the lateral nasal wall) **(Figure 26-7)**:

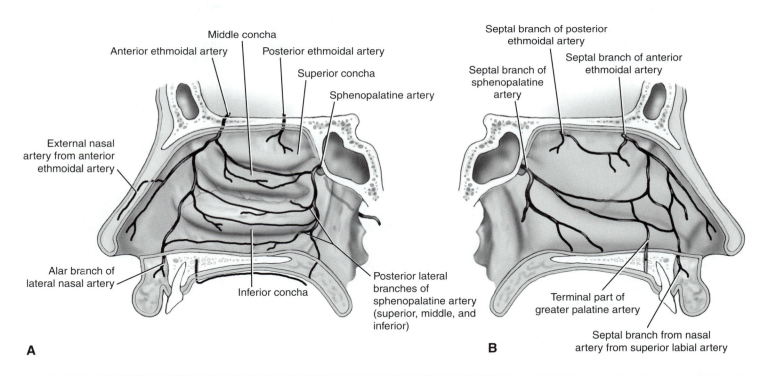

Figure 26-7 Arteries of the lateral nasal wall. **A,** Lateral wall of right nasal cavity. **B,** Septum (medial wall of left nasal cavity)   *Continued*

Vasculature of the Lateral Nasal Cavity Continued

Vasculature of the Lateral Nasal Cavity—cont'd

- **Sphenopalatine a.** — originates from the maxillary a. in the infratemporal fossa; enters the nasal cavity via the sphenopalatine foramen (accompanied by the posterior superior nasal nn.); bifurcates into lateral and septal (medial) posterior nasal aa.

    - **Posterior lateral nasal aa.** — originate from the sphenopalatine a.; divide into superior, middle, and inferior branches, giving each concha an arterial branch

- **Anterior ethmoidal a.** — originates from the ophthalmic a. and enters the nasal cavity via the anterior ethmoidal foramen; anastomoses with the posterior lateral and medial nasal branches of the sphenopalatine a.

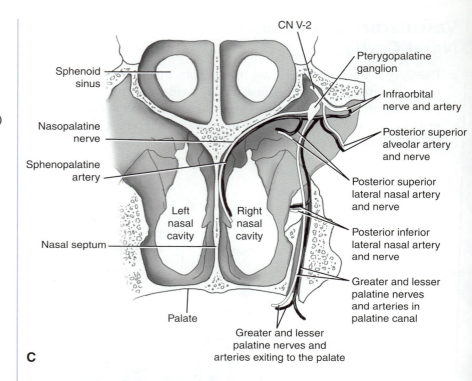

Figure 26-7, cont'd **C**, Coronal section through nasal cavities. (Adapted with permission from Augur AMR, Dalley AF: Grant's Atlas of Anatomy, 11th ed. Baltimore: Lippincott, Williams & Wilkins, 2005, Fig. 7.69C.)

Contents of the Palatine Canal

- If not already done, peel away the remaining mucous membrane from the lateral wall of the nasal cavity, posterior to the concha

- Use forceps to reveal and identify the following **(Figure 26-8)**:

  - **Palatine canal** — a vertical channel in the posterolateral wall of the nasal cavity; courses the height of the posterolateral nasal wall; its bony covering is translucent

    - Use forceps (or a blunt probe or scissors) to break through the translucent wall; the underlying channel is called the palatine canal, which contains the following, all of which are inside of a sleeve of periosteum (use a probe or tip of scissors to open the periosteal sleeve); carefully remove remaining fat lobules to clarify the dissection field:

      - **Pterygopalatine ganglion** (parasympathetic) — located at the superior end of the palatine canal

      - **Greater** and **lesser palatine nn.** — course through the palatine canal inferiorly from the pterygopalatine ganglion; follow both palatine nn. through the palatine foramina to enter the mucosal lining on the inferior surface of the hard palate of the maxilla and palatine bone; note the accompanying vessels, which are named the same as the nerves

- Bluntly dissect the mucous membrane from the oral part of the hard palate to identify the following (see Figures 26-7 and 26-8):

  - **Greater palatine n., a., and v.** — course in an anterior direction once they emerge from the palatine canal into the palate; branches meet with the palatine branches of the nasopalatine n. and sphenopalatine a. and v.

  - **Lesser palatine n., a., and v.** — course in a posterior direction over the soft palate and tonsillar fossa

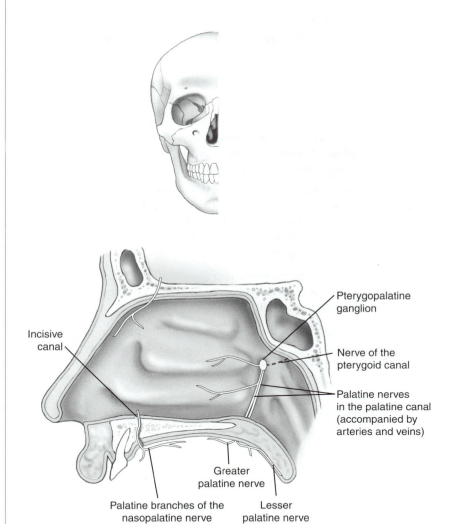

Figure 26-8 Palatine canal. View of the lateral wall of the nasal cavity

Greater Petrosal Nerve and Nerve to the Pterygoid Canal

- Peel away remaining dura mater from the medial portion of the middle cranial fossa; refer to a dry skull for reference to see the foramina clearly

- Use forceps to reveal and identify the following (**Figure 26-9A**):

  - **Greater petrosal n.** — emerges from the greater petrosal hiatus; courses anteriorly in a groove toward the foramen lacerum, where the nerve passes over the top of the foramen before it reaches the pterygoid canal

  - **N. of the pterygoid canal (Vidian n.)** — formed by union of the greater petrosal n. (parasympathetic) and the deep petrosal n. (sympathetic nerves that follow the internal carotid a.); courses through the pterygoid canal to enter the pterygopalatine ganglion

    - Look for the n. of the pterygoid canal in the floor of the sphenoid sinus by breaking away the bone covering the nerve (see Figure 26-9B)

    - A helpful approach is to follow the n. of the pterygoid canal posteriorly from the pterygopalatine ganglion by pulling the pterygopalatine ganglion anteriorly to locate the nerve

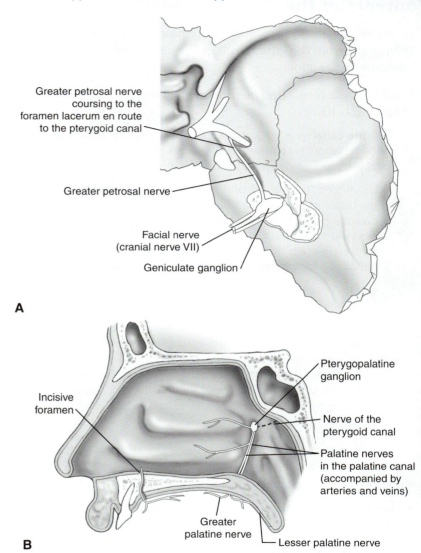

Figure 26-9 Greater petrosal nerve and nerve to the pterygoid canal. **A,** Superior view of the temporal bone with the tegmen tympani portion of the temporal bone removed. **B,** View of the lateral nasal wall

Dissection of the Infraorbital Canal

- Identify the following:

  - **Maxillary sinuses** — paired air sinuses on the lateral sides of the nasal cavity; to identify, remove mucous membrane and push a probe through the thin bone on the lateral wall of the nasal cavity (do this on the side with the removed conchae)

  - **Infraorbital canal** — a channel that courses from posterior to anterior along the roof of the opened maxillary sinus **(Figure 26-10A)**

  - **Infraorbital n., a., and v.** — course through the infraorbital canal; break open the roof of the opened maxillary sinus with a probe to expose the contents of the infraorbital canal; follow the infraorbital n. posteriorly to the foramen rotundum

    - **Anterior** and **middle superior alveolar n., a., and v.** — branches of the infraorbital n., a., and v. (see Figure 26-10B); they supply the corresponding maxillary teeth (often found within bony spurs inside the maxillary sinus); examine the floor of the maxillary air sinus to locate the roots of teeth that may project into the sinus

    - **Posterior superior alveolar n., a., and v.** — located in the infratemporal fossa; course along the lateral and posterior surface of the maxillary sinus to enter the posterior superior alveolar foramen in the infratemporal fossa

- The pharyngeal and zygomatico-orbital branches of CN V-2 will not be explored

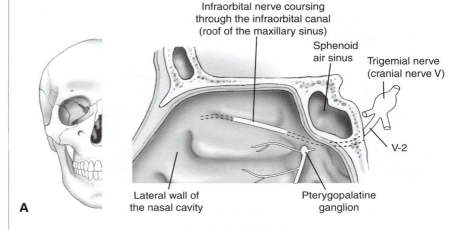

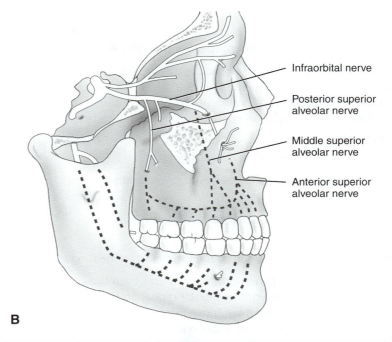

Figure 26-10 CN V-2. **A,** View of the lateral nasal wall. **B,** View of the maxilla from the infratemporal fossa

Palatal Structures

- Use forceps to reveal and identify the following **(Figure 26-11A)**:

  - **Palatine tonsils** (if present; usually atrophied in the aged) — located in the triangular (tonsillar) fossa, between the palatoglossal and palatopharyngeal arches
  - **Palatoglossal arch** — extends from the tip of the uvula to the base of the tongue
  - **Palatopharyngeal arch** — posterior to the palatoglossal arch; extends from the tip of the uvula posterolaterally to the pharynx

- Use forceps to reveal and identify the following muscles by removing remaining mucous membrane covering them (see Figure 26-11B):

  - **Levator veli palatini m.** — located between the floor of the auditory tube and the superior aspect of the soft palate
  - **Tensor veli palatini m.** — descends vertically; anterior and lateral to the levator veli palatini m.; the tensor veli palatini m. changes direction (90°) at the **pterygoid hamulus**, contributing to the palatine aponeurosis in the soft palate
    - **Palatine aponeurosis** — stabilizing foundation of the soft palate for palatine muscles to act upon
  - **Salpingopharyngeus m.** — courses from the auditory tube to the pharynx
  - **Palatopharyngeus m.** — courses from the soft palate to the pharynx
  - **Palatoglossus m.** — courses from the soft palate to the tongue
  - **Superior pharyngeal constrictor m.** — arises from the pterygoid hamulus, pterygomandibular raphe, and mylohyoid line of the mandible (posterior to the third molar); also attaches to the pharyngeal tubercle

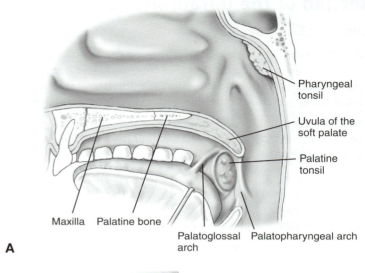

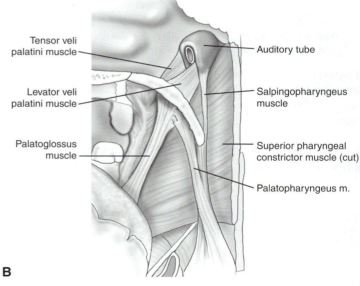

Figure 26-11 Palatal structures. **A,** Pharynx with the mucous membrane intact. **B,** Pharynx with the mucous membrane removed

Oral Cavity — Tongue

- Use either half of the cadaver's bisected head to identify the following muscles **(Figure 26-12)**:

  - **Genioglossus m.** — superior to the geniohyoid m.; largest extrinsic muscle of the tongue

  - **Geniohyoid m.** — superior to the mylohyoid m.

  - **Mylohyoid m.** — forms the floor of the oral cavity

  - **Intrinsic muscles of the tongue** — four groups: superior and inferior longitudinal, transverse, and vertical; the three directions in which these muscles course allow them to alter the shape and contour of the tongue

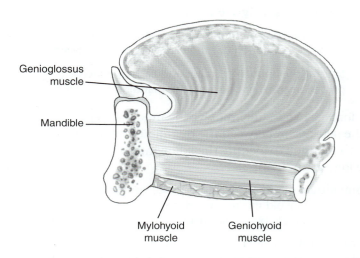

Figure 26-12 Medial view of the extrinsic tongue muscles (sagittal section)

Oral Cavity — Tongue Continued

Oral Cavity — Tongue—cont'd

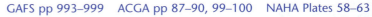

- To dissect deeper structures within the oral cavity, follow these instructions **(Figure 26-13A)**:

  - Incise the mucous membrane between the tongue and mandible, on either half of the cadaver's bisected head

    - Start at the lingual frenulum and carry the incision posteriorly, but not beyond the mandibular molar teeth

- Use forceps to carefully remove the mucous membrane in the depression between the mandibular molar teeth and the tongue to identify the following structures (see Figure 26-13B):

  - **Sublingual gland** — located superior to the anterior part of the mylohyoid m.; the gland is separated from the genioglossus m. by the lingual n. and submandibular duct

  - **Submandibular duct** — located in the deep part of the gland; courses diagonally across the medial aspect of the sublingual gland to the side of the lingual frenulum; the duct opens posterior to the anterior mandibular teeth and sublingual caruncle

  - **Lingual n.** — located posterior to the third molar of the mandible; courses between the ramus of the mandible and medial pterygoid m.; trace it anteriorly to observe it spiraled around the submandibular duct

    - **Submandibular ganglion** — suspended from the lingual n. on the surface of the hyoglossus m.

    - **Chorda tympani n.** — joins the lingual n. in the infratemporal fossa

  - **Hypoglossal n.** — courses anteriorly between the submandibular gland and the hyoglossus m., inferior to the lingual n.; follow the hypoglossal n. to the musculature of the tongue

  - **Lingual a.** — courses medial to the hyoglossus m.; divides into the **deep lingual a.** and **sublingual a.**

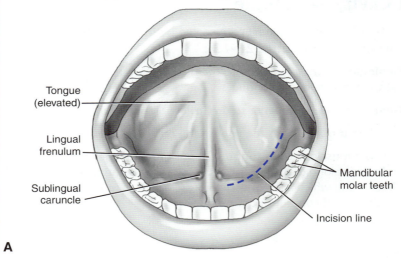

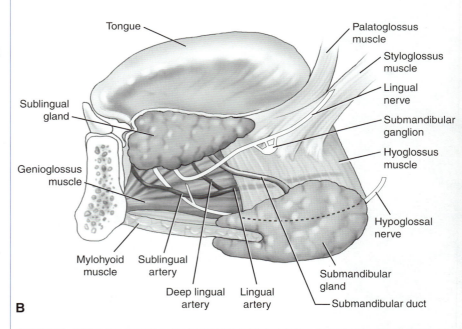

Figure 26-13 Oral cavity. **A**, Incisions. **B**, Nerves and vessels of the tongue; salivary glands (stylized drawing to illustrate anatomy)

Muscles of the Tongue

■ Identify the following extrinsic muscles of the tongue **(Figure 26-14)**:

- **Genioglossus m.** — arises from the internal surface of the mental symphysis; forms the bulk of the tongue

- **Hyoglossus m.** — attached to the hyoid bone and tongue; look for the **styloglossus m.**, which interdigitates with the posterior fibers of the hyoglossus m.

- **Styloglossus m.** — follow the muscle posterior to the styloid process of the temporal bone

- **Palatoglossus m.**

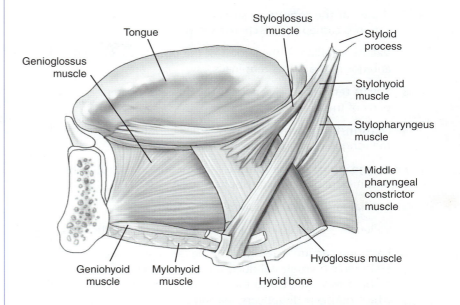

Figure 26-14 Extrinsic muscles of the tongue (mandibular ramus, angle, and body have been removed to provide a clear anatomic view)

Tongue

■ Identify the following **(Figure 26-15)**:

- **Oral part of the tongue** — anterior two thirds; taste sensation is carried by the chorda tympani n. (CN VII)
  - **Vallate papillae** — the largest of the taste buds; located anterior to the sulcus terminalis
  - **Sulcus terminalis** — separates the oral and pharyngeal parts of the tongue
  - **Filiform/fungiform papillae** — small elevations that give the tongue its rough surface
- **Pharyngeal part of the tongue** — posterior one third; taste sensation carried by the glossopharyngeal n. (CN IX)
  - **Medial and lateral glossoepiglottic folds**
  - **Vallecula** — depressions between the glossoepiglottic folds
  - **Foramen cecum** — remnant of the opening of the embryonic thyroglossal duct; the thyroid gland in the embryo was attached to the tongue by this duct, which normally disappears, leaving only this small pit in the tongue
  - **Lingual tonsils** — cause the surface elevations of the posterior one third of the tongue

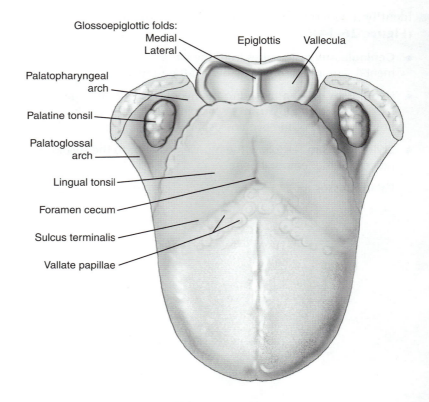

Figure 26-15 View of the superior surface of the tongue

Lab 27

Larynx

Prior to dissection, you should familiarize yourself with the following structures:

LARYNGEAL CARTILAGES AND JOINTS

- Thyroid cartilage
  - Laryngeal prominence
  - Right and left laminae
  - Superior and inferior thyroid notches
  - Oblique line
  - Superior and inferior horns
  - Thyrohyoid membrane
- Cricoid cartilage
- Cricothyroid joint
  - Median cricothyroid ligament
- Arytenoid cartilages
- Cricoarytenoid joint
  - Cricoarytenoid ligament
- Corniculate cartilages
- Cuneiform cartilages
- Epiglottic cartilage

LARYNGEAL MUSCLES

- Cricothyroid m.
- Posterior cricoarytenoid m.
- Lateral cricoarytenoid m.
- Vocalis m.
- Thyroarytenoid m.
- Transverse and oblique arytenoid mm.
- Aryepiglotticus m.
- Thyroepiglottic m.
- Thyrohyoid m.

LARYNGEAL NERVES

- Superior laryngeal n.
  - Internal laryngeal n.
  - External laryngeal n.
- Recurrent laryngeal n.

LARYNGEAL CAVITY

- Laryngeal inlet
  - Aryepiglottic fold
    - Corniculate tubercle
    - Cuneiform tubercle
- Laryngeal vestibule
  - Vestibular folds (false vocal cords)
- Laryngeal ventricle
  - Laryngeal saccule
- Glottis
  - Vocal folds (true vocal cords)
    - Rima glottidis
- Fibroelastic membrane of the larynx
  - Vocal ligament

MISCELLANEOUS

- Laryngopharynx
  - Piriform fossa/recess
    - Fold over the superior laryngeal n.

Lab 27 Dissection Overview

The purpose of this laboratory session is to learn the anatomy of the larynx through dissection. You will do so through the following suggested sequence:

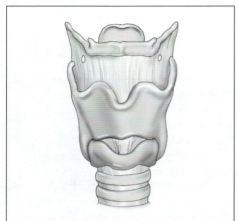

1. Using your cadaver and a model, study the cartilaginous skeleton of the larynx.

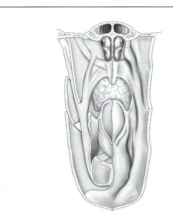

2. Make a vertical incision through the back of the pharynx to reveal the posterior aspect of the larynx.

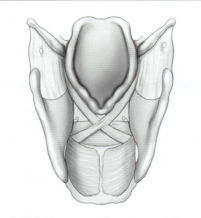

3. Strip the mucosa from the posterior aspect of the larynx.

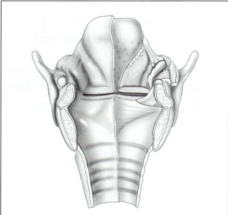

4. Make a vertical incision through the back of the cricoid cartilage to open the larynx.

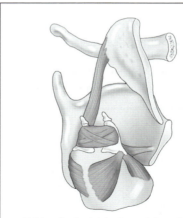

5. Identify the intrinsic muscles of the larynx.

Table 27-1 Muscles of the Larynx

Muscle	Attachments		Action	Innervation
Cricothyroid	Anterolateral part of the cricoid cartilage	Oblique part — lesser horn of the hyoid bone; straight part — inferior margin of the thyroid cartilage	Rotates the thyroid cartilage at the cricothyroid joint forward and downward	External branch of the superior laryngeal n. from the vagus n. (CN X)
Posterior cricoarytenoid	Posterior surface of the cricoid cartilage	Muscular process of the arytenoid cartilages	Abducts the vocal fold	Recurrent laryngeal branch of the vagus n. (CN X)
Lateral cricoarytenoid	Arch of the cricoid cartilage		Adducts the vocal fold (interligamentous region)	
Thyroarytenoid	Posterior surface of the thyroid cartilage		Relaxes the vocal fold	
Transverse and oblique arytenoids	The muscles course between the two arytenoid cartilages		Closes the intercartilaginous region of the rima glottidis	
Vocalis	Vocal processes of the arytenoid cartilages	Vocal ligaments	Adjusts tension in the vocal folds	

External Surface of the Larynx — Review

- Use forceps to reveal and identify the following **(Figure 27-1)**:

  - **Thyrohyoid mm.** — lateral to the larynx; paired muscles that attach the inferior border of the hyoid bone to the lateral surface of the thyroid cartilage

  - **Cricothyroid mm.** — anterior and lateral to the larynx; paired muscles that attach the inferior border and inferior horns of the thyroid cartilage to the cricoid cartilage

  - **Thyrohyoid membrane** — connective tissue sheet that spans between the inferior border of the hyoid bone and the superior border of the thyroid cartilage; deep to the thyrohyoid m.

  - **Cricothyroid membrane** — fan-shaped connective tissue sheet that spans between the superior border of the cricoid cartilage and the inferior border of the thyroid cartilage; deep to the cricothyroid mm.

  - **Superior laryngeal n. (CN X)** — descends between the carotid a. and internal jugular v., and divides into the following branches to the larynx:

    - **Internal laryngeal n.** — descends and pierces the thyrohyoid membrane; sensory nerve to the mucosa superior to the vocal folds

    - **External laryngeal n.** — descends and pierces the cricothyroid m.; motor nerve to cricothyroid m.

  - **Recurrent laryngeal n.** — ascends to reach the posteromedial aspect of the thyroid gland (inferior pole); ascends in the tracheoesophageal groove to supply the intrinsic laryngeal mm.

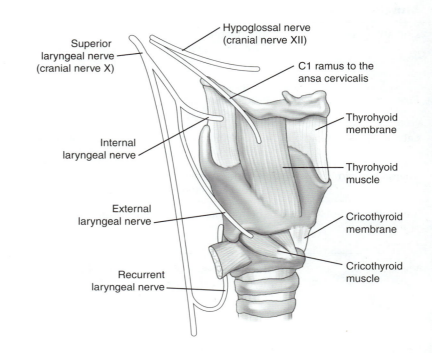

Figure 27-1 Lateral view of the laryngeal muscles and membranes

External Surface of the Larynx — Skeleton

- The larynx has a cartilaginous skeleton

- Refer to **Figure 27-2** and models of the larynx, if available, to identify the following structures:

  - **Thyroid cartilage** — shaped like a shield; largest of the cartilages

    - **Laryngeal prominence** — at the anterior median plane; union of the two laminae of the thyroid cartilage ("Adam's apple")

    - **Superior and inferior horns** — superior and inferior projections from the posterior surfaces of the thyroid cartilage

  - **Cricoid cartilage** — inferior to the thyroid cartilage; shaped like a signet ring, with the band facing anteriorly; the only complete ring of cartilage of the respiratory tract

  - **Arytenoid cartilages** — paired, pyramidal-shaped cartilages located on the superior border of the body of the cricoid cartilage (posterior surface of the larynx)

  - **Corniculate cartilages** — small cartilages attached to the apex of the arytenoid cartilages

  - **Epiglottic cartilage** — a leaf-shaped cartilage that extends superiorly from the thyroid cartilage, posterior to the hyoid bone and the base of the tongue; the base of the epiglottic cartilage is attached to the inside of the thyroid cartilage at the midline by the thyroepiglottic ligament

- The articulations between these cartilages are synovial joints, with joint capsules

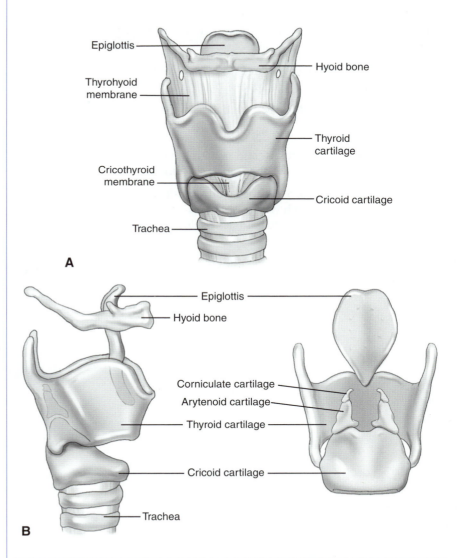

Figure 27-2 Laryngeal skeleton. **A,** Anterior view. **B,** Lateral and posterior views

Internal Features of the Larynx (Superior View)

- Inspect the interior of the larynx, from its superior aspect (as in looking down a tube) to identify the following **(Figure 27-3)**:

  - **Glottis** — the space superior to the vocal folds and posterior to the epiglottic cartilage space
    - **Rima glottis** — the aperture between the vocal folds
    - Vocal folds = true and false cords
      - **False vocal cords** — also named the vestibular folds; located superior to the true vocal folds
      - **True vocal cords** — these folds produce sound; the apex of each wedge-shaped vocal fold projects posteromedially; its base lies against the lamina of the thyroid cartilage
  - **Vocal ligament** — thickened edges of the cricothyroid ligament complex; forms the fibrous core of the true vocal folds

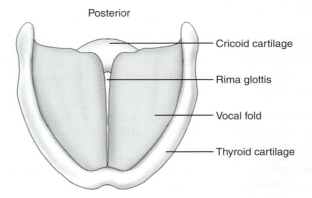

Figure 27-3 Superior view down into the larynx

Laryngopharynx

- The laryngopharynx is posterior to the larynx, extending from the superior border of the epiglottis to the inferior border of the cricoid cartilage

- View the posterior aspect of the larynx to identify the following **(Figure 27-4)**:

  - **Tongue** — the root is visible from this perspective
  - **Epiglottis** — a leaf-shaped plate of elastic cartilage covered with mucous membrane
  - **Greater horns of the hyoid bone** — project posterosuperiorly; the tips may be seen through the mucous membrane on the posterior aspect of the pharynx
  - **Thyroid cartilage** — superior horns; project posterosuperiorly and may be seen through the mucous membrane on the posterior aspect of the pharynx
  - **Cricoid cartilage** — prominence may be seen through the mucous membrane
  - **Piriform fossa** — located in the posterolateral sides of the laryngopharynx, lateral to the mucous membrane that covers the thyroid and cricoid cartilages
  - **Recurrent** and **internal laryngeal nn.** — strip the mucosa from the laryngopharyngeal aspect of the larynx; look for the recurrent and internal laryngeal nn. in the inferior and superior portions of the piriform recess, respectively

GAFS pp 945, 950–951, 964–965   ACGA pp 112–114, 116   NAHA Plates 77–80

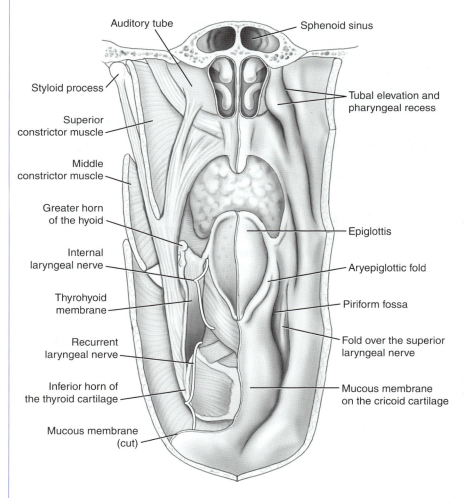

Figure 27-4 Posterior view of the pharynx and larynx

Larynx — Intrinsic Muscles: Posterior View

- Use forceps and scissors to peel and cut away the mucous membrane from the posterior surface of the larynx

- There is no fascial separation between the muscles on the internal wall of the larynx; the muscles are named by their attachments

- Identify the following **(Figure 27-5)**:

  - **Posterior cricoarytenoid mm.** — posterior to the larynx; paired muscles that attach the posterior lamina of the cricoid cartilage to the muscular processes of the arytenoid cartilages

  - **Oblique arytenoid mm.** — posterior to the larynx; paired muscles that course diagonally and attach to both arytenoid cartilages; the muscle fibers continue superiorly to the epiglottis (aryepiglotticus mm.)

  - **Transverse arytenoid mm.** — posterior to the larynx; paired muscles that attach horizontally to both arytenoid cartilages

  - **Aryepiglotticus mm.** — posterior to the larynx; paired muscles that course diagonally superiorly, as extensions of the oblique arytenoid mm., into the aryepiglottic folds

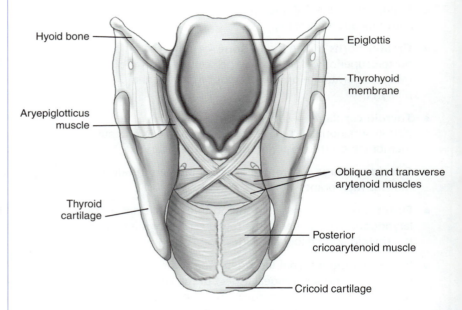

Figure 27-5 Posterior view of the laryngeal muscles

Internal Features of the Larynx

- Use a scalpel to make a longitudinal incision through the posterior aspect of the cricoid cartilage **(Figure 27-6A)** to identify the following (see Figure 27-6B):

  - **Vestibular folds** — false vocal cords; superior to the vocal folds (true vocal cords); they are not opposable and are more widely separated than the true vocal folds
  - **Vestibule** — the space superior to the vestibular folds
  - **Ventricle** — the space inferior to the vestibular folds; may extend laterally and superiorly, forming a recess called the **saccule**
  - **Vocal folds** — true vocal cords; inferior to the ventricle; more closely related than the false vocal folds; in life, they are movable and opposable
    - Vocal ligaments — connective tissue core deep to the vocal folds; superior, free rim of the cricothyroid membrane

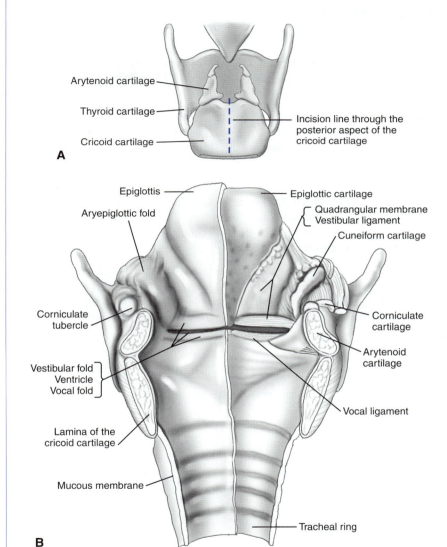

Figure 27-6 Posterior view of the internal features of the larynx. **A**, Cricoid cartilage incision. **B**, Internal view of the larynx

Larynx Intrinsic Muscles: Posterolateral View

■ Identify the following:

- **Cricothyroid joint (Figure 27-7A)** — lateral sides of the larynx; synovial articulation of the cricoid and thyroid cartilages

- Use a scalpel to cut through the cricothyroid joint on one side of the larynx; separate the two cartilages by reflecting the thyroid cartilage laterally (see Figure 27-7B) and anteriorly to identify the following two muscles that are internal to the thyroid and epiglottic cartilages:

  - **Lateral cricoarytenoid mm.** — lateral to the larynx; paired muscles that course from the superior border of the cricothyroid ligament to the muscular processes of the arytenoid cartilages

  - **Thyroarytenoid mm.** — lateral to the larynx; paired muscles that are superior to the lateral cricoarytenoid mm.; course from the thyroid cartilage anteriorly to the arytenoid cartilages posteriorly; their superior and most medial fibers are the **vocalis m.**

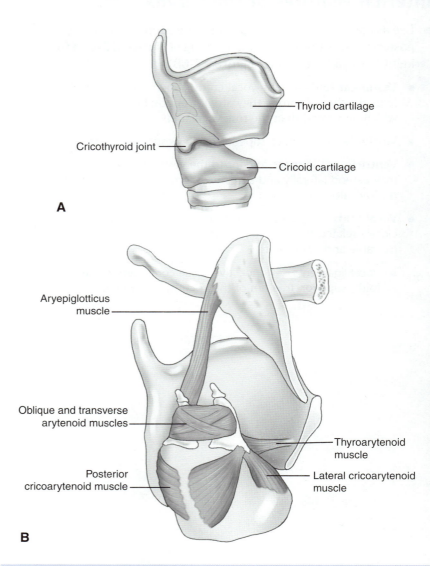

Figure 27-7 Laryngeal muscles. **A,** Lateral view. **B,** Posterolateral view; right side of thyroid cartilage is removed

Lab 28

Ear

Prior to dissection, you should familiarize yourself with the following structures:

EAR
- External ear
  - Auricle; pinna
    - Lobule of the auricle
    - Auricular cartilage
    - Helix
    - Antihelix
      - Triangular fossa
    - Scaphoid fossa
    - Concha of the auricle
    - Tragus
    - Antitragus
  - External auditory canal
  - Tympanic membrane

- Middle ear (tympanic cavity)
  - Tegmen tympani
    - Epitympanic recess
  - Aditus to the mastoid antrum
  - Mastoid antrum
    - Mastoid air cells
  - Ear ossicles
    - Malleus (hammer)
    - Incus (anvil)
    - Stapes (stirrup)
  - Muscles of the auditory tube
    - Stapedius m.
    - Tensor tympani m.

- Chorda tympani n. (CN VII)
- Mastoid air cells
- Auditory (pharyngotympanic) tube
  - Bony and cartilaginous parts
- Inner ear
  - Vestibule
  - Semicircular canals
  - Cochlea
  - Internal acoustic meatus
  - Vestibulocochlear n. (CN VIII)

Lab 28 Dissection Overview

The purpose of this laboratory session is to learn the anatomy of the ear through dissection. You will do so through the following suggested sequence:

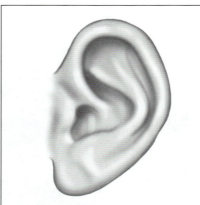

1. Study the external structures of the ear (pinna).

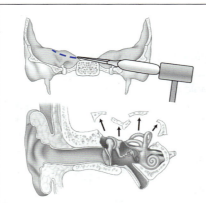

2. To study structures of the middle and inner ear, use a mallet and chisel to remove the roof of the petrous part of the temporal bone.

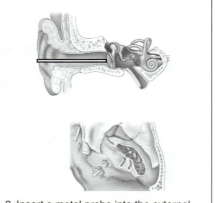

3. Insert a metal probe into the external auditory meatus and push against the tympanic membrane. By gently moving the tympanic membrane, you will observe the tiny ear ossicles move.

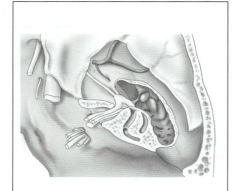

4. Identify the location of the semicircular canals and concha, and follow the course of the facial n. (CN VII) and vestibulocochlear n. (CN VIII).

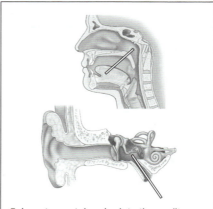

5. Insert a metal probe into the auditory tube to demonstrate the communication between the nasopharynx and middle ear.

Ear Dissection

- Check with your instructor before performing this dissection, to determine if you will dissect the ear

- Identify the following structures during this dissection **(Figure 28-1)**:
  - External ear (pinna)
    - External auditory canal
  - Middle ear
    - Tympanic membrane
    - Ear ossicles
      - Malleus
      - Incus
      - Stapes
    - Stapedius m.
    - Tensor tympani m.
    - Chorda tympani n. (CN VII)
    - Mastoid air cells
    - Auditory tube
  - Inner ear
    - Cochlea
    - Semicircular canals
    - Vestibule
    - Vestibulocochlear n. (CN VIII)

GAFS pp 854–871   ACGA p 72   NAHA Plate 92

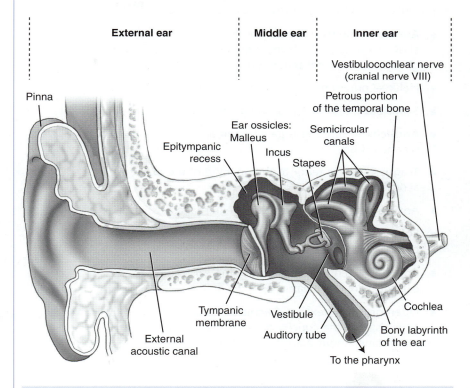

Figure 28-1 Coronal section through the ear

External Ear

- The external (outer) ear extends from the auricle (pinna) medially, via the external auditory canal, to the tympanic membrane

- Identify the following **(Figure 28-2)**:
  - **Auricle** — the shell-like part of the external ear; consists of elastic cartilage, skin, hairs, sweat glands, and sebaceous glands; acts as a collection funnel for sound waves
  - **Helix** — outer rim
  - **Scaphoid fossa** — depression anterior to the helix
  - **Antihelix** — rim that is parallel and anterior to the helix and scaphoid fossa
  - **Tragus** — rim anterior to the opening of the external acoustic canal
  - **Antitragus** — rim inferior to the external acoustic canal
  - **Lobule (ear lobe)** — consists of fibrous tissue, fat, and blood vessels
  - **Concha** — central depression of the ear leading to the external acoustic meatus
  - **Opening of the external acoustic canal** — the canal extends from the concha of the auricle to the tympanic membrane; about 2.5 cm long in the adult

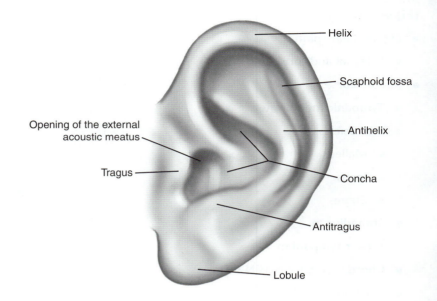

Figure 28-2   External ear

Middle Ear Dissection — Removal of the Tegmen Tympani

- The middle ear is an air-filled chamber sandwiched between the tympanic membrane (lateral) and the oval and round windows (medial) of the vestibulocochlear apparatus
  - Dissection of the middle ear is performed to demonstrate the spatial relationships of the external ear, middle ear, internal ear, auditory tube, and mastoid air cells

- To observe the contents of the middle ear, you will remove the **tegmen tympani** (bony roof of the middle ear [Figure 28-3]):
  - Use a mallet and chisel to break the tegmen tympani from the petrous portion of the temporal bone about:
    - 1.5 cm from the squamous part of the temporal bone
    - 2.5 cm from the posterior ridge of the petrous part of the temporal bone
  - Remove the bony fragments from the tegmen tympani to reveal the air-filled chamber of the middle ear

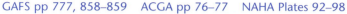
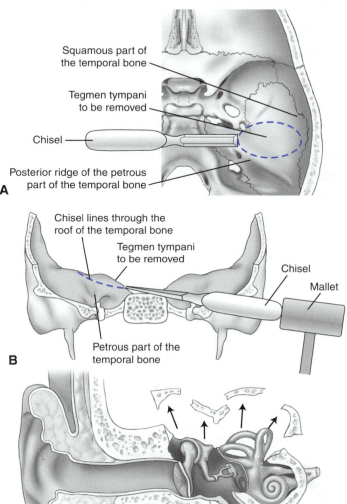

Figure 28-3 Removal of the tegmen tympani. **A**, Internal view of the skull base. **B**, Coronal section in an anterior view. **C**, Tegmen tympani of the temporal bone removed

Middle Ear Dissection — Ossicles

■ Identify the following (**Figure 28-4A** and **28-4B**):

- **Epitympanic recess** — the region between the ear ossicles and the tegmen tympani

- **Ossicles** — these three tiny bones form a chain across the middle ear (tympanic cavity), from the tympanic membrane to the oval widow; look for smooth, condylar surfaces in the exposed compartment; these structures are the malleus and incus bones; from lateral to medial, the bones are

    - **Malleus** — attached to the tympanic membrane; insert a probe into the external auditory canal to gently push against the tympanic membrane; because the malleus is attached to the tympanic membrane, and all of the ear ossicles are attached together, you will see the ossicles move when you gently push on and release the tympanic membrane with the probe

    - **Incus** — located between and attached to both the malleus and the stapes

    - **Stapes** — attached to the oval window; you will probably not see this ossicle

- **Tensor tympani m.** — look for the tensor tympani muscle's tendon passing anterior to the head of the malleus

- **Mastoid antrum** — the large cavity that continues into the mastoid air cells inferiorly; note the superior communication between the mastoid air cells and the middle ear

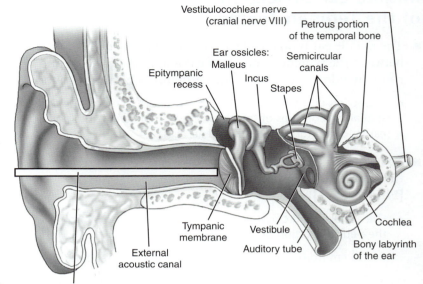

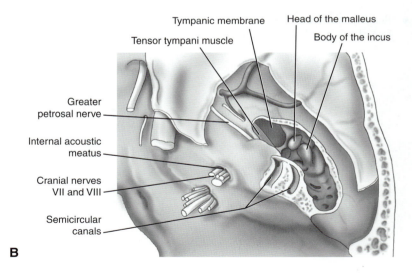

Figure 28-4 Middle ear dissection. **A,** Anterior view of a coronal section through the ear. **B,** Internal view of the skull base

Middle Ear Dissection — Geniculate Ganglion

- To identify the geniculate ganglion, follow these instructions **(Figure 28-5A)**:
  - Push a probe into the internal acoustic meatus to use as a guide
  - Use a mallet and chisel to break the bony roof above the probe
  - Remove the bone fragments to identify the facial n.

- Identify the following (see Figure 28-5B):
  - **Geniculate ganglion of the facial n.** — the facial n. enters the internal acoustic meatus and travels laterally through the petrous portion of the temporal bone into the cavity of the middle ear
    - Within the middle ear, the facial n. turns sharply posterior, forming a knee-shaped bend (genu), in which lies the geniculate (sensory) ganglion of CN VII
  - **Greater petrosal n.** — if the nerve is still intact, follow it posteriorly to the geniculate ganglion

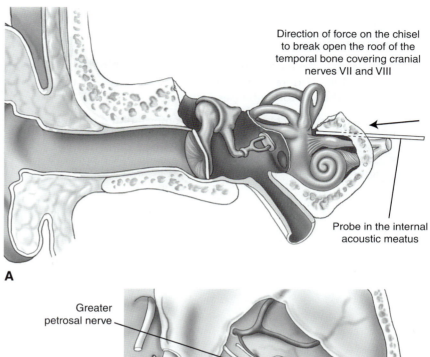

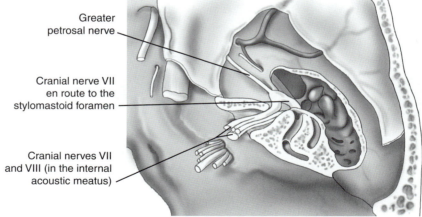

Figure 28-5 Dissection of CN VII and the geniculate ganglion. **A**, Anterior view of a coronal section through the middle ear. **B**, Internal view of the skull base, showing the course of CN VII

Middle Ear Dissection — Auditory Tube

GAFS p 861   ACGA pp 76–77   NAHA Plates 92–98

- To demonstrate the communication between the nasopharynx, middle ear, and mastoid air cells, follow these instructions:

  - Starting from the nasopharynx, push a probe into the auditory tube **(Figure 28-6A)** as far as you can to reveal the course of the auditory tube (see Figure 28-6B)

  - Using a mallet and chisel, extend the removal of the tegmen tympani anteriorly, until you see the tip of the probe

    - Look down at the stapes to identify the tip of the probe to appreciate where the auditory tube is located

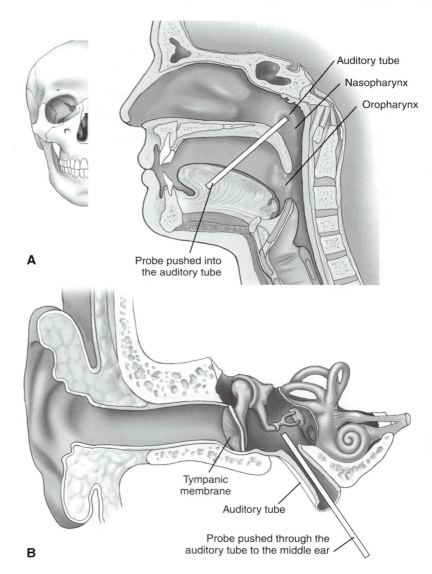

Figure 28-6 Dissection of the auditory tube. **A,** Medial view of a sagittal section through the head. **B,** Anterior view of a coronal section through the ear

Unit 4 Head and Neck Overview

At the end of Unit 4, you should be able to identify the following structures on cadavers, skeletons, and/or radiographs:

Osteology
- Parietal bone
  - Groove for the superior sagittal sinus
  - Grooves for the middle meningeal a.
- Frontal bone
  - Glabella
  - Supraorbital margin
    - Supraorbital foramen
  - Frontal sinus
  - Foramen cecum
- Occipital bone
  - Foramen magnum
  - Basioccipital region
    - Clivus
    - Pharyngeal tubercle
    - Grooves for the inferior petrosal sinuses
  - Occipital condyle
  - Hypoglossal canal
  - Condylar canal
  - Jugular notch (for the jugular foramen)
  - External occipital protuberance
  - Internal occipital crest
  - Internal occipital protuberance
  - Groove for the superior sagittal sinus
  - Grooves for the transverse sinuses
  - Groove for the occipital sinus
- Temporal bone
  - Petrous part
    - Mastoid process
    - Mastoid notch
    - Grooves for the sigmoid sinuses
    - Mastoid foramen
    - Facial canal
    - Carotid canal
    - Canal for the auditory tube
    - Tegmen tympani
    - Hiatus and groove for the greater petrosal n.
    - Internal acoustic meatus
    - Grooves for the inferior petrosal sinuses
    - Jugular notch (for the jugular foramen)
    - Styloid process
    - Stylomastoid foramen
  - External acoustic meatus
  - Groove for the middle meningeal a.
  - Zygomatic process
  - Mandibular fossa
  - Petrotympanic fissure
    - Foramen lacerum
- Sphenoid bone
  - Sella turcica
    - Hypophysial fossa
    - Dorsum sellae
    - Posterior clinoid processes
  - Carotid sulcus
  - Sphenoid sinus
  - Lesser wing
    - Optic canal
    - Anterior clinoid process
    - Supraorbital fissure
  - Greater wing
    - Foramen rotundum
    - Foramen ovale
    - Foramen spinosum
  - Pterygoid process
    - Lateral plate
    - Medial plate
  - Pterygoid notch and fossa
  - Pterygoid hamulus
  - Pterygoid canal
  - Sphenopalatine foramen
  - Inferior orbital fissure
  - Foramen lacerum
  - Sphenoethmoidal recess
- Ethmoid bone
  - Cribriform plate
    - Cribriform foramina
    - Crista galli
    - Perpendicular plate
    - Ethmoidal air cells
    - Anterior and posterior ethmoid foramina
  - Superior nasal concha
    - Superior meatus
  - Middle nasal concha
    - Middle meatus
  - Ethmoidal bulla
  - Uncinate process
  - Hiatus semilunaris
  - Sphenoethmoidal recess
  - Atrium

Continued

Osteology—cont'd

- Inferior nasal concha
  - Inferior meatus
- Lacrimal bone
- Nasal bone
- Vomer
- Zygomatic bone
  - Temporal process
  - Zygomaticofacial foramen
  - Zygomaticotemporal foramen
- Palatine bone
  - Perpendicular plate
    - Sphenopalatine notch
    - Greater and lesser palatine canals
  - Horizontal plate
    - Greater palatine foramen
    - Lesser palatine foramen
- Maxilla
  - Infraorbital foramen and canal
  - Alveolar foramen
  - Maxillary sinus
  - Incisive canal and foramen
  - Pterygomaxillary fissure
  - Anterior nasal spine
  - Palatine process
  - Greater palatine groove
  - Greater palatine foramen
- Mandible
  - Ramus, angle, neck, and body
  - Mental protuberance
  - Mental foramen
  - Oblique line
  - Digastric fossa
  - Superior and inferior mental spines
  - Mylohyoid line
  - Sublingual fossa
  - Mandibular foramen
  - Lingula
  - Mandibular canal
  - Coronoid and condylar processes
  - Mandibular notch
- Hyoid bone
  - Lesser horn
  - Greater horn
- Cranial fossae
  - Anterior
  - Middle
  - Posterior
- Sutures and landmarks
  - Sagittal
  - Coronal
  - Pterion
  - Lambdoidal
  - Squamous
  - Bregma/lambda
- Auditory ossicles
  - Malleus, incus, stapes
- Vertebral column
  - C1 (atlas)
  - C2 (axis)
    - Odontoid process (dens)
  - Transverse foramina
- Sternum
  - Manubrium
    - Jugular notch
- Clavicle
- Scapula
  - Acromion
  - Superior angle of the scapula

Joints

- Atlanto-occipital joint
- Atlantoaxial joint
- Temporomandibular joint
- Cricothyroid joint

Ligaments

- Cruciate ligament
  - Superior and inferior longitudinal bands
  - Transverse ligament of atlas (C1)
- Alar ligaments
- Sphenomandibular ligament
- Stylomandibular ligament

Muscles

- Trapezius m.
- Splenius capitis m.
- Levator scapulae m.
- Muscles of the neck
  - Platysma m.
  - Longus colli m.
  - Longus capitis m.
  - Scalene mm.
    - Anterior, middle, and posterior
  - Sternocleidomastoid m.
  - Suboccipital muscles
    - Rectus capitis lateralis m.
  - Suprahyoid muscles
    - Digastric m.
      - Anterior belly
      - Posterior belly
    - Stylohyoid m.
    - Mylohyoid m.
    - Geniohyoid m.
  - Infrahyoid muscles
    - Sternohyoid m.
    - Omohyoid m.
      - Superior belly
      - Inferior belly
    - Sternothyroid m.
    - Thyrohyoid m.
  - Prevertebral muscles

- Longus colli m.
- Rectus capitis anterior m.
- Longus capitis m.
- Muscles of mastication
  - Masseter m.
  - Temporalis m.
  - Lateral pterygoid m.
  - Medial pterygoid m.
- Facial muscles
  - Occipitofrontalis m.
  - Procerus m.
  - Nasalis m.
  - Orbicularis oculi m.
    - Palpebral part
    - Orbital part
  - Corrugator supercilii m.
  - Auricularis mm.
  - Orbicularis oris m.
- Depressor anguli oris m.
- Risorius m.
- Zygomaticus major m.
- Zygomaticus minor m.
  - Levator labii superioris m.
  - Levator labii superioris alaeque nasi m.
  - Depressor labii inferioris m.
  - Levator anguli oris m.
  - Buccinator m.
  - Mentalis m.
- Extraocular muscles and associated structures
  - Levator palpebrae superioris m.
  - Superior and inferior oblique mm.
  - Medial, lateral, superior, and inferior rectus mm.
  - Common tendinous ring
  - Trochlea
- Muscles of the soft palate
  - Levator veli palatini m.
  - Tensor veli palatini m.
- Musculus uvulae m.
- Palatoglossus m.
- Palatopharyngeus m.
- Structures associated with the palate
  - Uvula
  - Palatoglossal arch
  - Palatopharyngeal arch
  - Palatine aponeurosis
- Pharyngeal muscles and related structures
  - Superior, middle, and inferior pharyngeal constrictor mm.
  - Stylopharyngeus m.
  - Salpingopharyngeus m.
  - Palatopharyngeus m.
  - Buccopharyngeal fascia
  - Pharyngeal raphe
  - Pterygomandibular raphe
- Muscles of the tongue
  - Genioglossal m.
  - Hyoglossus m.
  - Styloglossus m.
  - Superior and inferior longitudinal and oblique mm.
  - Palatoglossus m.
- Intrinsic muscles of the larynx
  - Cricothyroid m.
  - Posterior cricoarytenoid m.
  - Lateral cricoarytenoid m.
  - Vocalis m.
  - Thyroarytenoid m.
  - Oblique arytenoid m.
  - Transverse arytenoid m.

Nerves

- 12 pairs of cranial nerves (CN)
  - Olfactory n. (CN I)
  - Optic n. (CN II)
  - Oculomotor n. (CN III)
    - Branch to the ciliary ganglion (parasympathetic root of the ciliary ganglion)
    - Long (sensory) and short (parasympathetic) ciliary nn.
  - Trochlear n. (CN IV)
  - Trigeminal n. (CN V)
    - Motor root
    - Sensory root
      - Trigeminal ganglion
    - V-1 — ophthalmic division of the trigeminal n.
      - Lacrimal n.
      - Frontal n.
        - Supraorbital n.
        - Supratrochlear n.
      - Nasociliary n.
      - External nasal n.
      - Anterior and posterior ethmoidal nn.
      - Infratrochlear n.
    - V-2 — maxillary division of the trigeminal n.
      - Pterygopalatine ganglion
      - Nasopalatine n.
      - Greater and lesser palatine nn.
      - Superior, middle, and posterior superior alveolar nn.
      - Zygomatic n.
        - Zygomaticotemporal n.
        - Zygomaticofacial n.
      - Infraorbital n.
    - V-3 — mandibular division of the trigeminal n.
      - Meningeal n.
      - Nerves to the masseter and medial and lateral pterygoid mm.
      - Deep temporal nn.
      - Buccal n.
      - Auriculotemporal n.
        - Superficial temporal nn.

Continued

Nerves—cont'd

- 12 pairs of cranial nerves (CN)—cont'd
  - V-3 — mandibular division of the trigeminal n.—cont'd
    - Lingual n.
    - Inferior alveolar n.
      - Nerve to the mylohyoid m.
      - Inferior dental plexus
  - Abducens n. (CN VI)
  - Facial n. (CN VII)
    - Posterior auricular n.
    - Temporal branch(es)
    - Zygomatic branch(es)
    - Buccal branch(es)
    - Mandibular branch(es)
    - Cervical branches
    - Intermediate n.
      - Geniculate ganglion
      - Greater petrosal n. (parasympathetic root to the pterygopalatine ganglion)
        - Joins with the deep petrosal (sympathetic) nerve to become the nerve of the pterygoid canal (Vidian n.)
      - Chorda tympani n. (carries the parasympathetic root to the submandibular ganglion)
  - Vestibulocochlear n. (CN XIII)
  - Glossopharyngeal n. (CN IX)
    - Carotid body
    - Lesser petrosal n. (parasympathetic root to the otic ganglion)
  - Vagus n. (CN X)
    - Superior ganglion of the vagus n.
    - Inferior ganglion of the vagus n.
    - Pharyngeal n.
    - Superior laryngeal n.
      - Internal laryngeal n.
      - External laryngeal n.
    - Right and left recurrent laryngeal nn.
  - Spinal accessory n. (CN XI)
  - Hypoglossal n. (CN XII)
- Cervical plexus
  - Ansa cervicalis
    - Superior and inferior roots
  - Lesser occipital n.
  - Great auricular n.
  - Transverse cervical n.
  - Supraclavicular nn.
  - Phrenic n.
- Brachial plexus
  - Suprascapular n.
- Autonomics
  - Sympathetic
    - Superior cervical sympathetic ganglion
      - Deep petrosal n. (sympathetic root)
    - Middle cervical sympathetic ganglion
    - Inferior cervical sympathetic ganglion
  - Parasympathetic
    - Oculomotor n. (CN III)
    - Facial n. (CN VII)
    - Glossopharyngeal n. (CN IX)
    - Vagus n. (CN X)

Arteries

- Common carotid a.
  - Carotid body
- Common carotid a.
  - External carotid a.
    - Superior thyroid a.
      - Superior laryngeal a.
    - Ascending pharyngeal a.
    - Lingual a.
      - Sublingual a.
      - Deep lingual a.
    - Facial a.
      - Submental a.
      - Superior labial a.
      - Inferior labial a.
      - Angular a.
    - Occipital a.
    - Posterior auricular a.
    - Superficial temporal a.
      - Transverse facial a.
    - Maxillary a.
      - Inferior alveolar a.
      - Middle meningeal a.
      - Masseteric a.
      - Deep temporal aa.
      - Buccal a.
      - Posterior superior alveolar a.
      - Infraorbital a.
      - Anterior and middle superior alveolar aa.
      - Descending palatine a.
      - Greater and lesser palatine aa.
      - Sphenopalatine a.
      - Posterior lateral nasal aa.
      - Posterior septal aa. (superior, middle, inferior)
- Common carotid a.
  - Internal carotid a.
    - Carotid sinus
    - Ophthalmic a.
      - Central retinal a.
      - Lacrimal a.
      - Ciliary aa. (long and short)
      - Supraorbital a.
      - Anterior and posterior ethmoidal aa.
      - Supratrochlear a.
  - Subclavian a.
    - Thyrocervical trunk
      - Transverse cervical a.
      - Suprascapular a.
      - Inferior thyroid a.
    - Vertebral a.
    - Costocervical trunk
      - Supreme intercostal a.
      - Deep cervical a.

- Cerebral arterial circle (of Willis)
  - Internal carotid a.
    - Anterior cerebral a.
    - Anterior communicating a.
    - Middle cerebral a.
    - Posterior communicating a.
  - Basilar a.
    - Posterior cerebral a.
  - Vertebral a.
    - Posterior meningeal a.
    - Posterior inferior cerebellar a.
    - Posterior spinal a.
    - Anterior spinal a.
  - Basilar a.
    - Anterior inferior cerebellar a.
    - Labyrinthine a.
    - Pontine aa.
    - Superior cerebellar a.
    - Posterior cerebral a.
- Subclavian a.
  - Vertebral a.
  - Thyrocervical trunk
    - Inferior thyroid a.
      - Inferior laryngeal a.
    - Ascending cervical a.
    - Suprascapular a.
    - Transverse cervical a.
      - Superficial cervical a.
      - Dorsal scapular a.
  - Costocervical trunk
    - Deep cervical a.

Lymphatics
- Submental lymph nodes
- Submandibular lymph nodes
- Superficial cervical lymph nodes
- Deep cervical lymph nodes
- Thoracic lymphatic duct

- Palatine tonsil
- Lingual tonsils
- Pharyngeal tonsils (adenoids)

Veins
- Superior vena cava
  - Brachiocephalic v.
    - Inferior thyroid v.
    - Inferior laryngeal v.
    - Vertebral v.
    - Deep cervical v.
  - Internal jugular v.
    - Superior bulb of the jugular v.
    - Superior thyroid v.
    - Middle thyroid v.
    - Superior laryngeal v.
    - Facial v.
      - Supratrochlear, supraorbital, superior labial, inferior labial, and deep facial vv.
    - Retromandibular v.
      - Superficial temporal, middle, temporal, transverse facial, and maxillary vv.
      - Pterygoid plexus of veins
  - External jugular v.
    - Posterior auricular v.
    - Anterior jugular v.
      - Jugular venous arch
    - Suprascapular v.
    - Transverse cervical v.
- Cerebral veins
  - Superficial cerebral vv.
  - Deep cerebral vv.
  - Veins of the brainstem
  - Cerebellar vv.
- Orbital veins
  - Superior ophthalmic v.
  - Ciliary vv.
  - Central vein of the retina
  - Inferior ophthalmic v.

Dural Venous Sinuses
- Superior sagittal sinus
- Inferior sagittal sinus
- Straight sinus
- Transverse sinuses
- Occipital sinus
- Confluence of sinuses
- Sigmoid sinuses
- Inferior petrosal sinuses
- Superior petrosal sinuses
- Basilar plexus
- Cavernous sinuses
- Sphenoparietal sinus

Pharynx
- Nasopharynx
  - Choanae
  - Pharyngeal tonsil
  - Openings of the auditory tubes
  - Torus tubarius
    - Salpingopharyngeal fold
    - Salpingopalatine fold
- Oropharynx
  - Epiglottic vallecula
- Laryngopharynx
  - Piriform recess/fossa
    - Fold over the superior laryngeal n.
  - Pharyngobasilar fascia
- Pharyngeal muscles (see previously)

Glands
- Thyroid gland
  - Right lobe, left lobe, and isthmus

Continued

Glands—cont'd
- Parathyroid glands
- Submandibular glands
- Parotid glands (parotid ducts)
  - Sublingual glands

Tongue
- Frenulum
- Filiform papillae
- Fungiform papillae
- Vallate papillae
- Sulcus terminalis
- Foramen cecum
- Lingual tonsil
- Median and lateral glossoepiglottic folds
- Vallecula
- Extrinsic muscles of the tongue (see previously)
- Plica sublingualis

Larynx
- Laryngeal inlet
  - Aryepiglottic fold
  - Vestibular folds (false vocal cords)
  - Glottis
    - Vocal folds (true vocal cords)
      - Rima glottis
  - Quadrangular membrane
    - Vestibular ligament
    - Vocal ligament
- Laryngeal skeleton
  - Thyroid cartilage
    - Laryngeal prominence
    - Superior and inferior horns
  - Cricoid cartilage
  - Arytenoid cartilages
  - Corniculate cartilages
  - Cuneiform cartilages
- Thyrohyoid membrane
- Cricothyroid ligament
- Intrinsic muscles of the larynx (see previously)

Eye and Related Structures
- Sclera and cornea
- Choroid
  - Ciliary body
    - Ciliary mm. (meridional fibers)
- Iris and pupil
- Retina
- Central artery and vein of the retina
- Lens
- Chambers of the eyeball
  - Aqueous humor
    - Anterior and posterior chambers
  - Vitreous body
    - Vitreous chamber
- Periorbita
- Conjunctiva
- Lacrimal glands (nasolacrimal ducts)
- Tarsal glands
- Extraocular muscles (see previously)

Brain
- Cerebrum
  - Frontal, temporal, and occipital poles
  - Frontal, temporal, parietal, and occipital lobes
  - Lateral sulcus and central sulcus
  - Cerebral gyri and sulci
- Corpus callosum
- Diencephalon
- Midbrain
- Pons
- Medulla oblongata
- Cerebellum and vermis
- Ventricular system
  - Lateral ventricles
    - Interventricular foramen
  - Third ventricle
    - Cerebral aqueduct
  - Fourth ventricle
  - Central canal

Ear
- Outer ear
  - Auricle; pinna
  - Lobule
  - Helix
  - Antihelix
    - Triangular fossa
  - Scapha and concha of the auricle
  - Antitragus and tragus
  - External auditory canal
  - Tympanic membrane
- Middle ear
  - Tegmen tympani
    - Epitympanic recess
  - Mastoid antrum
    - Mastoid air cells
  - Auditory ossicles
    - Malleus, incus, and stapes
  - Muscles of the auditory ossicles
    - Stapedius m.
    - Tensor tympani m.
  - Auditory tube

- Tympanic opening
- Bony and cartilaginous parts
- Inner ear
  - Vestibule
  - Semicircular canals
  - Cochlea
  - Internal acoustic meatus

Meninges
- Dura mater
  - Falx cerebri and cerebelli
  - Tentorium cerebelli
- Arachnoid mater
  - Subarachnoid space
  - Arachnoid granulations (villi)
- Pia mater

Fascia/Membranes
- Cervical fascia
  - Investing fascia; superficial fascia
  - Pretracheal fascia
  - Prevertebral fascia
  - Carotid sheath
- Alar fascia
- Palatine aponeurosis
- Pterygomandibular raphe
- Retropharyngeal space
- Thyrohyoid membrane
- Cricothyroid membrane
- Tectorial membrane
- Buccopharyngeal fascia
- Parotid fascia
- Temporal fascia

Miscellaneous
- Buccal fat pad
- Triangles of the neck
  - Anterior triangle of the neck
    - Muscular triangle
    - Submandibular triangle
    - Submental triangle
    - Carotid triangle
  - Posterior triangle of the neck
    - Supraclavicular triangle
    - Suboccipital triangle
    - Interscalene triangle

Unit 5
Upper Limb

The purpose of this unit is to learn the anatomic structure of the upper limb through dissection.

Lab 29 Osteology of the Upper Limb 425

Lab 30 Superficial Structures of the Upper Limb, Shoulder, and Axilla 435

Lab 31 Arm 454

Lab 32 Forearm 466

Lab 33 Hand 477

Lab 34 Joints of the Upper Limb 490

Unit 5 Upper Limb Overview 498

Muscles of the Upper Limb

Muscle	Proximal Attachment	Distal Attachment	Action	Innervation
Subclavius	Rib 1 and costal cartilage	Inferior medial surface of the clavicle	Depresses the clavicle; stabilizes the sternoclavicular joint	Nerve to the subclavius (C5–C6)
Trapezius	Occipital bone, nuchal ligament, C7–T12 vertebrae	Spine, acromion, and lateral end of the clavicle	Acts as powerful elevator of the scapula; middle fibers retract the scapula; lower fibers depress the scapula	Spinal accessory n. and C3 and C4 spinal nerves
Latissimus dorsi	Spinous processes of vertebrae T7–T12, sacrum, thoracolumbar fascia	Intertubercular groove of the humerus	Adducts, extends, and medially rotates the humerus at the glenohumeral joint	Thoracodorsal n. (C6–C8)
Levator scapulae	Transverse processes of C1–C4 vertebrae	Superior angle of the scapula	Elevates the scapula	Dorsal scapular n. (C5) and C3 and C4 spinal nerves
Rhomboid minor	Spinous processes of C7–T1 vertebrae	Medial margin of the scapula	Retract and elevate the scapula	Dorsal scapular n. (C4–C5)
Rhomboid major	Spinous processes of T2–T5 vertebrae	Medial margin of the scapula	Retract and elevate the scapula	Dorsal scapular n. (C4–C5)
Serratus anterior	External and lateral surfaces of ribs 1–8	Medial margin of the scapula	Protracts and rotates the scapula; keeps the scapula opposed to the thoracic wall	Long thoracic n. (C5–C7)
Pectoralis major	Clavicle, sternum, and costal cartilage	Intertubercular groove of the humerus (lateral lip)	Adducts, medially rotates, extends, and flexes the humerus	Medial and lateral pectoral nn. (C5–T1)
Pectoralis minor	Ribs 3–5	Coracoid process of the scapula	Protracts the scapula; pulls the tip of the shoulder down	Medial pectoral n. (C6–C8)
Deltoid	Spine, acromion, and lateral end of the clavicle	Deltoid tuberosity of the humerus	Flexes, abducts, and extends the humerus	Axillary n. (C5–C6)

Muscles of the Upper Limb—cont'd

Muscle	Proximal Attachment	Distal Attachment	Action	Innervation
Supraspinatus	Supraspinous fossa	Greater tubercle of the humerus	Stabilizes the shoulder joint and abducts the humerus to 15 degrees at the glenohumeral joint	Suprascapular n. (C5–C6)
Infraspinatus	Infraspinous fossa		Stabilizes the shoulder joint and laterally rotates the humerus	Suprascapular n. (C5–C6)
Teres minor	Lateral margin of the scapula		Stabilizes the shoulder joint and laterally rotates the humerus	Axillary n. (C5–C6)
Teres major	Inferior angle of the scapula	Intertubercular groove of the humerus (lateral lip)	Medially rotates and extends the humerus at the glenohumeral joint	Lower subscapular n. (C5–C7)
Subscapularis	Subscapular fossa	Lesser tubercle of the humerus	Stabilizes the shoulder joint and medially rotates the humerus	Upper and lower subscapular nn. (C5–C7)
Biceps brachii	Long head: supraglenoid tubercle Short head: coracoid process	Radial tuberosity	Flexes and supinates the elbow	Musculocutaneous n. (C5–C6)
Brachialis	Anterior aspect of the humerus	Tuberosity of the ulna	Flexes the elbow	
Coracobrachialis	Coracoid process of the scapula	Medial surface of the humerus	Flexes and adducts the humerus	Musculocutaneous n. (C5–C7)
Triceps brachii	Long head: infraglenoid tubercle Lateral head: posterior surface of the humerus Medial head: posterior surface of the humerus	Olecranon process of the ulna	Extends the elbow and extends and adducts the arm at the shoulder joint	Radial n. (C6–C8)
Anconeus	Lateral epicondyle of the humerus	Olecranon process of the ulna	Extends the elbow	Radial n. (C7–T1)
Pronator teres	Medial epicondyle of the humerus	Middle of the lateral surface of the radius	Pronates and flexes the elbow	Median n. (C6–C7)
Flexor carpi radialis		Base of the second metacarpal bone	Flexes and abducts the wrist	

Continued

Muscles of the Upper Limb—cont'd

Muscle	Proximal Attachment	Distal Attachment	Action	Innervation
Palmaris longus	Medial epicondyle of the humerus	Flexor retinaculum and palmar aponeurosis	Flexes the wrist and tightens the palmar aponeurosis	Median n. (C7–C8)
Flexor carpi ulnaris	Medial epicondyle and olecranon process	Pisiform, hamate, and fifth metacarpal bones	Flexes and adducts the wrist	Ulnar n. (C7–T1)
Flexor digitorum superficialis	Medial epicondyle, coronoid process of the ulna, and anterior border of the radius	Bodies of the middle phalanx of digits 2–5	Flexes the wrist, metacarpophalangeal joints, and proximal interphalangeal joints	Median n. (C8–T1)
Flexor digitorum profundus	Proximal three fourths of the medial surfaces of the ulna and interosseous membrane	Distal phalanx of digits 2–5	Flexes the wrist and distal interphalangeal joints	Medial part: ulnar n. (C8–T1) Lateral part: median n. via the anterior interosseous n. (C8–T1)
Flexor pollicis longus	Anterior surface of the radius	Distal phalanx of digit 1	Flexes the thumb	Anterior interosseous n. from the median n. (C7–C8)
Pronator quadratus	Distal anterior surface of the ulna	Distal anterior surface of the radius	Pronates the elbow	
Brachioradialis	Lateral supracondylar ridge of the humerus	Styloid process of the radius	Flexes the elbow	Radial n. (C5–C6)
Extensor carpi radialis longus		Base of the second metacarpal bone	Extends and abducts the wrist	Radial n. (C6–C7)
Extensor carpi radialis brevis	Lateral epicondyle of the humerus	Base of the third metacarpal bone	Extends the wrist	Posterior interosseous n. (C7–C8), the continuation of the deep branch of the radial n.
Extensor digitorum		Extensor expansion of digits 2–5	Extends the wrist and fingers	
Extensor digiti minimi		Extensor expansion of digit 5	Extends digit 5	
Extensor carpi ulnaris		Base of the fifth metacarpal bone	Extends and adducts the wrist	

Muscles of the Upper Limb—cont'd

Muscle	Proximal Attachment	Distal Attachment	Action	Innervation
Supinator	Lateral epicondyle and supinator crest of the ulna	Distal to the radial tuberosity	Supinates the forearm	Deep branch of the radial n. (C6–C7)
Abductor pollicis longus	Posterior surface of the ulna, radius, and interosseous membrane	Base of the first metacarpal bone	Abducts and extends the thumb	Posterior interosseous n. (C7–C8), the continuation of the deep branch of the radial n. (C7–C8)
Extensor pollicis brevis	Posterior surface of the radius and interosseous membrane	Base of the proximal phalanx of digit 1	Extends the thumb at the carpometacarpal joint	
Extensor pollicis longus	Posterior surface of the ulna and interosseous membrane	Distal phalanx of digit 1	Extends the thumb	
Extensor indicis		Extensor expansion of digit 2	Extends digit 2	
Palmaris brevis	Palmar aponeurosis and flexor retinaculum	Dermis on the ulnar side of the hand	Tenses the skin over the hypothenar muscles	Ulnar n., superficial branch (C8–T1)
Thenar muscles of the hand				
• Abductor pollicis brevis	Flexor retinaculum and tubercles of the scaphoid and trapezium bones	Base of the proximal phalanx of digit 1	Abducts and opposes the thumb	Median n., recurrent branch (C8–T1)
• Flexor pollicis brevis			Flexes the thumb	
• Opponens pollicis		Base of the first metacarpal bone	Opposes the thumb to the other digits	
Adductor pollicis	Oblique head: base of the second and third metacarpal bones, capitate bone Transverse head: palmar surface of the third metacarpal bone	Base of the proximal phalanx of digit 1	Adducts the thumb	Ulnar n., deep branch (C8–T1)

Continued

Muscles of the Upper Limb—cont'd

Muscle	Proximal Attachment	Distal Attachment	Action	Innervation
Hypothenar muscles of the hand				
• Abductor digiti minimi	Pisiform bone	Proximal phalanx of digit 5	Abducts digit 5	Ulnar n., deep branch (C8–T1)
• Flexor digiti minimi brevis	Hook of the hamate bone and flexor retinaculum		Flexes the proximal phalanx of digit 5	
• Opponens digiti minimi		Fifth metacarpal	Opposes digit 5 to the thumb	
Lumbricals 1 and 2	Lateral two tendons of the flexor digitorum profundus m.	Lateral sides of the extensor expansion for digits 2–5	Flex the metacarpophalangeal joints and extend the interphalangeal joints	Median n. (C8–T1)
Lumbricals 3 and 4	Medial two tendons of the flexor digitorum profundus m.			Ulnar n. (C8–T1)
Dorsal interossei 1–4	Adjacent sides of two metacarpals	Extensor expansion and base of the proximal phalanges of digits 2–4	Abducts the digits	Ulnar n., deep branch (C8–T1)
Palmar interossei 1–3	Anterior surface of metacarpals 2, 4, and 5	Extensor expansion of the digits and proximal phalanges 2, 4, and 5	Adducts the digits	

Osteology of the Upper Limb

Lab 29

Prior to dissection, you should familiarize yourself with the following structures:

OSTEOLOGY
- Clavicle
  - Acromial and sternal ends
  - Conoid tubercle
- Scapula
  - Subscapular fossa
  - Spine
  - Supraspinous fossa
  - Infraspinous fossa
  - Acromion
  - Medial and lateral borders
  - Superior angle
    - Suprascapular notch
  - Inferior angle
  - Glenoid cavity
  - Supraglenoid and infraglenoid tubercles
  - Coracoid process
- Humerus
  - Head
  - Anatomic and surgical necks
  - Greater and lesser tubercles
  - Intertubercular (bicipital) groove
  - Radial groove
  - Deltoid tuberosity
  - Lateral and medial supracondylar ridges
  - Lateral and medial epicondyles
  - Trochlea
  - Capitulum
  - Coronoid and olecranon fossae
- Radius
  - Head
  - Neck
  - Radial tuberosity
  - Interosseous border
  - Radial styloid process
  - Ulnar notch
- Ulna
  - Olecranon
  - Coronoid process
    - Radial notch
  - Trochlear notch
  - Interosseous border
  - Supinator crest
  - Ulnar head
    - Ulnar styloid process
- Hand
  - Carpals (8)
    - Proximal row
      - Pisiform
      - Triquetrum
      - Lunate
      - Scaphoid
    - Distal row
      - Trapezium
      - Trapezoid
      - Capitate
      - Hamate
        - Hook of the hamate
  - Metacarpals (5)
  - Phalanges (14)
    - Proximal, middle, and distal phalanges

Lab 29 Dissection Overview

The purpose of this laboratory session is to learn the osteology of the upper limb through dissection. You will do so through the following suggested sequence:

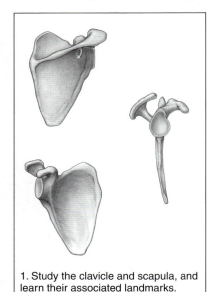

1. Study the clavicle and scapula, and learn their associated landmarks.

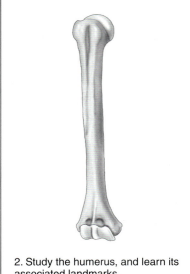

2. Study the humerus, and learn its associated landmarks.

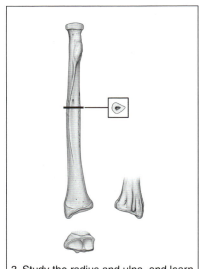

3. Study the radius and ulna, and learn their associated landmarks.

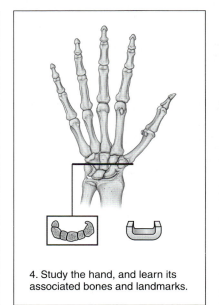

4. Study the hand, and learn its associated bones and landmarks.

Table 29-1 Osteology of the Upper Limb

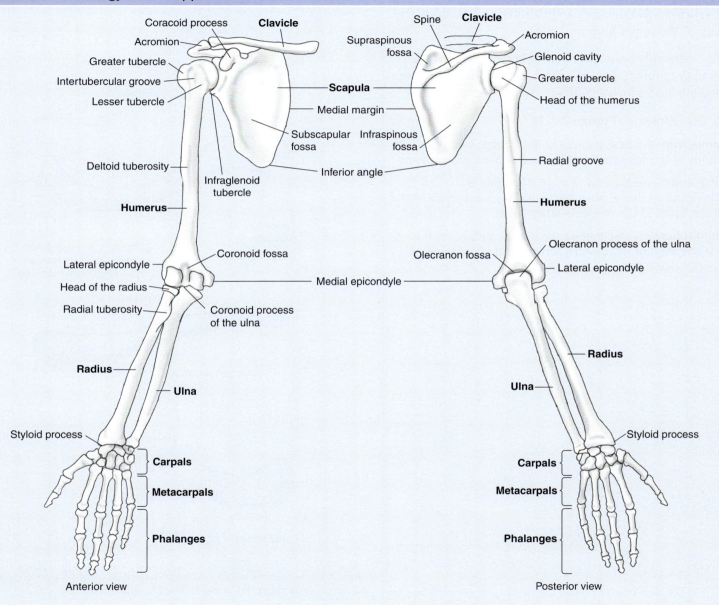

Upper Limb Osteology — Clavicle

- Use an articulated skeleton or individual bones to study the osteology of the upper limb

- Clavicle — the only bony attachment between the trunk and the upper limb; S shaped, with a forward-facing convex part medially and a forward-facing concave part laterally

- Identify the following **(Figure 29-1)**:
  - **Acromial end** — lateral, flat end of the clavicle; articulates with the spine of the scapula, forming the acromioclavicular joint
  - **Sternal end** — medial end of the clavicle that is quadrangular in shape; articulates with the manubrium of the sternum, forming the sternoclavicular joint
  - **Conoid tubercle** — located on the inferior surface on the lateral one third of the clavicle; serves as an attachment for the coracoclavicular joint

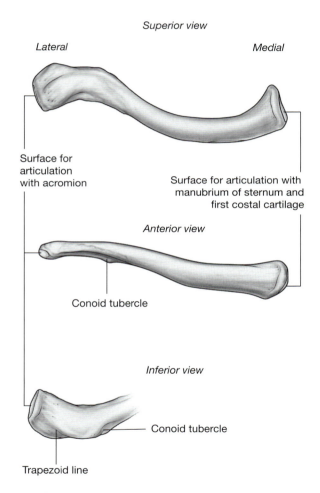

Figure 29-1 Clavicle. (Redrawn from Drake R, Vogl W, Mitchell A: Gray's Anatomy for Students. Philadelphia: Elsevier, 2005, Fig. 7.20)

Upper Limb Osteology — Scapula

- **Scapula** — a large, flat triangular bone; identify the following landmarks **(Figure 29-2)**:

  - **Lateral border** — lateral edge of the scapula; also known as the axillary border

  - **Glenoid cavity** — shallow, comma-shaped fossa that articulates with the head of the humerus to form the glenohumeral joint

  - **Infraglenoid tubercle** — triangular-shaped roughening inferior to the glenoid cavity; attachment for the long head of the triceps brachii m.

  - **Supraglenoid tubercle** — a less distinct roughening superior to the glenoid cavity; attachment for the long head of the biceps brachii m.

  - **Spine** — subdivides the posterior surface of the scapula into a small, superior supraspinous fossa and a larger, inferior infraspinous fossa

  - **Acromion** — anterolateral projection of the spine; arches over the glenohumeral joint and articulates, via a small oval facet on its distal end, with the clavicle

  - **Greater scapular notch (spinoglenoid notch)** — a notch between the lateral angle of the scapula and the attachment of the spine to the posterior surface of the scapula

  - **Subscapular fossa** — also known as the costal surface; characterized by a shallow concave space over much of its extent

  - **Coracoid process** — a hooklike structure that projects anterolaterally and is positioned directly inferior to the lateral part of the clavicle

  - **Suprascapular notch** — medial to the coracoid process

  - **Medial border** — medial edge of the scapula; also known as the vertebral border

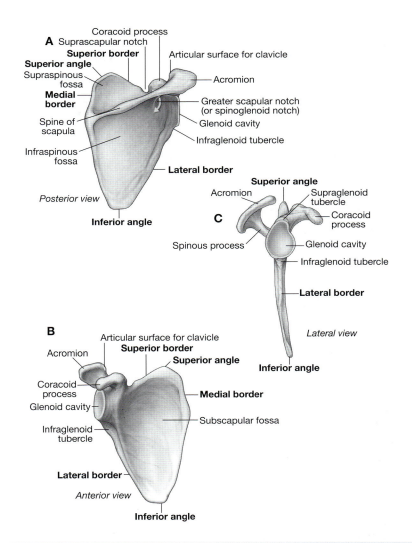

Figure 29-2 Scapula. **A,** Posterior view. **B,** Anterior view. **C,** Lateral view. (Redrawn from Drake R, Vogl W, Mitchell A: Gray's Anatomy for Students. Philadelphia: Elsevier, 2005, Fig. 7.21)

Upper Limb Osteology — Humerus

- **Humerus** — the long bone of the arm; identify the following landmarks **(Figure 29-3)**:
  - **Head** — half-spherical in shape; projects medially and somewhat superiorly to articulate with the glenoid cavity of the scapula
  - **Anatomical neck** — short, narrow constriction immediately distal to the humeral head
  - **Greater tubercle** — proximal and lateral; serves as attachment site for the rotator cuff muscles (supraspinatus m., infraspinatus m., and teres minor m.)
  - **Lesser tubercle** — proximal and anterior; serves as attachment site for the subscapularis m.
  - **Intertubercular (bicipital) groove** — a narrow groove that separates the greater and lesser tubercles; the tendon of the long head of the biceps brachii m. passes through this groove
  - **Surgical neck** — between the head, anatomical neck, and tubercles of the humerus and the narrower shaft; the axillary n. and posterior humeral circumflex a. pass posterior to the surgical neck
  - **Deltoid tuberosity** — V-shaped protrusion on the lateral surface of the humerus midway along its length where the deltoid muscle inserts on the humerus
  - **Radial groove** — posterior surface of the humerus; the radial n. and deep brachial a. lie in this groove
  - **Capitulum** — distal end of the humerus; lateral and oval in shape; articulates with the radius
  - **Trochlea** — distal end of the humerus; medial and pulley shaped; articulates with the ulna
  - **Coronoid fossa** — distal end of the humerus; superior to the trochlea on the anterior surface of the humerus

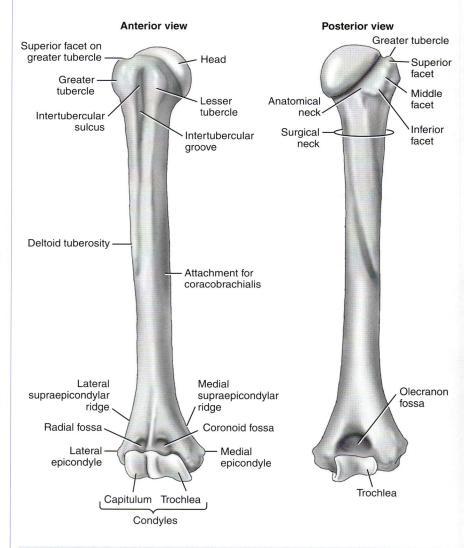

Figure 29-3 Humerus. (Redrawn from Drake R, Vogl W, Mitchell A: Gray's Anatomy for Students. Philadelphia: Elsevier, 2005, Figs. 7.22, 7.60)

Upper Limb Osteology — Humerus—cont'd

- **Olecranon fossa** — distal end of the humerus; superior to the trochlea on the posterior surface of the humerus

- **Medial epicondyle** — distal end of the humerus; large, bony protuberance on the medial side of the elbow; serves for muscle attachment in the anterior compartment of the forearm

- **Lateral epicondyle** — distal end of the humerus; on the lateral side of the elbow; not as large as the medial epicondyle; serves for muscle attachment in the posterior compartment of the forearm

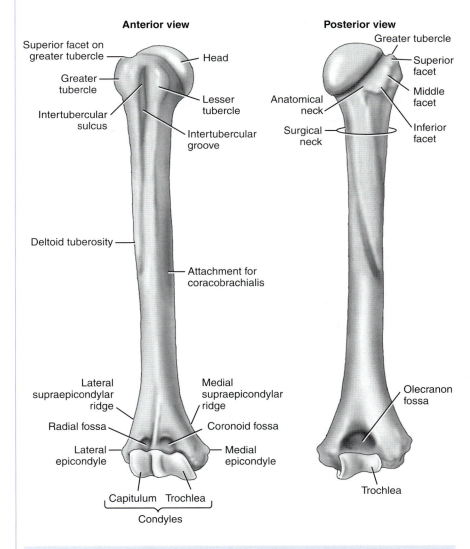

Figure 29-3 Humerus. (Redrawn from Drake R, Vogl W, Mitchell A: Gray's Anatomy for Students. Philadelphia: Elsevier, 2005, Figs. 7.22, 7.60)

Upper Limb Osteology — Radius and Ulna

■ Identify the following bones and landmarks **(Figure 29-4)**:

- **Radius** — in the anatomic position, the radius is the lateral bone of the forearm; articulates with the ulna

  - **Head of the radius** — thick, disc-shaped structure on the proximal end of the radius

  - **Neck of the radius** — short and narrow cylinder of bone

  - **Radial tuberosity** — a large, blunt projection on the medial surface of the radius inferior to the neck; serves as insertion for the biceps brachii m.

  - **Interosseous crest** — attachment for the interosseous membrane

  - **Styloid process of the radius** — attachment for the brachioradialis m.

  - **Ulnar notch** — a notch on the medial, distal surface of the radius for articulation with the ulna

- **Ulna** — in the anatomic position, the ulna is the medial bone of the forearm; articulates with the radius

  - **Olecranon process** — large projection that extends proximally from the ulna; contributes to the trochlear notch; articulates with the humerus in the olecranon fossa

  - **Coronoid process** — projects anteriorly from the proximal end of the ulna; contributes to the trochlear notch

  - **Trochlear notch** — formed by the olecranon and coronoid processes; articulates with the trochlea on the humerus

  - **Radial notch** — articulates with the head of the radius

  - **Supinator crest** — a crest on the proximal, lateral surface of the ulna that serves as an attachment for the supinator m.

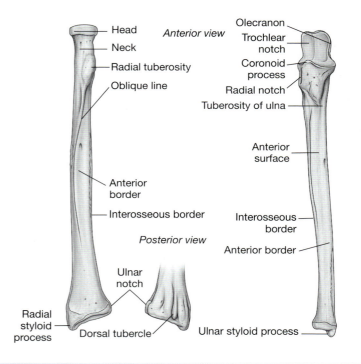

Figure 29-4 Radius and ulna. (Redrawn from Drake R, Vogl W, Mitchell A: Gray's Anatomy for Students. Philadelphia: Elsevier, 2005, Figs. 7.77, 7.78)

Upper Limb Osteology — Hand

- Hand — subdivided into the wrist (carpus), metacarpus, and digits

- The carpal bones form an arch; the flexor retinaculum (transverse carpal ligament) spans the distance between the medial and lateral ends of the bony arch to form the carpal tunnel

- Identify the following bones and landmarks of the carpus **(Figure 29-5)**:

  • **Carpal bones — Proximal row;** lateral to medial
    • **Scaphoid** — boat shaped; has a prominent tubercle on its lateral, palmar surface
    • **Lunate** — crescent shaped
    • **Triquetrum** — three-sided bone
    • **Pisiform** — pea-shaped sesamoid bone in the tendon of the flexor carpi ulnaris m.; articulates with the triquetrum

  • **Carpal bones — Distal row;** lateral to medial
    • **Trapezium** — irregular, four-sided bone that articulates with the metacarpal bone of the thumb; has a prominent tubercle
    • **Trapezoid** — four-sided bone
    • **Capitate** — bone with a head; largest of the carpal bones; articulates with the base of the third metacarpal
    • **Hamate** — bone with a hook; positioned lateral and distal to the pisiform bone; has a prominent hook (hook of hamate) on its palmar surface

GAFS pp 708–710   ACGA pp 247, 256, 266, 270   NAHA Plates 452, 456

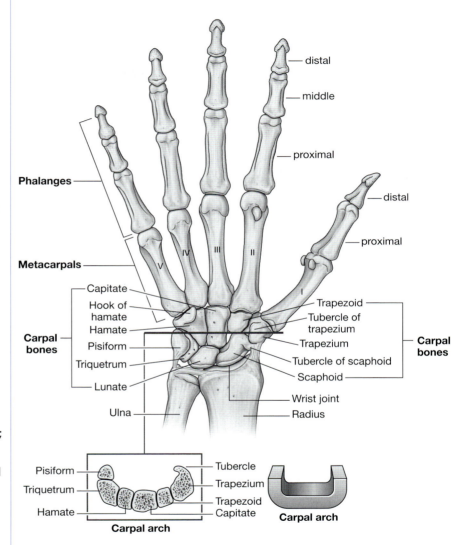

Figure 29-5   Hand. (Redrawn from Drake R, Vogl W, Mitchell A: Gray's Anatomy for Students. Philadelphia: Elsevier, 2005, Fig. 7.91A)

Upper Limb Osteology — Hand Continued

Upper Limb Osteology — Hand—cont'd

- Each of the five metacarpal bones consists of a base (proximal end), shaft, and head (distal end); all of the bases articulate with the carpal bones and the heads each relate to one digit (see Figure 29-5):
  - **Metacarpal 1** is related to the thumb
  - **Metacarpals 2 to 5** are related to the index, middle, ring, and little fingers, respectively
- Identify the following regarding the digits (phalanges):
  - The **phalanges** are the bones of the digits and consist of the following:
    - Thumb — two phalanges; a proximal and a distal phalanx
    - Digits 2 through 5 — three phalanges; a proximal, middle, and distal phalanx

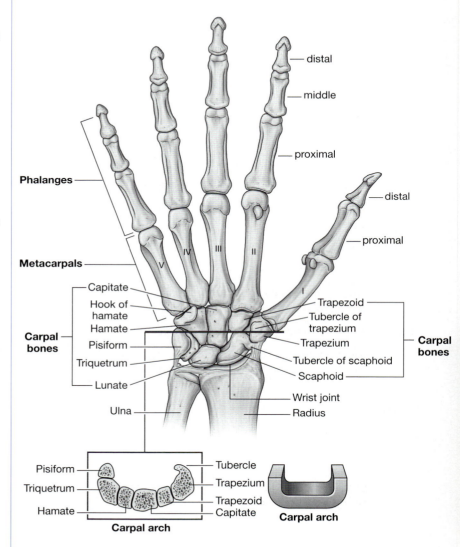

Figure 29-5 Hand. (Redrawn from Drake R, Vogl W, Mitchell A: Gray's Anatomy for Students. Philadelphia: Elsevier, 2005, Fig. 7.91A)

Lab 30

Superficial Structures of the Upper Limb, Shoulder, and Axilla

Prior to dissection, you should familiarize yourself with the following structures:

SUPERFICIAL STRUCTURES OF THE UPPER LIMB

- Superficial veins
  - Cephalic v.
    - Thoracoacromial v.
  - Basilic v.
  - Median cubital v.
  - Dorsal venous arch
  - Superficial venous palmar arch
- Lymphatic system
  - Axillary lymph nodes
- Superficial nerves
  - Intercostobrachial n.
  - Medial cutaneous n. of the arm*
  - Lateral cutaneous n. of the arm
  - Posterior cutaneous n. of the arm
  - Medial cutaneous n. of the forearm*
  - Lateral cutaneous n. of the forearm
  - Posterior cutaneous n. of the forearm

*Note: Arm and brachium refer to the same region of the upper limb, as do forearm and antebrachium. For example, the medial cutaneous n. of the forearm is the same as the medial antebrachial cutaneous n.

MUSCLES

- Shoulder
  - Deltoid m.
  - Trapezius m.
  - Levator scapulae m.
  - Serratus anterior m.
  - Rhomboid major m.
  - Rhomboid minor m.
  - Subclavius m.
  - Rotator cuff muscles
    - Supraspinatus m.
    - Infraspinatus m.
    - Teres minor m.
    - Subscapularis m.
  - Teres major m.
  - Pectoralis major m.
  - Pectoralis minor m.
  - Latissimus dorsi m.

FASCIA

- Supraspinous fascia
- Infraspinous fascia
- Axillary fascia
  - Suspensory ligament of the axilla

INNERVATION

Five Roots (C5, C6, C7, C8, T1)

- Dorsal scapular n. and long thoracic n.

Three Trunks

- Superior — suprascapular n. and n. to the subclavius m.
- Middle
- Inferior

Six Divisions

- Three anterior and three posterior divisions

Three Cords

- Lateral
  - Lateral pectoral n.
- Medial
  - Medial pectoral n.
  - Medial cutaneous n. of the arm
  - Medial cutaneous n. of the forearm

Continued

INNERVATION—cont'd

Three Cords—cont'd

- Posterior
  - Upper subscapular n.
  - Thoracodorsal n.
  - Lower subscapular n.
- Branches
  - Radial n.
  - Ulnar n.
  - Median n.
  - Musculocutaneous n.

VASCULATURE

- Subclavian a.
  - Thyrocervical trunk
    - Transverse cervical a.
      - Superficial branch
      - Deep branch (dorsal scapular a.)
    - Suprascapular a.
- Axillary a.
  - Superior thoracic a.
  - Thoracoacromial a.
    - Acromial branch
    - Deltoid branch
    - Pectoral branch
    - Clavicular branch
  - Lateral thoracic a.
  - Subscapular a.
    - Circumflex scapular a.
    - Thoracodorsal a.
  - Anterior humeral circumflex a.
  - Posterior humeral circumflex a.

Lab 30 Dissection Overview

The purpose of this laboratory session is to learn the anatomy of the superficial structures of the upper limb, the shoulder, and the axilla through dissection. You will do so through the following suggested sequence:

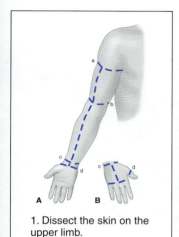

1. Dissect the skin on the upper limb.

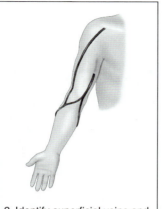

2. Identify superficial veins and nerves.

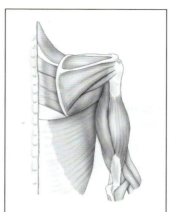

3. Dissect the deltoid and posterior regions of the shoulder to identify muscles acting on the posterior shoulder joint.

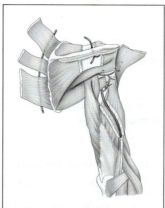

4. Dissect the nerves and vessels associated with the posterior region of the shoulder.

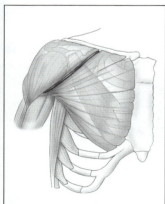

5. Dissect the anterior region of the shoulder to identify muscles acting on the shoulder joint.

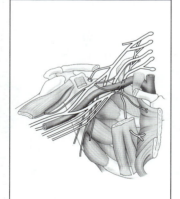

6. Dissect through the axillary sheath and identify the roots, trunks, divisions, and cords of the brachial plexus.

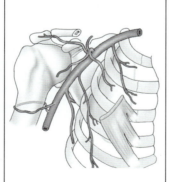

7. Dissect and identify the three divisions of the axillary artery and its associated branches.

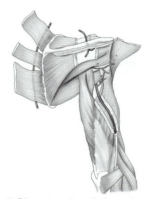

8. Dissect and study branches of the posterior division of the brachial plexus.

Upper Limb — Skin Removal

- Use a scalpel to make the following circular incisions through the skin on both upper limbs; do *not* cut the superficial veins and nerves in the superficial fascia **(Figure 30-1)**:

  - Proximal on the arm (brachium); *a*
  - Proximal to the elbow (antebrachium); *b*
  - Wrist *(c)*
  - About 5 cm distal to the wrist on the palmar surface of the hand and along the metacarpophalangeal joints on the posterior surface of the hand *(d)*

- Join the four circular incisions with a longitudinal incision on the anterior aspect of the upper limb *(a–d)*

- Remove the skin of the upper limb *but* leave the superficial fascia, with the superficial nerves and veins, intact; this may be difficult to accomplish on emaciated bodies

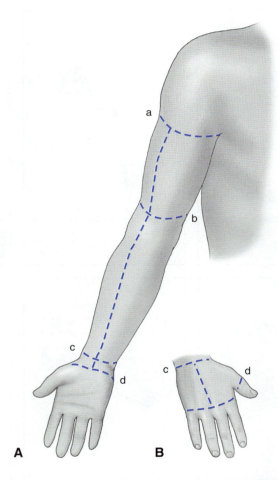

Figure 30-1 Right upper limb skin incisions. **A,** Anterior view. **B,** Posterior view of the hand

Upper Limb — Cutaneous Veins

■ Use forceps to reveal and identify the following veins in the superficial fascia; use the scraping technique and blunt dissection to remove fat and follow the veins' continuity; you may want to prop up the shoulder to improve the view of structures on both the anterior and posterior surfaces:

- **Cephalic v.** — find it coursing from the **dorsal venous arch** (network of veins) on the posterior aspect (dorsum) of the hand **(Figure 30-2B)** to the posterior, lateral side of the forearm (see Figure 30-2A)
  - Anterior to the elbow, communicates with the **basilic v.** via the **median cubital v.**
  - Ascends on the lateral surface of the biceps brachii m.; pierces the deep fascia of the deltopectoral triangle, emptying into the **axillary v.**
- **Basilic v.** — courses from the dorsal venous arch of the hand to the posterior, medial side of the forearm (see Figure 30-2B), and then to the anterior side of the elbow, where it communicates with the cephalic v. via the median cubital v.
  - Courses superiorly on the medial surface of the arm, then pierces the deep fascia at midarm to become the **axillary v.** (see Figure 30-2A)

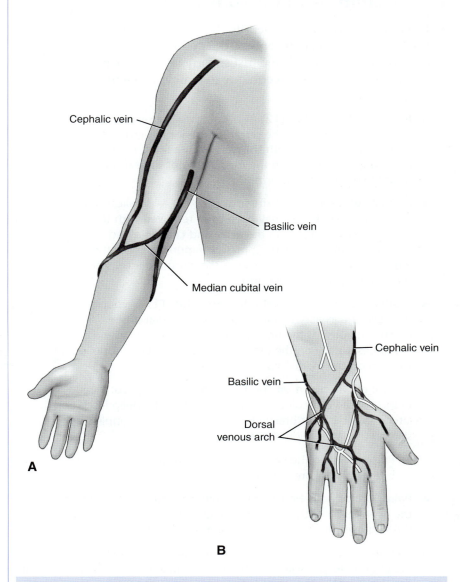

Figure 30-2 Cutaneous veins of the right upper limb. **A,** Anterior view. **B,** Posterior view

Upper Limb — Cutaneous Nerves

- Use forceps to reveal and identify the following nerves in the superficial fascia; in general, the main trunks of cutaneous nerves are found just superficial to the deep fascia; use the scraping technique to remove remaining fat **(Figure 30-3)**:

  - **Intercostobrachial n. (T2)** — arises from the second intercostal n., piercing the serratus anterior m.; crosses the axilla; communicates with the medial cutaneous n. of the arm; supplies the skin on the medial side of the axilla and upper two thirds of the arm

  - **Medial cutaneous n. of the arm (C8, T1)** — smallest branch of the brachial plexus (may have been removed with the skin); pierces the fascia in the axilla and courses along the medial side of the axillary v.; may communicate with the intercostobrachial n.; supplies the skin on the medial side of the distal one third of the arm

  - **Medial cutaneous n. of the forearm (C8, T1)** — courses between the axillary a. and v.; descends medial to the brachial a., pierces the deep fascia with the basilic v. and continues distally on the ulnar aspect of the elbow; supplies the skin on the medial side of the forearm

  - **Lateral cutaneous n. of the forearm (C5–C7)** — cutaneous branch of the musculocutaneous n.; pierces the deep fascia lateral to the biceps brachii tendon at the elbow; supplies the skin on the lateral side of the forearm
    - Passes deep to the cephalic v., descends along the radial border of the forearm to the wrist

  - **Palmar cutaneous branch of the ulnar n. (C8–T1)** — pierces the deep fascia of the forearm, proximal to the wrist; supplies the skin over the hypothenar compartment of the hand

  - **Palmar cutaneous branch of the median n. (C6–T1)** — pierces the deep fascia near the flexor retinaculum; supplies the skin over the thenar compartment of the hand

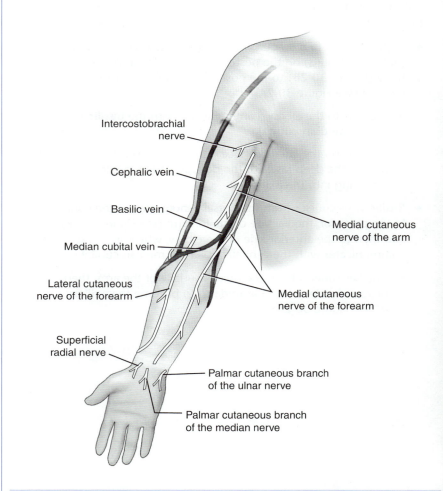

Figure 30-3 Cutaneous nerves of the right upper limb

Upper Limb — Cutaneous Nerves—cont'd

- Identify the following cutaneous nerves along the posterior aspect of the upper limb **(Figure 30-4)**:

  - **Superior lateral cutaneous n. of the arm** — the terminal branch of the axillary n.; emerges from the posterior border of the deltoid m. to supply the skin over the lower border of the deltoid m. and the skin around the deltoid tuberosity

  - **Posterior cutaneous n. of the arm** — a branch of the radial n.; pierces the deep fascia on the posterior aspect of the arm, inferior to the posterior border of the deltoid m.; supplies skin over the upper lateral part of the arm

  - **Inferior lateral cutaneous n. of the arm** — a branch of the radial n.; perforates the lateral head of the triceps brachii m., distal to the deltoid tuberosity; supplies the inferior lateral skin of the arm

  - **Posterior cutaneous n. of the forearm** — a branch of the radial n.; perforates the lateral, distal surface of the lateral head of the triceps brachii m.; descends along the lateral aspect of the forearm and then along the posterior surface of the hand; supplies the skin over the posterior aspect of the forearm

  - **Superficial branch of the radial n.** — descends in the forearm, deep to the brachioradialis m.; emerges at the distal part of the forearm and crosses over the anatomical snuff box (a landmark at the wrist) to provide cutaneous innervation to the posterolateral surface of the hand

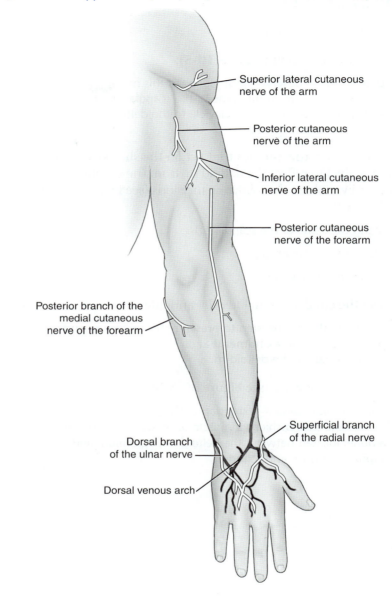

Figure 30-4 Posterior view of the cutaneous nerves of the right upper limb

Deltoid Muscle

- Turn the cadaver prone

- Identify the following **(Figure 30-5)**:

  - **Deltoid m.** — observe the striations of this multipennate muscle; courses from the spine of the scapula, acromion, and lateral one third of the clavicle to the deltoid tuberosity of the humerus

- To better study the muscles that act on the shoulder joint, use a scalpel to reflect the deltoid m. from the scapula and clavicle by making the following incisions (see Figure 30-5A and 30-5B):

  - Along the spine of the scapula *(a)*
  - Along the acromion *(b)*
  - Along the clavicle *(c)*

- Reflect the cut deltoid m. laterally and inferiorly

  - Be careful during this step to preserve the **axillary n.** and **posterior circumflex humeral a.** on the deep surface of the posterior part of the deltoid m.

- Identify the following (see Figure 30-5C):

  - **Subacromial bursa** — extension of the joint's synovial membrane that cushions a muscle or tendon that crosses a bone; located between the deltoid m., acromion, and supraspinatus m. and tendon

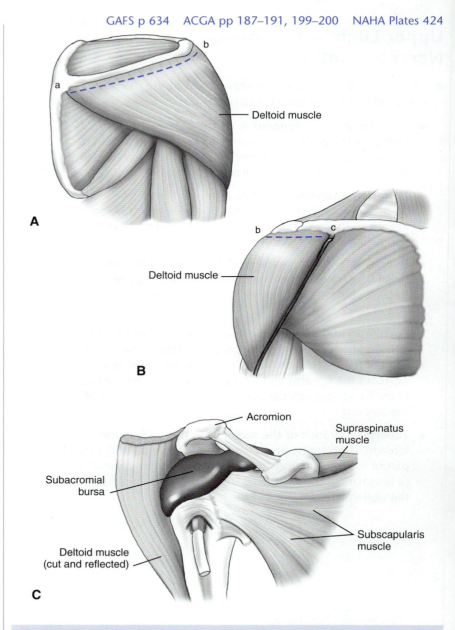

Figure 30-5 Right deltoid muscle. **A,** Posterior view. **B,** Anterior view. **C,** Anterior view of the shoulder with the deltoid muscle cut and reflected

Posterior Scapular Region — Muscles

- Identify the following muscles on the posteromedial border of the scapula **(Figure 30-6)**:

  - **Levator scapulae m.** — attached near the superior angle of the scapula

  - **Rhomboid minor m.** — attached at the level of the spine of the scapula

  - **Rhomboid major m.** — attached to the medial border of the scapula, inferior to the spine; inferior to the rhomboid minor m.

- Identify the following ("rotator cuff" muscles are designated with *):

  - **Supraspinatus m.*** — named according to its location in the supraspinous fossa

  - **Infraspinatus m.*** — named according to its location in the infraspinous fossa

  - **Teres minor m.*** — located inferior to the infraspinatus m.; may blend with the infraspinatus m.

  - **Teres major m.** — located inferior to the teres minor m.

  - **Latissimus dorsi m.** — located inferior to the teres major m.; note its superior attachment wraps around the teres major m. to attach near the intertubercular groove of the humerus

  - **Subscapularis m.*** — studied further in another laboratory session

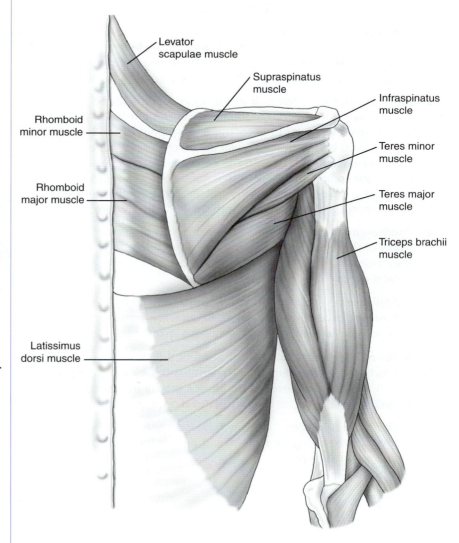

Figure 30-6 Posterior view of the right shoulder muscles

Posterior Scapular Region — Nerves

- Use forceps to reveal and identify the following nerves derived from the brachial plexus **(Figure 30-7)**:

  - **Dorsal scapular n.** — after piercing the middle scalene m. in the neck, descends with the deep branch of the transverse cervical a., deep to the levator scapulae and rhomboid mm., along the medial (vertebral) border of the scapula

  - **Suprascapular n.** — follow it to the superior trunk of the brachial plexus in the root of the neck; courses inferior to the suprascapular ligament to enter the supraspinous fossa accompanied by the suprascapular a., which courses superior to the suprascapular ligament; the nerve and artery course around the spinoglenoid notch to enter the infraspinous fossa; use a scalpel to make a vertical incision through the supraspinatus and infraspinatus mm. to verify their course

  - **Quadrangular space** — a four-sided space on the posterior aspect of the shoulder bordered by the teres minor m., teres major m., long head of the triceps brachii m., and surgical neck of the humerus

    - **Axillary n.** — courses posteriorly, accompanied by the posterior circumflex humeral a., to enter the posterior region of the arm through the quadrangular space

  - **Radial n.** — enters the posterior region of the arm, accompanied by the deep a. of the arm; find it by separating the long and medial heads of the triceps brachii m., inferior to the teres major m., to follow the radial groove

    - The radial n. descends between the long and medial heads of the triceps brachii m. and pierces the lateral intermuscular septum

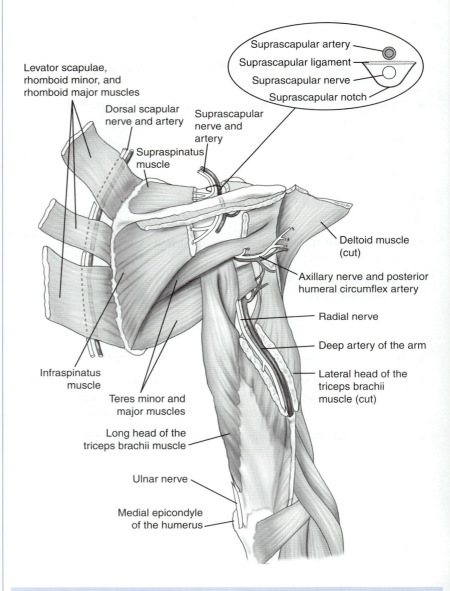

Figure 30-7 Posterior view of the nerves of the right shoulder

Posterior Scapular Region — Vessels

- Use forceps to reveal and identify the following vessels (Figure 30-8):

  - **Deep branch of the transverse cervical a.** — also known as the dorsal scapular a.; follow it to the thyrocervical trunk in the root of the neck; descends with the dorsal scapular n., deep to the levator scapulae and rhomboid mm., along the medial (vertebral) border of the scapula

  - **Suprascapular a.** — follow it to the thyrocervical trunk in the root of the neck; courses superior to the suprascapular ligament; enters the supraspinous fossa accompanied by the suprascapular n., which courses inferior to the suprascapular ligament; the nerve and artery course around the spinoglenoid notch to enter the infraspinous fossa

  - **Quadrangular space** — a four-sided space on the posterior aspect of the shoulder bordered by the teres minor m., teres major m., long head of the triceps brachii m., and surgical neck of the humerus

    - **Posterior circumflex humeral a.** — courses through the quadrangular space accompanied by the axillary n.

  - **Deep a. of the arm** — enters the posterior region of the arm, accompanied by the radial n.; find it by separating the long and medial heads of the triceps brachii m., inferior to the teres major m., to follow the radial groove

    - The deep a. of the arm descends between the long and medial heads of the triceps brachii m. and pierces the lateral intermuscular septum

  - **Circumflex scapular a.** — a branch of the subscapular a.; find it as it courses through a triangular space bordered by the teres minor, teres major, and long head of the triceps brachii mm.

- Note: The dorsal scapular a. anastomoses with the suprascapular and circumflex scapular aa., forming collateral circulation around the scapula

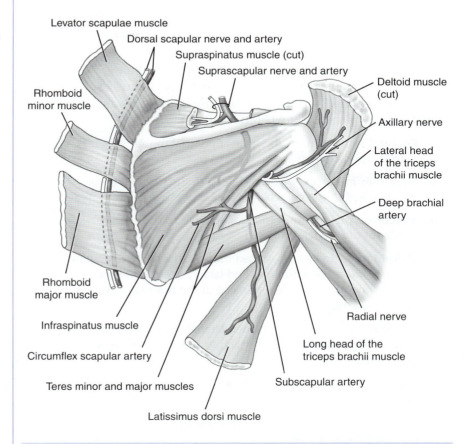

Figure 30-8 Arteries of the posterior region of the right shoulder

Anterior Region of the Shoulder

- *Note:* If the pectoralis major m. has not yet been dissected, please go to page 65, Unit 2, Lab 6, and follow the instructions

- Turn the cadaver supine

- Use your fingers or forceps to separate the following muscles. (*Note:* If you flex the joint[s] that each muscle crosses, the muscles will have less tension on them and will therefore be more pliable) **(Figure 30-9)**:

  - **Pectoralis major m.** — the most superficial muscle on the anterior thoracic wall

  - **Pectoralis minor m.** — located deep to the pectoralis major m.; attached to the coracoid process and ribs 3–5

  - **Subclavius m.** — a small muscle attached to the inferior border of the clavicle and rib 1

  - **Deltoid m.** — triangular-shaped muscle attached to the spine of the scapula, the acromion, and lateral one third of the clavicle; the deltoid m. is superficial to the brachial and rotator cuff muscles

  - **Serratus anterior m.** — attached laterally along the first 8 ribs; courses posteriorly to attach to the medial margin of the scapula

  - **Teres major m.** — distal attachment is on the intertubercular groove

  - **Latissimus dorsi m.** — distal attachment is on the intertubercular groove

  - **Subscapularis m.** — a deep muscle attached to the subscapular fossa; the brachial plexus and axillary a. course anterior to this muscle

- The remainder of this laboratory session will be discovering structures in the axillary fat that presently obscures your view of the subscapularis m.

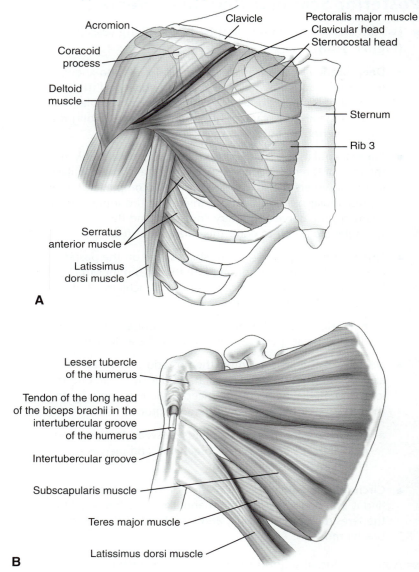

Figure 30-9 Anterior muscles of the right shoulder. **A,** Superficial view. **B,** Deep view

Brachial Plexus — Roots

- The roots are the **ventral rami of C5–T1** spinal segments
  - Find the roots as they pass between the anterior and middle scalene mm. and eventually flank the subclavian a.

- Identify the following branches from the roots **(Figure 30-10)**:
  - **Dorsal scapular n. (C5)** — pierces the middle scalene m., descends deep to the levator scapulae m., and enters the deep surface of the rhomboid mm.; accompanied by the dorsal scapular a. (deep branch of the transverse cervical a.)
  - **Long thoracic n. (C5–C7)** — descends posterior to C8 and T1 rami and courses inferiorly on the external surface of the serratus anterior m.

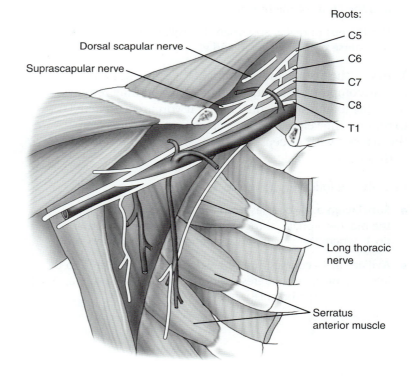

Figure 30-10 Right brachial plexus roots

Axillary Artery and Veins

- Turn the cadaver supine and move the pectoralis major and minor mm. from the axilla to expose the underlying structures

  - **Axillary sheath** — located about 2 cm inferior to the coracoid process; contains the axillary a., the axillary v., and the cords of the brachial plexus

  - Use forceps to reveal and open the axillary sheath to follow the course of the axillary a. and v.

- **Veins** — the deep veins are named the same as the arteries they accompany; ask your instructor if you may remove the veins to improve visual clarity; if you are instructed to remove the veins, do so by separating the veins from the arteries with forceps and then cut away the veins with scissors

- Identify the following **(Figure 30-11)**:

  - **Subclavian a.** — courses from the aortic arch (left side) or the brachiocephalic a. (right side) to the external border of rib 1, where the subclavian a. continues as the axillary a.

  - **Axillary a.** — courses from the external border of rib 1 to the inferior border of the teres major m., where the axillary a. continues as the brachial a.

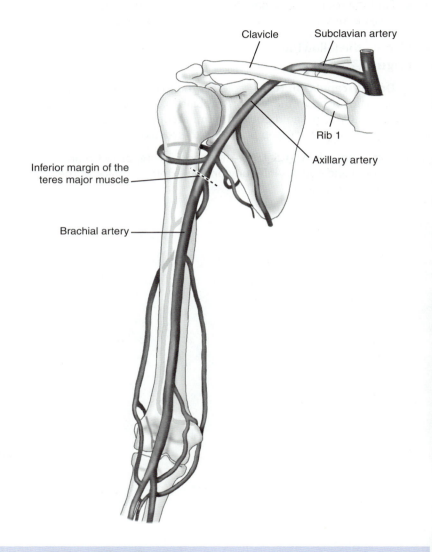

Figure 30-11   Right axillary artery

Brachial Plexus — Trunks

- At the root of the neck, the roots of the brachial plexus unite to form three trunks

- Use forceps to reveal and identify the following (**Figure 30-12**):

  - **Brachial plexus — Trunks**

    - **Superior trunk** — union of C5 and C6 roots; the union is usually sandwiched between the scalene mm.

      - **Suprascapular n.** — passes posterolaterally across the posterior triangle of the neck, superior to the brachial plexus, to pass through the scapular notch

    - **Middle trunk** — continuation of the root of C7; usually sandwiched between the scalene mm.

    - **Inferior trunk** — union of C8 and T1 roots; the union is usually sandwiched between the scalene mm.

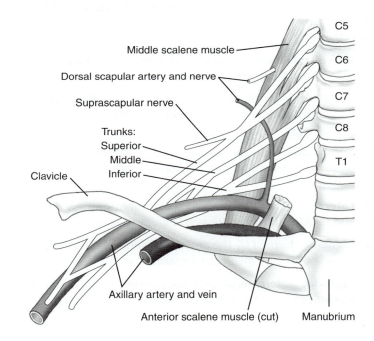

Figure 30-12 Right brachial plexus trunks

Brachial Plexus — Divisions and Cords

- Use forceps or the open-scissors technique to reveal and identify the following **(Figure 30-13A)**:

  - **Brachial plexus — Divisions** — each trunk (superior, middle, and inferior) of the brachial plexus divides into an anterior and posterior division as the plexus passes posterior to the clavicle

    - **Anterior divisions** — supply the muscles of the anterior (flexor) compartment of the upper limb

    - **Posterior divisions** — supply the muscles of the posterior (extensor) compartment of the upper limb

  - **Brachial plexus — Cords** (see Figure 30-13B) — the three anterior divisions and three posterior divisions form three cords that are named by their anatomic position relative to the axillary a.

    - **Lateral** — formed by the anterior divisions of the superior and middle trunks; positioned lateral to the axillary a.

    - **Medial** — formed by the anterior division of the inferior trunk; positioned medial to the axillary a.

    - **Posterior** — formed by the posterior divisions of all three trunks; positioned posterior to the axillary a.

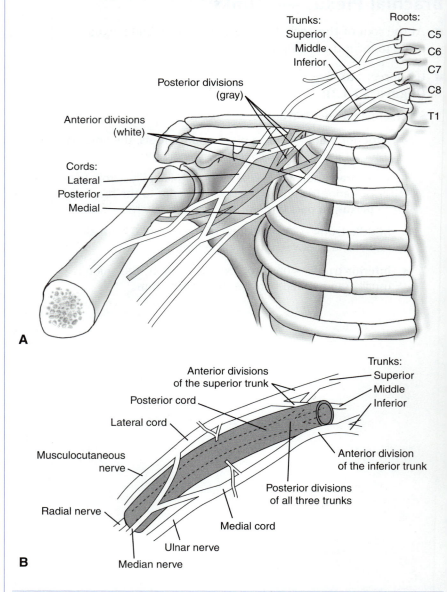

Figure 30-13 Right brachial plexus divisions and cords. **A,** Divisions and cords. **B,** Cords in situ

Brachial Plexus — Branches from the Lateral and Medial Cords

■ Use forceps to reveal and identify the following **(Figure 30-14)**:

- **Lateral cord** — lateral to the axillary a.
  - **Lateral pectoral n.** — innervates the pectoralis major m.; there may be a communicating branch between the lateral and medial cords
- **Medial cord** — medial to the axillary a.
  - **Medial pectoral n.** — innervates the pectoralis major and minor mm.
  - **Medial cutaneous n. of the arm** — a small branch that courses along the medial surface of the axillary v.; communicates with the intercostobrachial n.
  - **Medial cutaneous n. of the forearm** — courses between the axillary a. and v. along the side of the ulnar n.

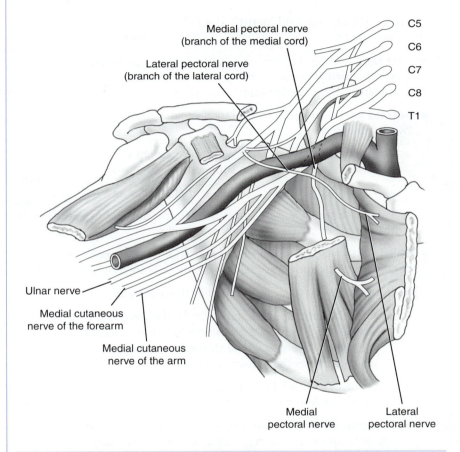

Figure 30-14 Right brachial plexus nerves from the lateral and medial cords

Axillary Artery — Branches

- The axillary a. is subdivided into three parts by its relationship to the pectoralis minor m.

- Use forceps to reveal and identify the following **(Figure 30-15)**:

  - **First part** — medial to the pectoralis minor m.; between rib 1 and the medial border of the pectoralis minor m.; one branch, the **superior (supreme) thoracic a.**

  - **Second part** — deep to the pectoralis minor m.; two branches:
    - **Thoracoacromial a.** — follow its four branches (each named for the region supplied):
      - **Acromial, deltoid, pectoral, and clavicular aa.**
    - **Lateral thoracic a.** — supplies the serratus anterior m.; in the female, it provides mammary branches

  - **Third part** — lateral to the pectoralis minor m.; between the pectoralis minor and teres major mm.; three branches:
    - **Subscapular a.** — largest branch of the axillary a.
      - After the subscapular a. gives rise to the **circumflex scapular a.** (seen on the posterior side of the scapula), the artery continues as the **thoracodorsal a.**, which supplies the latissimus dorsi m.
    - **Anterior circumflex humeral a.** — courses anterior to the surgical neck of the humerus
    - **Posterior circumflex humeral a.** — usually larger than the anterior circumflex humeral a.; courses posteriorly through the quadrangular space with the axillary n.

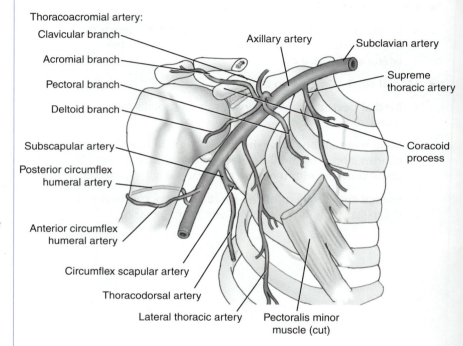

Figure 30-15 Branches of the right axillary artery

Brachial Plexus — Branches from the Posterior Cord

- Use forceps to remove the remaining axillary fat and lift up the axillary artery to expose the following branches of the posterior cord

- Use forceps to identify the following **(Figure 30-16)**:

  - **Upper subscapular n.** — courses posteriorly to enter the subscapularis m.

  - **Thoracodorsal n.** — courses along the posterior axillary wall to enter the deep surface of the latissimus dorsi m.

  - **Lower subscapular n.** — passes inferolaterally, deep to the subscapular a. and v., to the subscapularis and teres major mm.

  - **Radial n.** — a terminal branch of the posterior cord; enters the radial groove with the deep a. of the arm to pass between the long and medial heads of the triceps brachii m.

  - **Axillary n.** — the other terminal branch of the posterior cord; courses through the quadrangular space to innervate the deltoid and teres minor mm.

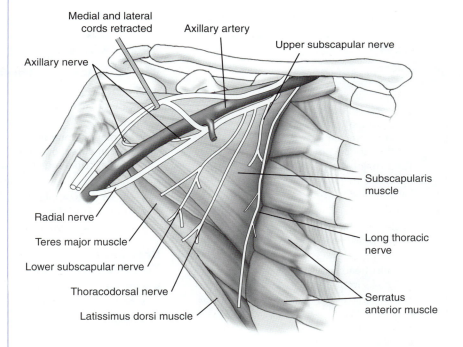

Figure 30-16 Right brachial plexus nerves from the posterior cord

Arm

Lab 31

Prior to dissection, you should familiarize yourself with the following structures:

MUSCLES
- Shoulder
  - Deltoid m.
  - Rotator cuff muscles
    - Supraspinatus m.
    - Infraspinatus m.
    - Teres minor m.
    - Subscapularis m.
  - Teres major m.
  - Pectoralis major m.
  - Latissimus dorsi m.
- Arm
  - Coracobrachialis m.
  - Biceps brachii m.
    - Long head
    - Short head
  - Brachialis m.
  - Triceps brachii m.
    - Long head
    - Lateral head
    - Medial head

INNERVATION

Brachial Plexus — Three Cords
- Lateral
  - Lateral pectoral n.
- Medial
  - Medial pectoral n.
  - Medial cutaneous n. of the arm*
  - Medial cutaneous n. of the forearm*
- Posterior
  - Upper subscapular n.
  - Thoracodorsal n.
  - Lower subscapular n.

Brachial Plexus — Five Terminal Branches
- Musculocutaneous n.
  - Muscular branches
- Median n.
  - Muscular branches
- Ulnar n.
  - Muscular branches
- Radial n.
  - Muscular branches
  - Posterior cutaneous nn. of the arm
  - Inferior lateral cutaneous n. of the arm
- Axillary n.
  - Muscular branches
  - Superior lateral cutaneous n. of the arm

*Note: Arm and *brachium* refer to the same region of the upper limb, as do *forearm* and *antebrachium*. For example, the medial cutaneous n. of the forearm is the same as the medial antebrachial cutaneous n.

VASCULATURE
- Brachial a.
  - Deep artery of the arm
    - Radial collateral a.
    - Middle collateral a.
  - Superior ulnar collateral a.
  - Inferior ulnar collateral a.
- Radial a.
- Ulnar a.

Lab 31 Dissection Overview

The purpose of this laboratory session is to learn the anatomy of the arm through dissection. You will do so through the following suggested sequence:

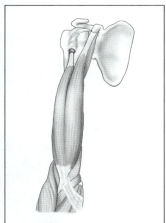

1. Dissect the anterior muscles of the arm.

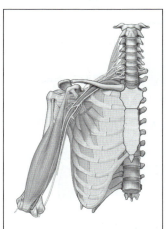

2. Identify anterior division cords and branches of the brachial plexus.

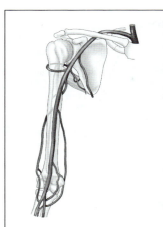

3. Dissect and identify the brachial artery and its associated branches.

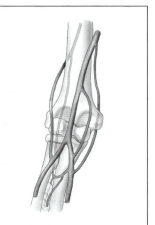

4. Dissect and identify the brachial artery, proximal radial and ulnar arteries, and their associated branches.

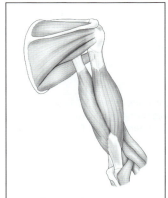

5. Dissect the posterior muscles of the arm.

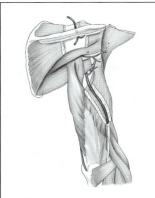

6. Dissect the arteries of the posterior aspect of the arm.

Table 31-1 Brachial Plexus

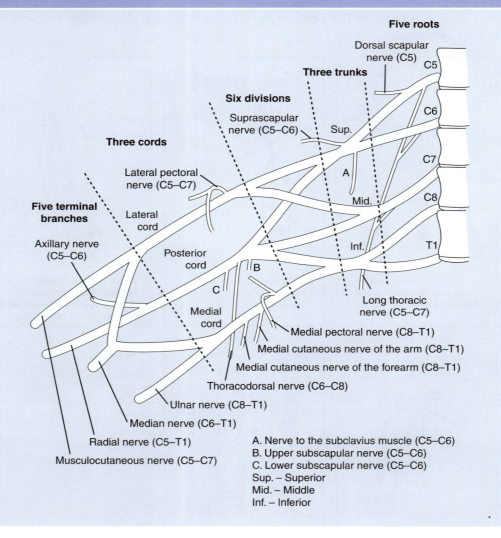

Anterior Muscles of the Arm

- Use your fingers and/or forceps to separate and identify the following (if necessary to separate one muscle from another, use a scalpel or scissors to incise the deep fascia at the border of two adjoining muscles, and then slide your fingers up and down the adjoining borders to free one muscle from another; keep in mind that many neurovascular bundles run between adjoining muscle bellies):

  - **Biceps brachii m. (Figure 31-1A):**

    - **Long head** — the tendon of the long head courses through the intertubercular groove of the humerus and arches over the head of the humerus to attach to the supraglenoid tubercle of the scapula

      - **Transverse humeral ligament** — the tendon of the long head passes through an opening in the capsular ligament called the transverse humeral ligament; this ligament tethers the tendon

    - **Short head** — attaches to the coracoid process of the scapula

  - **Coracobrachialis m.** — medial to the short head of the biceps m.; its belly is pierced by the musculocutaneous n.

- Flex the upper limb at the shoulder to reduce tension on the biceps brachii m. so that you can push it aside to reveal the brachialis m. (see Figure 31-1B):

  - **Brachialis m.** — located deep to the biceps brachii m.; attaches distally to the coronoid process of the ulna

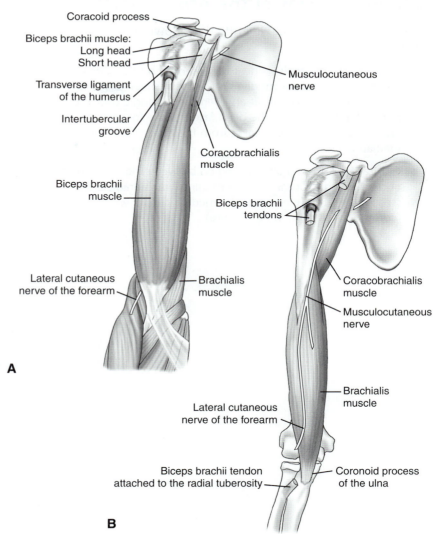

Figure 31-1 Anterior muscles of the right arm. **A,** Superficial view. **B,** Deep view; the biceps brachii m. is removed *Continued*

Anterior Muscles of the Arm Continued

Anterior Muscles of the Arm—cont'd

- Use forceps to reveal and identify the following (**Figure 31-1C**):

  - **Bicipital aponeurosis** — near the insertion on the radial tuberosity, the biceps m. gives off a fascial sheet (bicipital aponeurosis) that passes at an inferomedial angle over the brachial a. to fuse with the deep fascia of the forearm; this fascia separates the brachial a. from the more superficial median cubital vein

  - **Cubital fossa** — a triangular region between the epicondyles of the humerus, pronator teres m., and brachioradialis m. (see Figure 31-1C); contains the median cubital v. (commonly used for venipuncture)

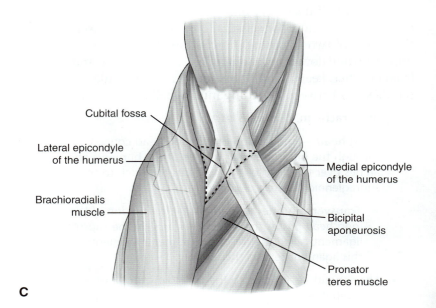

Figure 31-1, cont'd   C, Bicipital fossa

Brachial Plexus — Five Terminal Branches in the Arm

- Review the lateral and medial cords of the brachial plexus

  - Observe that the medial and lateral cords bifurcate and converge in a form that resembles the letter M; use forceps to remove remaining fat to reveal and identify the five terminal branches (Figure 31-2):

- **Musculocutaneous n.** — terminal branch of the lateral cord; pierces the coracobrachialis m. and descends between the biceps and brachialis mm.

  - The musculocutaneous n. continues distally as the lateral cutaneous n. of the forearm

- **Median n.** — terminal branch formed by the convergence of the medial branch of the lateral cord and the lateral branch of the medial cord

  - In the proximal part of the arm, the median n. courses lateral to the brachial a.

  - At the insertion of the coracobrachialis m. to the humerus, the median n. crosses anterior to the brachial a. and courses distally on the medial side of the brachial a., deep to the bicipital aponeurosis

- **Ulnar n.** — terminal branch of the medial cord

  - Courses medial to the brachial a. to the middle of the arm, where the ulnar n. pierces the medial intermuscular septum to enter the posterior compartment

  - Courses anterior to the medial head of the triceps brachii m.

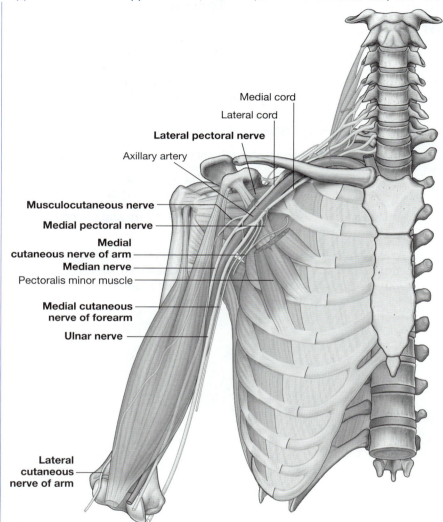

Figure 31-2 Right brachial plexus terminal branches — arm. (From Drake R, Vogl W, Mitchell A: Gray's Anatomy for Students. Philadelphia: Elsevier, 2005, Fig. 7.54)

Brachial Plexus — Five Terminal Branches in the Arm Continued

Brachial Plexus — Five Terminal Branches in the Arm—cont'd

- Review the posterior cords of the brachial plexus

- Reflect the anterior division of the brachial plexus (M shaped) to observe the posterior division of the brachial plexus; use forceps to remove remaining fat to reveal and identify the following **(Figure 31-3)**:

    - **Radial n.** — one of two terminal branches of the posterior cord
        - Courses posterior to the axillary and brachial aa. and enters the radial groove with the deep a. of the arm
        - Descends between the heads of the triceps m. and pierces the lateral intermuscular septum
    - **Axillary n.** — the second terminal branch of the posterior cord; passes posteriorly through the quadrangular space, with the posterior circumflex humeral a., en route to the deltoid and teres minor mm.

GAFS pp 676–679 ACGA pp 175–176, 178–180, 217 NAHA Plates 477–478

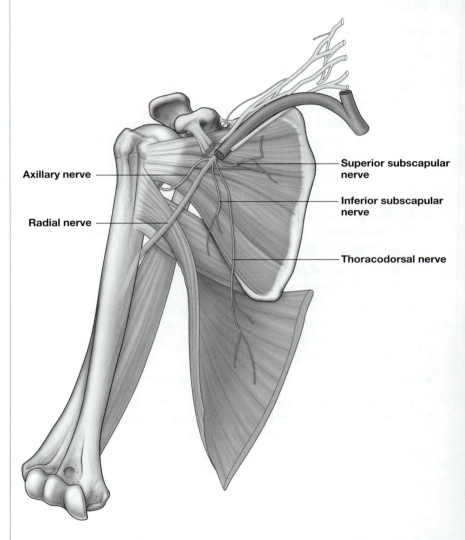

Figure 31-3 Right brachial plexus terminal branches — arm. (From Drake R, Vogl W, Mitchell A: Gray's Anatomy for Students. Philadelphia: Elsevier, 2005, Fig. 7.55)

Brachial Artery

■ Use forceps to reveal and identify the following **(Figure 31-4)**:

- **Venae comitantes** — observe that the brachial a. is accompanied by smaller paired veins called venae comitantes; ask your instructor if you may remove the venae comitantes

- **Brachial a.** — begins at the inferior border of the teres major m. as the continuation of the axillary a.; courses on the medial aspect of the biceps brachii m. to the cubital fossa under the protection of the bicipital aponeurosis; has the following branches:

  - **Deep a. of the arm** — courses in the radial groove (accompanied by the radial n.) on the posterior aspect of the humerus (described in more detail later on in this laboratory session)

    ◆ *Note:* The anastomotic connections around the elbow are often difficult to demonstrate; limit the time spent in pursuit of these anastomoses

  - **Superior ulnar collateral a.** — arises midway along the brachial a.; accompanies the ulnar n.; courses posterior to the medial epicondyle of the humerus; anastomoses with the posterior ulnar recurrent a.

  - **Inferior ulnar collateral a.** — arises from the brachial a. about 5 cm superior to the elbow; courses anterior to the medial epicondyle of the humerus, between the median n. and the brachialis m.; anastomoses with the anterior ulnar recurrent a.

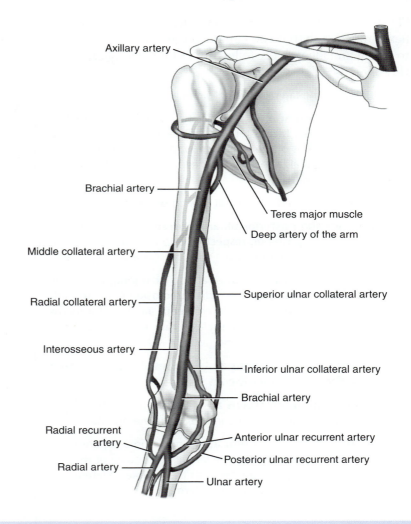

Figure 31-4 Right brachial artery

Proximal Portions of the Radial and Ulnar Arteries

■ Flex the forearm at the elbow to reduce tension on the flexor muscles so that you can push them aside; use forceps to reveal and identify the following distal to the elbow **(Figure 31-5)**:

- **Radial a.** — the lateral terminal branch of the brachial a.
  - **Radial recurrent a.** — arises in the cubital fossa; crosses anterior to the biceps tendon, between the superficial and deep branches of the radial n.; anastomoses with the radial collateral branch of the deep a. of the arm and follows the radial n.
- **Ulnar a.** — the medial terminal branch of the brachial a.
  - **Anterior** and **posterior ulnar recurrent aa.** — located anterior and posterior, respectively, to the medial epicondyle of the humerus
  - **Common interosseous a.** — about 1 cm long; arises from the ulnar a., medial to the radial tuberosity; bifurcates into the anterior and posterior interosseous aa.; look for its two branches by parting the muscles it runs between, but do not follow them at this time
    - ◆ **Anterior interosseous a.** — courses along the anterior surface of the interosseous membrane
    - ◆ **Posterior interosseous a.** — courses along the posterior surface of the interosseous membrane
    - ◆ **Interosseous recurrent a.** — courses in a superior direction, posterior to the lateral epicondyle of the humerus, to anastomose with the middle collateral branch of the deep a. of the arm

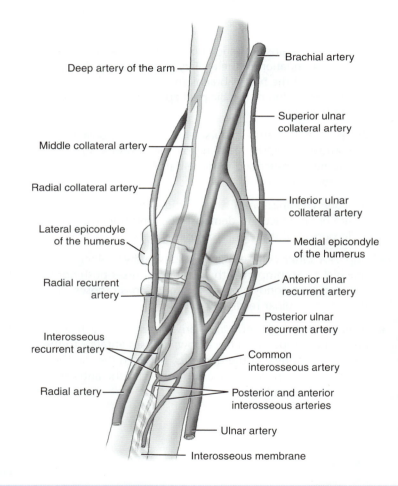

Figure 31-5 Collateral arterial circulation around the right elbow

Posterior Muscles of the Arm

- Extend the arm at the shoulder to reduce tension on the extensor muscles so that you can push them aside; use your fingers or forceps to reveal and identify the following **(Figure 31-6)**:

  - **Triceps brachii m.** — positioned on the posterior aspect of the humerus; has three heads:
    - **Long head** — separates the teres major and minor mm.
      - Teres major m. is anterior to the long head of the triceps brachii m.
      - Teres minor m. is posterior to the long head of the triceps brachii m.
    - **Lateral head** — the most lateral head of the three proximal attachments
    - **Medial head** — deep to the long and lateral heads
  - The distal attachment of the triceps brachii m. is to the olecranon process of the ulna

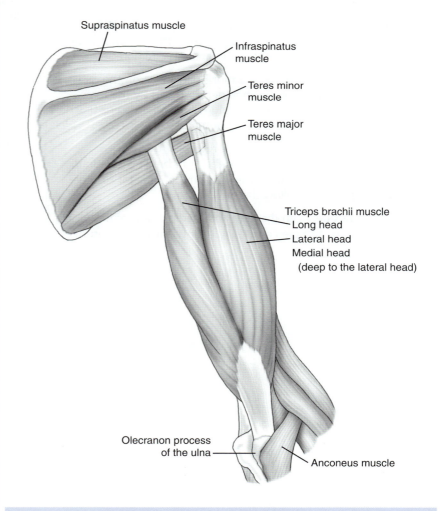

Figure 31-6 Posterior view of the right arm muscles

Brachial Plexus — Posterior Branches of the Shoulder Region

- Turn the cadaver prone; review the following **(Figure 31-7)**:

  - **Axillary n.** — courses posteriorly, accompanied by the posterior circumflex humeral a., to enter the posterior region of the arm through the following anatomic region:

    - **Quadrangular space** — a four-sided space on the posterior aspect of the shoulder bordered by the teres minor m., teres major m., long head of the triceps brachii m., and surgical neck of the humerus

  - **Radial n.** — enters the posterior region of the arm, accompanied by the deep a. of the arm, between the long and medial heads of the triceps brachii m., inferior to the teres major m., to follow the radial groove

    - Descends between the long and medial heads of the triceps brachii m. and pierces the lateral intermuscular septum

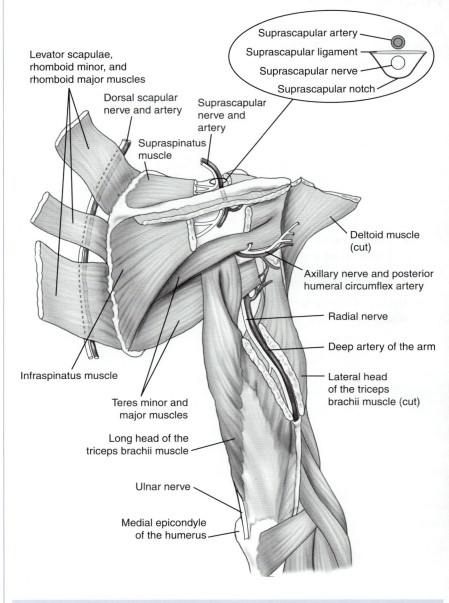

Figure 31-7 Posterior view of the nerves of the right shoulder

Arteries of the Posterior Region of the Arm

- The brachial a. courses within the anterior compartment of the arm; however, a few of its branches course in the posterior compartment of the arm

- Use forceps to reveal and identify the following **(Figure 31-8)**:

  - **Superior ulnar collateral a.** — courses posterior to the medial epicondyle of the humerus; anastomoses with the **posterior ulnar recurrent a.**

  - **Deep a. of the arm** — courses in the radial groove along the posterior aspect of the humerus (accompanied by the radial n.), between the long head of the triceps brachii m. and the medial head of the triceps brachii m.; has the following branches:

    - **Middle collateral a.** — descends in the medial head of the triceps brachii m., posterior to the lateral epicondyle of the humerus; anastomoses with the **interosseous recurrent a.**

    - **Radial collateral a.** — accompanies the radial n. between the brachioradialis and brachialis mm.; anterior to the lateral epicondyle of the humerus, anastomoses with the **radial recurrent a.**

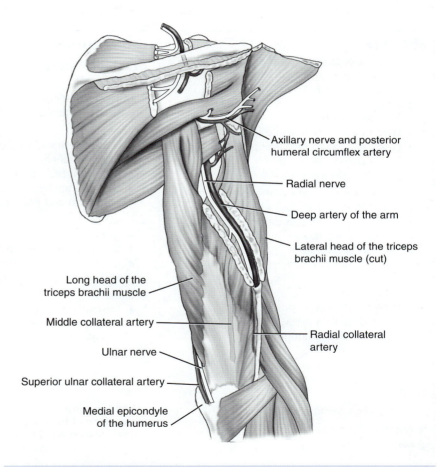

Figure 31-8 Arteries of the posterior region of the right arm

Forearm

Lab 32

Prior to dissection, you should familiarize yourself with the following structures:

MUSCLES

- Anterior compartment of the forearm
  - Pronator teres m.
  - Flexor carpi radialis m.
  - Flexor carpi ulnaris m.
  - Palmaris longus m.
  - Flexor digitorum superficialis m.
  - Flexor digitorum profundus m.
  - Flexor pollicis longus m.
  - Pronator quadratus m.
- Posterior compartment of the forearm
  - Brachioradialis m.
  - Extensor carpi radialis longus m.
  - Extensor carpi radialis brevis m.
  - Extensor digitorum m.
  - Extensor digiti minimi m.
  - Extensor carpi ulnaris m.
  - Extensor indicis m.
  - Extensor pollicis longus m.
  - Extensor pollicis brevis m.
  - Abductor pollicis longus m.
  - Anconeus m.
  - Supinator m.

FASCIA

- Interosseous membrane
- Antebrachial fascia
- Extensor retinaculum

INNERVATION

Brachial Plexus — Terminal Branches*

- Musculocutaneous n.
  - Lateral cutaneous n. of the forearm
- Median n.
  - Muscular branches
  - Palmar branch
  - Recurrent branch of the median n.
  - Digital branches of the median n. (common and proper palmar digital nn.)
- Ulnar n.
  - Muscular branches
  - Superficial and deep branches of the ulnar n.
  - Digital branches of the ulnar n. (common and proper palmar digital nn.)
- Radial n.
  - Muscular branches
  - Posterior cutaneous n. of the forearm
  - Superficial and deep branches of the radial n.

*Note: Forearm and antebrachium refer to the same region of the upper limb. For example, the medial cutaneous n. of the forearm is the same as the medial antebrachial cutaneous n.

VASCULATURE†

- Deep a. of the arm
  - Radial collateral a.
  - Middle collateral a.
- Superior ulnar collateral a.
- Inferior ulnar collateral a.
- Radial a.
  - Radial recurrent a.
- Ulnar a.
  - Anterior ulnar recurrent a.
  - Posterior ulnar recurrent a.
  - Common interosseous a.
    - Anterior interosseous a.
    - Posterior interosseous a.
      - Interosseous recurrent a.

†Note: Deep veins are named the same as the arteries they accompany. Vasculature of the hand will be dissected in another laboratory session.

Lab 32 Dissection Overview

The purpose of this laboratory session is to learn the anatomy of the forearm through dissection. You will do so through the following suggested sequence:

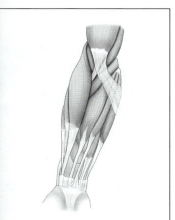

1. Dissect and identify the superficial anterior muscles of the forearm.

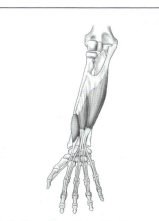

2. Dissect and identify the intermediate anterior muscles of the forearm.

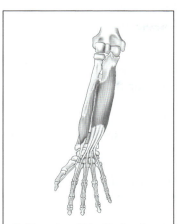

3. Dissect and identify the deep anterior muscles of the forearm.

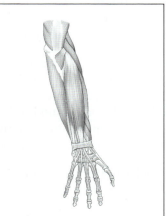

4. Dissect and identify the superficial and deep posterior muscles of the forearm.

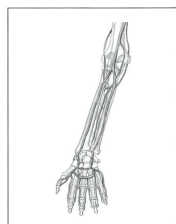

5. Dissect and identify the proximal and distal ends of the radial and ulnar arteries and their associated branches.

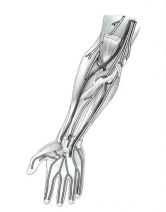

6. Dissect and identify the distal branches of the brachial plexus in the forearm.

Anterior Muscles of the Forearm — Superficial Layer

- Depending on whether you are dissecting flexor or extensor muscles, flex or extend, respectively, the joint across which the muscle(s) of interest span to reduce tension on them so that the muscles can be more easily identified

- Turn the forearm supine; if necessary, to separate one muscle from another, use a scalpel to incise the deep fascia at the border of two adjoining muscles, then slide your fingers up and down the adjoining borders to free one muscle from another; keep in mind that many neurovascular bundles run between adjoining muscle bellies

- Many of the muscles in the anterior compartment of the forearm attach to the medial epicondyle of the humerus

- Use your fingers or forceps to separate and identify the following, from superior to inferior, from the medial epicondyle of the humerus to the wrist and hand **(Figure 32-1)**:

  - **Pronator teres m.** — forms the medial border of the cubital fossa; deep to the bicipital aponeurosis; identify the superior border of the pronator teres m. by locating the tendon of the biceps brachii m.

  - **Flexor carpi radialis m.** — medial to the pronator teres m.; attaches distally to the base of the second and third metacarpals on the palmar surface of the hand

  - **Palmaris longus m.** — if present, it is medial to the flexor carpi radialis m.; attached distally in the transverse fibers of the palmar aponeurosis (palmar carpal ligament) and the flexor retinaculum

  - **Flexor carpi ulnaris m.** — the most medial muscle on the anterior surface of the forearm; attached distally to the pisiform bone and base of the fifth metacarpal bone on its palmar surface

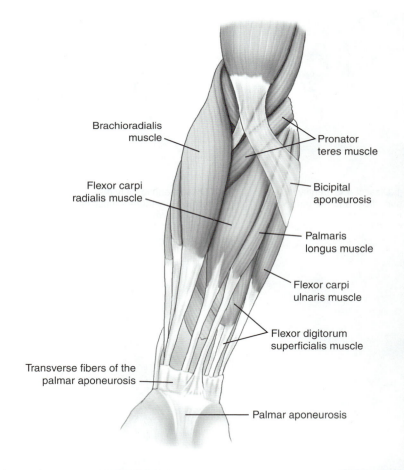

Figure 32-1 Anterior view of the superficial muscles of the right forearm

Anterior Muscles of the Forearm — Intermediate Layer

- To reveal the flexor digitorum superficialis m., you may follow either of these instructions:

  1. Flex the hand at the wrist, and flex the forearm at the elbow; the intervening muscles will bow and therefore may be pushed away from the deeper muscles

  2. With a scalpel, transect the flexor carpi radialis, palmaris longus, and flexor carpi ulnaris mm. on one forearm and reflect them to reveal deeper structures

- Be careful to leave vessels and nerves intact

- Use your fingers or forceps to separate and identify the muscles in the intermediate layer of the anterior region of the forearm **(Figure 32-2)**:

  - **Flexor digitorum superficialis m.** — deep to the flexor carpi radialis, palmaris longus, and flexor carpi ulnaris mm.
    - Inserts distally on the middle phalanx of digits 2–5 on the palmar surface; you will not study the distal attachments until the hand dissection

  - **Flexor pollicis longus m.** — attached to the distal phalanx of digit 1 (thumb); located lateral and deep to the flexor digitorum superficialis m. on the radial side of the forearm

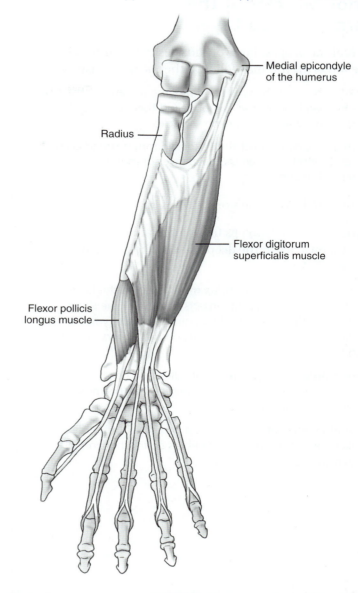

Figure 32-2 Anterior view of the intermediate muscles of the right forearm

Anterior Muscles of the Forearm — Deep Layer

- To reveal the deepest layer of muscles in the anterior region of the forearm, you may follow either of these instructions:

  1. Flex the hand at the wrist, and flex the forearm at the elbow; the intervening muscles will bow and therefore may be pushed away from the deeper muscles

  2. With a scalpel, transect the flexor digitorum superficialis m. and reflect it to see the deep layer of muscles in the anterior forearm

- Be careful to leave vessels and nerves intact

- Use your fingers or forceps to separate and identify the following muscles in the deep layer of the forearm **(Figure 32-3)**:

  - **Flexor digitorum profundus m.** — deep to the flexor digitorum superficialis m.; inserts distally on the distal phalanx of digits 2–5 on their palmar surface; you will not study the tendinous attachments on the fingers until the hand dissection

  - **Flexor pollicis longus m.** — lateral to the flexor digitorum profundus m.; the radial a. is superficial to this muscle; avoid damaging this artery

  - **Pronator quadratus m.** — deep and distal to the flexor pollicis longus m.; the muscle fibers course horizontally and attach to both the radius and ulna

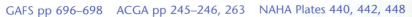

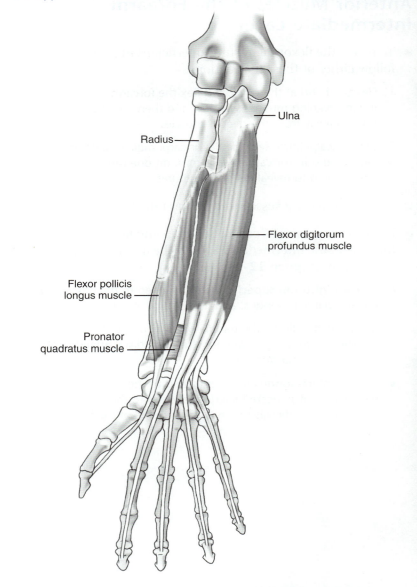

Figure 32-3 Anterior view of the deep muscles of the right forearm

Posterior Muscles of the Forearm — Superficial Layer

- Turn the forearm prone; if necessary, to separate one muscle from another, use a scalpel to incise the deep fascia at the border of two adjoining muscles, then slide your fingers up and down the adjoining borders to free one muscle from another; keep in mind that many neurovascular bundles run between adjoining muscle bellies

- Identify the lateral epicondyle of the humerus; this is a common attachment for many of the posterior forearm muscles

- Use your fingers or forceps to separate and identify the following forearm muscles **(Figure 32-4)**:

  - **Brachioradialis m.** — crosses the elbow joint on its lateral side; has the most superior attachment on the humerus of the extensor group of forearm muscles

  - **Extensor carpi radialis longus m.** — on the lateral aspect of the forearm; parallel and medial to the brachioradialis m.

  - **Anconeus m.** — short triangular muscle; closely associated with the distal end of the triceps brachii m.

  - **Extensor carpi radialis brevis m.** — deep and medial to the extensor carpi radialis longus m.

  - **Extensor digitorum m.** — medial to the extensor carpi radialis brevis m.; four tendons arise from the muscle belly to attach to digits 2–5

  - **Extensor digiti minimi m.** — medial to the extensor digitorum m. and courses to the little finger

  - **Extensor carpi ulnaris m.** — most medial of the superficial posterior muscles of the forearm

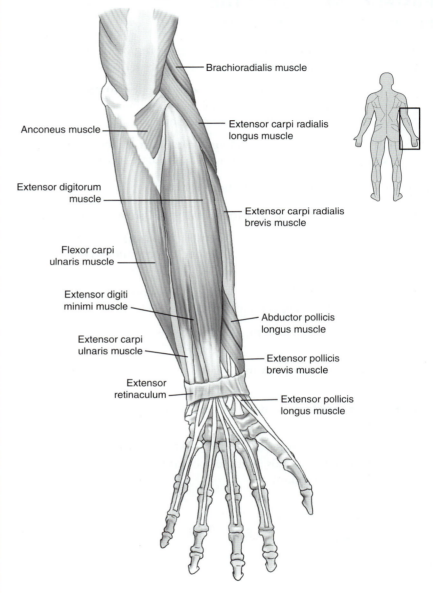

Figure 32-4 Posterior view of the superficial muscles of the right forearm

Posterior Muscles of the Forearm — Deep Layer

- To reveal the deep muscles of the posterior region of the forearm, you may follow either of these instructions:

  1. Extend the hand at the wrist, and extend the forearm at the elbow; the intervening muscles will bow and therefore may be pushed away from the deeper muscles
  2. With a scalpel, transect the extensor digitorum m. about 6 cm proximal to the wrist and reflect the cut muscle superiorly

- Be careful to leave vessels and nerves intact

- Use your fingers to identify the following **(Figure 32-5A)**:

  - **Supinator m.** — deep to the extensor carpi radialis brevis and extensor digitorum mm.; attached to both the ulna and radius
  - **Abductor pollicis longus m.** — lateral and parallel to the extensor pollicis longus m.; distal to the supinator m.
  - **Extensor pollicis brevis m.** — distal to the abductor pollicis longus m.
  - **Extensor pollicis longus m.** — distal to the extensor pollicis brevis m.
  - **Extensor indicis m.** — distal to the extensor pollicis longus m.
  - **Anatomical snuff box** (see Figure 32-5B) — bordered by the abductor pollicis longus, extensor pollicis brevis, and extensor pollicis longus tendons

GAFS pp 703–706, 715   ACGA p 254   NAHA Plates 440–441, 445

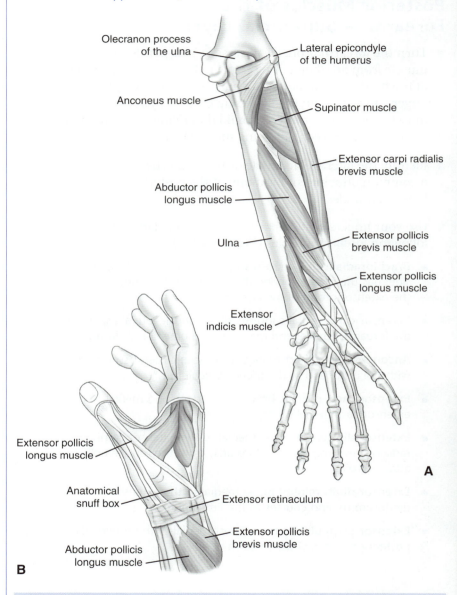

Figure 32-5 Posterior muscles of the right forearm. **A,** Posterior view. **B,** Lateral view.

Proximal Portions of the Radial and Ulnar Arteries

■ Use forceps to reveal and identify the following **(Figure 32-6)**:

- **Radial a.** — the lateral terminal branch of the brachial a.; arises in the cubital fossa
  - **Radial recurrent a.** — arises in the cubital fossa; crosses anterior to the biceps tendon, between the superficial and deep branches of the radial n.; anastomoses with the radial collateral branch of the deep a. of the arm
- **Ulnar a.** — the medial terminal branch of the brachial a.; arises in the cubital fossa
  - **Anterior** and **posterior ulnar recurrent aa.** — located anterior and posterior, respectively, to the medial epicondyle of the humerus; contribute to collateral circulation around the elbow joint
  - **Common interosseous a.** — about 1 cm long; arises from the ulnar a., medial to the radial tuberosity; bifurcates into the anterior and posterior interosseous aa.
    - **Anterior interosseous a.** — courses along the anterior surface of the interosseous membrane
    - **Posterior interosseous a.** — courses along the posterior surface of the interosseous membrane
      - **Interosseous recurrent a.** — courses in a superior direction, posterior to the lateral epicondyle of the humerus, to anastomose with the middle collateral branch of the deep a. of the arm

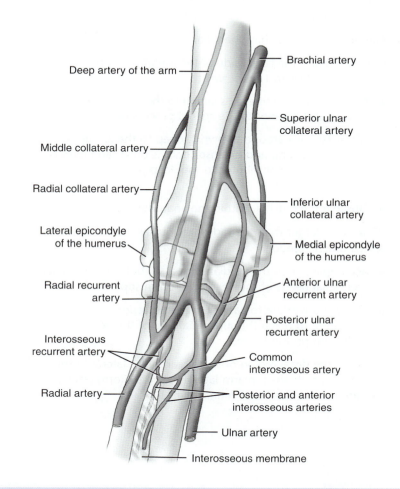

Figure 32-6 Collateral arterial circulation around the right elbow

Distal Portion of the Radial and Ulnar Arteries

- Use forceps to reveal and trace the following arteries distally through the forearm **(Figure 32-7)**:

  - **Radial a.** — smaller than the ulnar a.
    - Passes along the radial side of the forearm (deep to brachioradialis m.) to the wrist
    - At the wrist, the radial a. is lateral to the flexor carpi radialis tendon and anterior to the styloid process of the radius
    - Winds laterally around the wrist, deep to the abductor pollicis longus m. and extensor pollicis brevis and longus mm.; principal contributor to the deep palmar arterial arch of the hand
    - Observe the radial a. within the anatomical snuff box
  - **Ulnar a.** — larger than the radial a.; courses medial to the biceps brachii tendon
    - Accompanied by the median n.; passes between the ulnar and radial heads of the flexor digitorum superficialis m.
    - Midway down the forearm, crosses posterior to the median n. to reach the superficial side of the flexor digitorum profundus m.
    - Along the distal region of the forearm, lies lateral to the ulnar n.; exits the forearm lateral to the pisiform bone and superficial to the flexor retinaculum

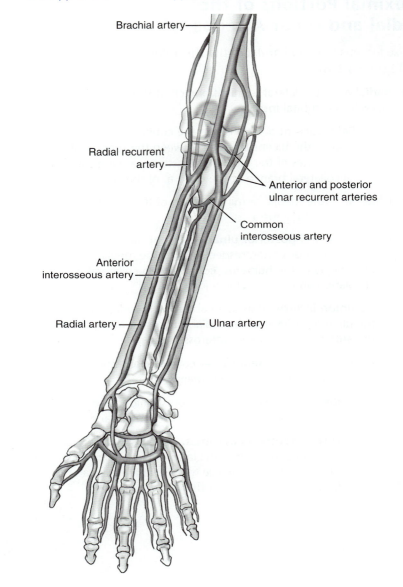

Figure 32-7 Distal portion of the right radial and ulnar arteries

Brachial Plexus — Branches in the Forearm

- Use forceps to reveal and identify the terminal branches of the median and ulnar nn.; follow each nerve distally to the wrist **(Figure 32-8)**:

  - **Median n.** — enters the forearm by coursing between the humeral and ulnar heads of the pronator teres m.; descends between the flexor digitorum superficialis and profundus mm. in the forearm, entering the carpal tunnel of the wrist; divides into the following:

    - **Anterior interosseous n.** — originates between the two heads of the pronator teres m. and courses distally down the forearm with the anterior interosseous a.; innervates the deeper muscles of the anterior compartment of the forearm (flexor pollicis longus m., lateral half of the flexor digitorum profundus m., and pronator quadratus m.)

    - **Palmar cutaneous branch** — originates from the median n. in the distal forearm, proximal to the flexor retinaculum; courses superficially into the hand and innervates the skin over the base and central palm

  - **Ulnar n.** — courses posterior to the medial epicondyle of the humerus ("funny bone") to enter the forearm

    - Enters the forearm between the two heads of the flexor carpi ulnaris m.; courses down the medial side of the forearm, between the flexor carpi ulnaris and flexor digitorum profundus mm.; courses under the lateral lip of the tendon of the flexor carpi ulnaris m. proximal to the wrist

    - Observe a palmar branch that originates in the middle of the forearm and passes into the hand superficial to the flexor retinaculum to supply skin on the medial side of the palm

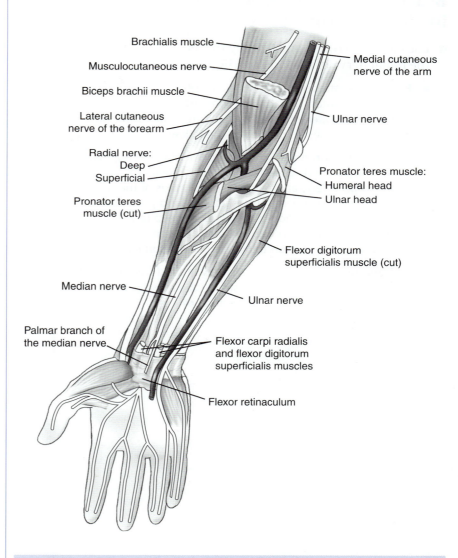

GAFS pp 699–700   ACGA pp 227, 244, 246, 253   NAHA Plates 447–448

Figure 32-8   Right brachial plexus terminal branches — forearm

Brachial Plexus — Branches in the Forearm Continued

Brachial Plexus — Branches in the Forearm—cont'd

- Use forceps to reveal and identify the terminal branches of the radial nerve in the forearm **(Figure 32-9)**:

  - **Radial n.** — after piercing the lateral intermuscular septum, the radial n. enters the anterior compartment of the forearm and descends lateral to the brachialis m., anterior to the lateral epicondyle; branches into the following:

    - **Superficial branch** — passes superficial to the supinator m. and descends deep to the brachioradialis m., alongside the radial artery; approximately two thirds of the way down the forearm, it courses laterally and posteriorly around the radial side of the forearm deep to the brachioradialis m.; continues into the hand, where it innervates the skin on the posterolateral surface

    - **Deep branch** — wraps posteriorly around the radius and pierces the supinator m. to supply the muscles in the posterior compartment of the forearm

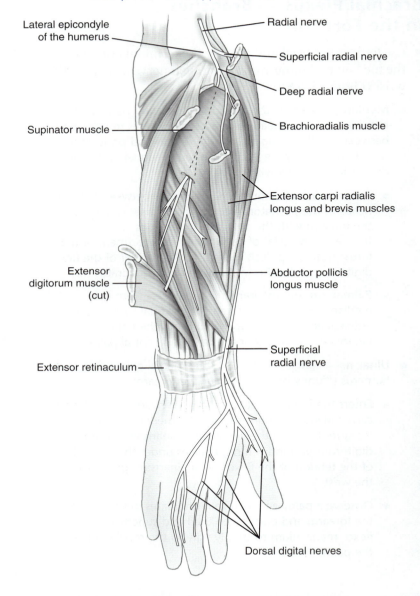

Figure 32-9 Posterior view of the nerves of the right forearm

Hand

Lab 33

Prior to dissection, you should familiarize yourself with the following structures:

OSTEOLOGY
- Hand
  - Carpal bones (8)
    - Proximal row
      - Pisiform
      - Triquetrum
      - Lunate
      - Scaphoid
    - Distal row
      - Trapezium
      - Trapezoid
      - Capitate
      - Hamate
        - Hook of the hamate
  - Metacarpals (5)
  - Phalanges (14)
    - Proximal, middle, and distal phalanges

VASCULATURE
- Radial and ulnar aa.
  - Superficial palmar arch
    - Common palmar digital aa.
      - Proper palmar digital aa.
  - Deep palmar arch
    - Palmar metacarpal aa.
    - Princeps pollicis a.

HAND
- Tendons and muscles
  - Flexor digitorum superficialis tendons
  - Flexor digitorum profundus tendons
  - Palmaris longus m.
  - Palmaris brevis m.
  - Thenar mm.
    - Abductor pollicis brevis m.
    - Opponens pollicis m.
    - Flexor pollicis brevis m.
  - Adductor pollicis m.
  - Hypothenar mm.
    - Abductor digiti minimi m.
    - Opponens digiti minimi m.
    - Flexor digiti minimi m.
  - Lumbrical mm. (4)
  - Dorsal interossei mm. (4)
  - Palmar interossei mm. (3)

NERVES
- Median n.
  - Superficial palmar branch of the median n.
  - Recurrent branch of the median n.
  - Common palmar digital nn.
    - Proper palmar digital nn.
- Ulnar n.
  - Superficial branch of the ulnar n.
  - Common palmar digital nn.
    - Proper palmar digital nn.
  - Deep branch of the ulnar n.
- Radial n.

MISCELLANEOUS
- Flexor retinaculum
- Anatomical snuff box
- Palmar aponeurosis
- Carpal tunnel
- Fibrous digital sheaths
- Extensor expansion hood

Lab 33 Dissection Overview

The purpose of this laboratory session is to learn the anatomy of the hand through dissection. You will do so through the following suggested sequence:

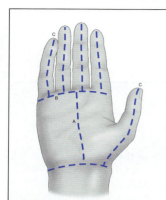

1. Dissect and reflect the skin covering the hand.

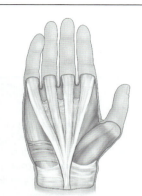

2. Dissect and reflect the palmar aponeurosis.

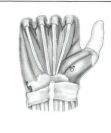
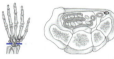

3. Dissect and identify the flexor retinaculum and study the carpal tunnel, its borders, and the structures that traverse the tunnel.

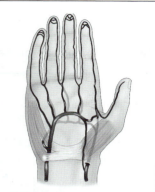

4. Dissect and identify the arterial supply of the hand.

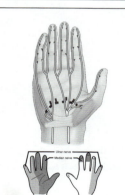

5. Dissect and identify the nerves of the hand, primarily the ulnar and median nerves.

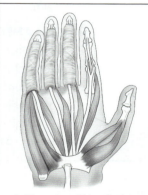

6. Dissect and identify the muscles of the thenar and hypothenar compartments, as well as the central compartment of the hand.

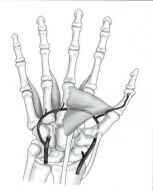

7. Dissect the adductor pollicis muscle and deep palmar arterial arch from the radial artery.

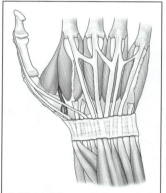

8. Dissect the posterior aspect of the hand and extensor expansion hood over the digits.

Hand — Skin Removal

- Use a scalpel to make the following incisions to remove the skin from the palmar surface of the hand; leave the palmar aponeurosis intact **(Figure 33-1)**:
  - If the hand is clenched, have a partner hold it open as much as possible while you make a longitudinal incision along the middle of the palm *(A)* and transversely across the palm *(B)*
  - Use a sharp scalpel to remove the skin from the hand; note that the skin is bound to the palmar aponeurosis (a tough fascia), which may require time and patience to separate
  - Make a longitudinal incision along the length of each finger and the thumb *(C)*
  - Remove the skin, being careful to not damage the underlying nerves, vessels, and fibrous sheaths
  - Ask your instructor about the number of fingers to dissect

- Use a scalpel to remove the skin on the dorsal surface of the hand, leaving the superficial fascia intact

- The palmar structures are customarily grouped into the following compartments:
  - **Thenar** — lateral compartment
  - **Hypothenar** — medial compartment
  - **Intermediate** — central compartment
  - **Adductor** — deep compartment

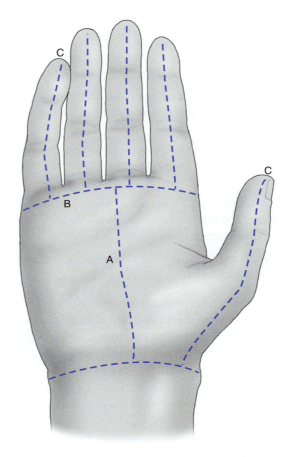

Figure 33-1 Right hand skin incisions

Palmar Aponeurosis

- Use forceps to reveal and identify the following structures **(Figure 33-2)**:
  - **Palmar aponeurosis** — a thick, well-defined part of the deep fascia of the palm
    - The proximal end is continuous with the flexor retinaculum and the palmaris longus tendon
    - **Fibrous digital sheaths of the hand** — ligamentous tubes that enclose the synovial sheaths of tendons en route to the digits
  - **Thenar eminence** — the lateral eminence on the palmar surface; the palmar aponeurosis is thin over the thenar eminence
  - **Hypothenar eminence** — the medial eminence on the palmar surface; the palmar aponeurosis is also thin over the hypothenar eminence
  - **Palmaris brevis m.** — muscle fibers course transversely over the hypothenar eminence

- Use a scalpel to detach the palmaris brevis m. from the palmar aponeurosis and then carefully remove the palmar aponeurosis; do not damage the **common** and **proper digital nn., aa.,** and **vv.** deep to the palmar aponeurosis; removal of the palmar aponeurosis requires lifting up the palmar aponeurosis and cutting, with scalpel or scissors, connections to the underlying tendons and bones

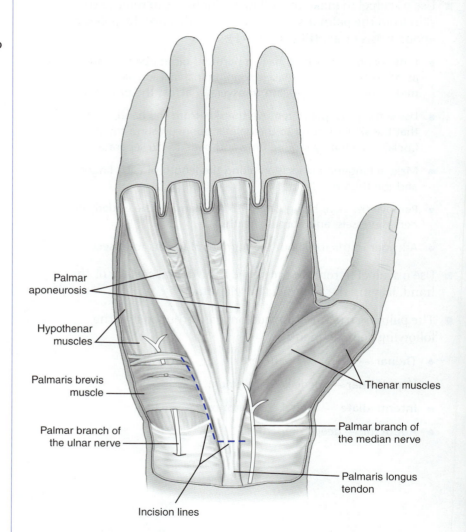

Figure 33-2 Palmar aponeurosis of the right hand

Carpal Tunnel

■ Use forceps to reveal and identify the following **(Figure 33-3)**:

● **Flexor retinaculum** (transverse carpal ligament) — attached medially to the pisiform bone and hook of the hamate bone; attached laterally to the trapezium and scaphoid bones (see Figure 33-3A)

● **Carpal tunnel** — the carpal bones form an anterior concavity, which is converted into a tunnel by the overlying flexor retinaculum (see Figure 33-3B)

  • Contains the flexor pollicis longus tendon, all of the flexor digitorum tendons, and the median n.

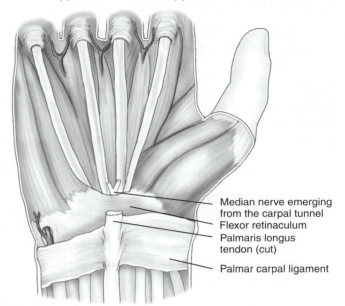

Figure 33-3 Right flexor retinaculum and carpal tunnel. **A,** Anterior view. **B,** Cross-section through the distal row of carpal bones

Vessels of the Palm of the Hand

- Use forceps to reveal and identify the following arteries; the veins have the same names and may be removed **(Figure 33-4)**:

  - **Ulnar a.** — lateral to the pisiform bone and superficial to the flexor retinaculum; major contributor to the superficial palmar arch
    - **Deep branch of the ulnar a.** — branch of the ulnar a.; courses deep to the hypothenar mm.; do not follow the deep branch at this time
      - **Common palmar digital aa.** — arise from the superficial palmar arch and bifurcate into the proper palmar digital aa.; course over the metacarpal bones
      - **Proper palmar digital aa.** — bifurcation of the common palmar digital aa.; course along the medial and lateral surfaces of each finger
  - **Superficial palmar branch of the radial a.** — courses deep to the thenar mm.
    - **Superficial palmar arch** — formed by the superficial anastomosis between the radial and ulnar aa.
      - **Princeps pollicis a.** — arterial supply to the thumb; usually a branch from the deep radial a.

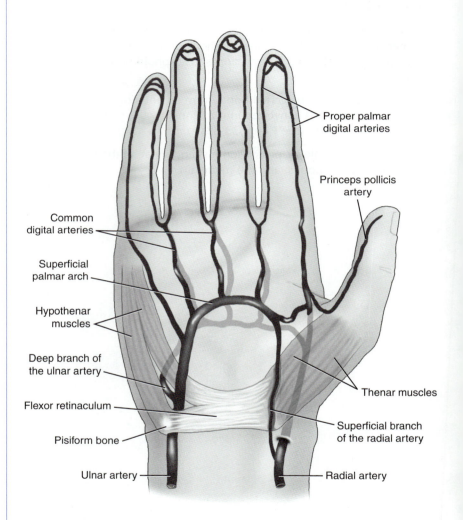

Figure 33-4 Vessels of the palm of the right hand

Nerves of the Palm of the Hand

- Use forceps to reveal and identify the following nerves:

  - **Median n.** — enters the palmar surface of the hand, deep to the flexor retinaculum, and divides into a number of branches **(Figure 33-5A)**

    - **Recurrent median n.** — supplies the thenar mm.; accompanies the princeps pollicis a. and v.

    - **Common palmar digital nn.** — course distally through the hand and terminate by dividing into proper palmar digital nn.; accompany the common palmar digital aa. and vv.

      - **Proper palmar digital nn.** — supply digits 1, 2, 3, and the lateral (radial) side of digit 4 (see Figure 33-5B); accompany the proper palmar digital aa. and vv.

  - **Ulnar n.** — enters the palmar surface of the hand with the ulnar a., superficial to the flexor retinaculum, and divides into superficial and deep branches (see Figure 33-5A)

    - **Superficial branch of the ulnar n.**

      - **Common palmar digital nn.** — course distally through the hand and terminate by dividing into proper palmar digital nn.

      - **Proper palmar digital nn.** — supply digit 5 and the medial (ulnar) side of digit 4 (see Figure 33-5B); accompany proper palmar digital aa. and vv.

    - **Deep branch of the ulnar n.** — disappears through the hypothenar mm., in company with the deep ulnar a.; do not follow the deep branch at this time

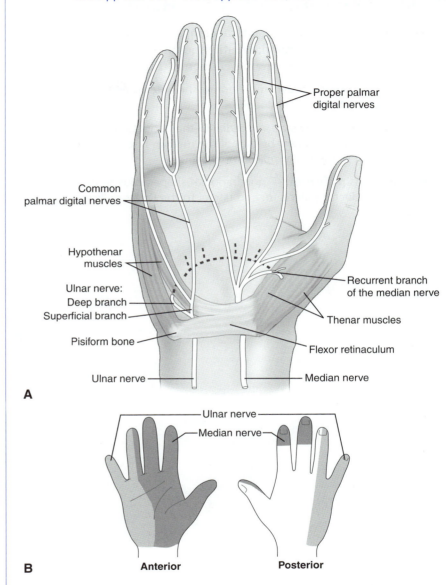

Figure 33-5 Nerves of the palm of the right hand. **A,** Nerves. **B,** Cutaneous fields

Thenar Compartment of the Hand

- **Thenar compartment** — lateral compartment of the palmar surface of the hand; identify the three muscles of the thumb that form the thenar eminence **(Figure 33-6)**:

  - **Abductor pollicis brevis m.** — forms the anterolateral portion of the thenar eminence

  - **Flexor pollicis brevis m.** — medial to the abductor pollicis brevis m.; the recurrent branch of the median n. crosses superficial to the flexor pollicis brevis m.

  - **Opponens pollicis m.** — quadrangular-shaped muscle deep to the abductor pollicis m. and lateral to the flexor pollicis brevis m.

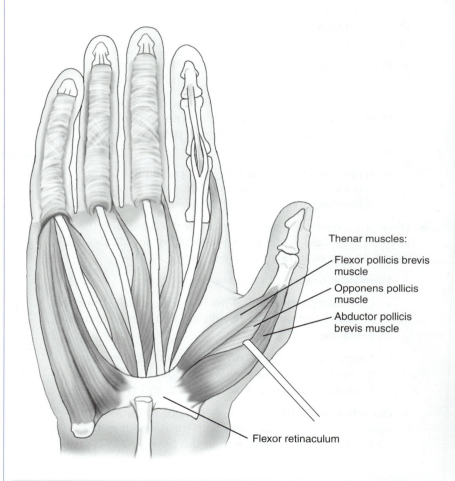

Figure 33-6 Right thenar muscles

Hypothenar Compartment of the Hand

- **Hypothenar compartment** — medial compartment of the palmar surface of the hand; identify the three muscles of digit 5 that form the hypothenar eminence (Figure 33-7):

  - **Abductor digiti minimi m.** — most superficial and medial of the three muscles

  - **Flexor digiti minimi m.** — lateral to the abductor digiti minimi m.

  - **Opponens digiti minimi m.** — quadrangular-shaped muscle deep to the abductor and flexor digiti minimi mm.

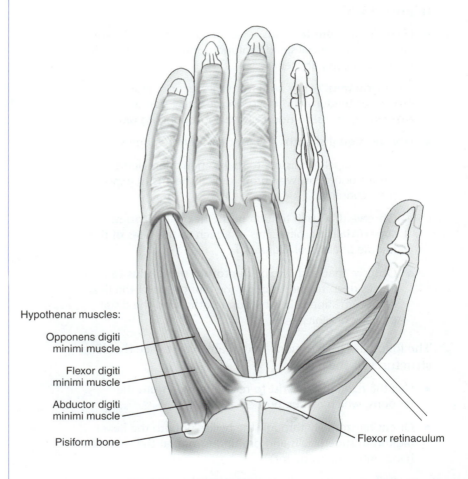

Figure 33-7 Right hypothenar muscles

Central Compartment of the Palm of the Hand

- Use forceps to reveal and identify the following **(Figure 33-8)**:

  - **Flexor digitorum tendons** — tendons of both the flexor digitorum superficialis and profundus mm. course through the central compartment

  - **Lumbrical mm.** (4) — arise from the flexor digitorum profundus tendons and insert on the radial side of the **extensor expansion hood** of the corresponding digit

  - **Fibrous digital sheaths** — cover each of the fingers
    - Use a scalpel or scissors to make an incision along the length of one or two fibrous digital sheaths to expose their contents
    - Observe that each tendon of the **flexor digitorum superficialis m.** bifurcates to attach to the sides of the middle phalanx of digits 2–5
    - Observe that each **flexor digitorum profundus tendon** passes deep to and through the bifurcation of the flexor digitorum superficialis tendon to attach on the distal phalanx of digits 2–5

- The following instructions will enable you to see the deep structures of the palm:

  - Flex the hand at the wrist to relieve tension from the tendons, which can be pushed aside

  - Or cut horizontally through the bellies of both the flexor digitorum superficialis and profundus mm. at the wrist of one hand only (ask instructor)
    - Reflect the flexor digitorum superficialis and profundus tendons from the wrist toward the fingertips

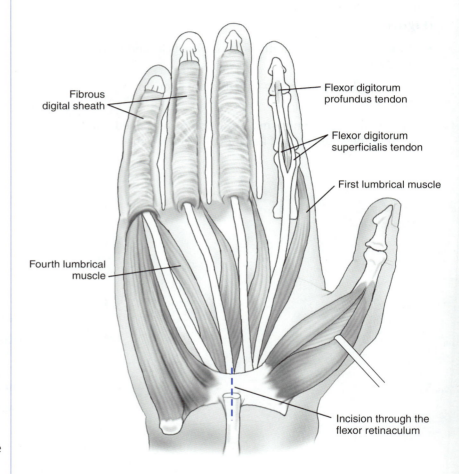

Figure 33-8 Central compartment of the right palm

Adductor Compartment

- Use forceps to reveal and identify the following **(Figure 33-9)**:

  - **Adductor pollicis m.** — a fan-shaped muscle; it has two heads (oblique and transverse) that are separated by the radial a. as the artery enters the palm to form the deep palmar arterial arch
    - Follow the muscle's tendon to the base of the proximal phalanx of the thumb
  - **Deep palmar arch** — direct continuation of the radial a.; anastomoses with the deep branch of the ulnar a., deep to the long flexor tendons and in contact with the bases of the metacarpal bones
    - **Palmar metacarpal aa.** — anastomose with the common palmar digital aa. from the superficial palmar arterial arch
  - **Princeps pollicis a.** — courses along the medial side of the thumb
  - **Deep ulnar n.** — courses deep to the abductor digiti minimi and flexor digiti minimi mm.; perforates the opponens digiti minimi m.
  - **Palmar interossei mm.** (3) — three muscles located between the metacarpal bones on the palmar surface of the hand (adduct digits 2, 4, and 5)

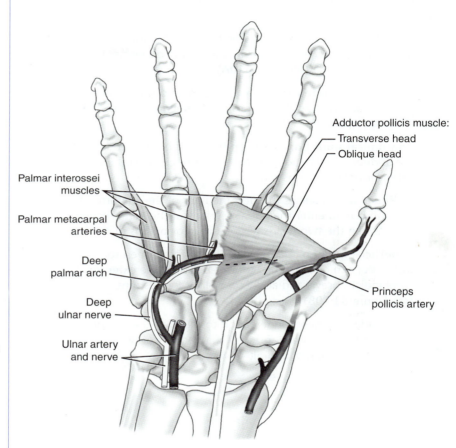

Figure 33-9 Deeper structures of the central compartment of the right palm

Dorsal Surface of the Hand

■ Turn the hand prone and use forceps to reveal and identify the following:

- **Dorsal interossei mm.** (4) — the four muscles that occupy the intervals between the dorsal metacarpal bones (abduct digits 2, 3, and 4) **(Figure 33-10A)**

  - **First dorsal interosseus m.** — the most obvious; the radial a. separates its two proximal attachments between metacarpals 1 and 2

- **Anatomical snuff box** — region bounded by the tendons of the abductor pollicis longus, extensor pollicis brevis, and extensor pollicis longus mm.

  - **Radial a.** — courses through the floor of the anatomical snuff box to enter the palmar surface of the hand; courses between the two heads of the adductor pollicis m.

- **Superficial radial n.** — usually exits the forearm en route to the dorsum of the hand; courses between the extensor carpi radialis brevis and abductor pollicis longus mm. (see Figure 33-10B)

  - Provides cutaneous innervation to much of the dorsum of the hand, thumb, and proximal regions of digits 2, 3, and the radial half of digit 4

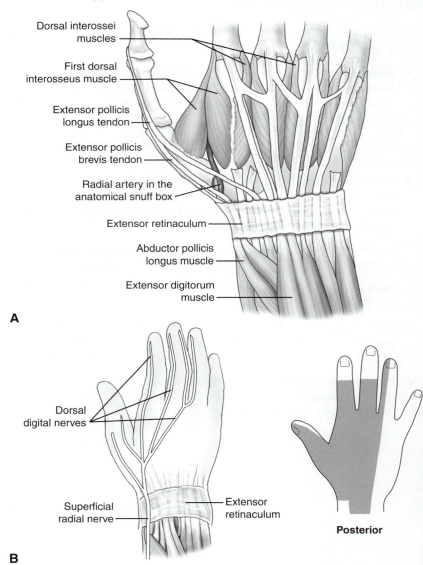

Figure 33-10 Dorsal surface of the right hand. **A,** Structures. **B,** Superficial radial nerve

Dorsal Hood and Extensor Expansion of the Digits

- Use forceps to reveal and identify the following **(Figure 33-11)**:

  - **Dorsal hood** — associated with the metacarpophalangeal joint; stabilizes the lumbrical and interossei tendons and provides leverage to the extensor digitorum tendons

  - **Extensor expansion** — the four tendons from the extensor digitorum m. spread out over the metacarpophalangeal joint to form the extensor expansion

    - Triangular shaped, with the base facing proximally and the apex facing distally

    - The extensor expansions of digit 2 (index finger) and digit 5 are joined by the tendons of the extensor indicis and extensor digiti minimi mm., respectively

    - The lumbrical and interosseous mm. attach to the proximal sides of the extensor expansion

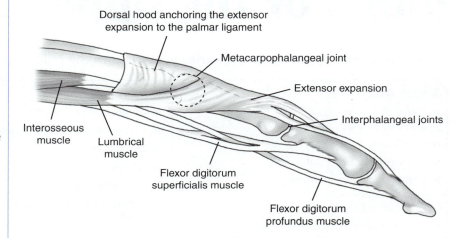

Figure 33-11 Lateral view of digit 3

Joints of the Upper Limb

Lab 34

Prior to dissection, you should familiarize yourself with the following structures:

SHOULDER
- Sternoclavicular joint
  - Articular disc
- Costoclavicular ligament
- Acromioclavicular joint
- Coracoclavicular ligaments
  - Conoid ligament
  - Trapezoid ligament
- Glenohumeral joint capsule
  - Posterior region of the joint capsule
  - Superior glenohumeral ligament
  - Middle glenohumeral ligament
  - Inferior glenohumeral ligament
- Subscapular bursa
- Coracohumeral ligament
- Transverse humeral ligament
- Glenoid labrum
- Articular cartilage
- Glenoid cavity
- Tendon of the long head of the biceps brachii m.

ELBOW
- Joint capsule
- Radial collateral ligament of the elbow
- Ulnar collateral ligament of the elbow
- Annular ligament

WRIST
- Radial collateral ligament of the wrist
- Ulnar collateral ligament of the wrist
- Intercarpal ligaments

HAND AND DIGITS
- Metacarpophalangeal joints
- Interphalangeal joints
- Medial collateral digital ligaments
- Lateral collateral digital ligaments

Lab 34 Dissection Overview

The purpose of this laboratory session is to learn the anatomy of the joints of the upper limb through dissection. You will do so through the following suggested sequence:

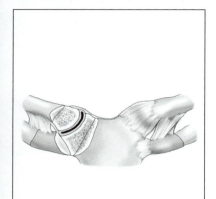

1. To ensure that the limb dissections are not completely destroyed, choose one or two joints to dissect on the upper limb. Other dissection tables will choose another limb joint. All should dissect the sternoclavicular joint.

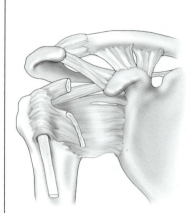

2. Dissect and cut away the muscles that cross the shoulder joint. Dissect and reveal the structures associated with the shoulder joint.

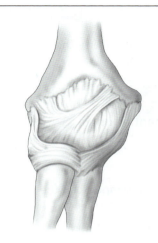

3. Dissect and cut away the muscles that cross the elbow joint. Dissect and reveal the structures associated with the elbow joint.

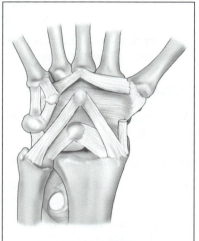

4. Dissect and cut away the muscles that cross the wrist and finger joints. Dissect and reveal the structures associated with the wrist and finger joints.

UPPER LIMB — JOINT DISSECTION

- Select one upper limb on which to dissect the joints; using a scalpel and forceps, dissect using the following steps:
  - First, muscles that surround each joint will be removed from the joint to reveal the joint capsule
  - Second, the joint capsule and tendons that traverse the capsule will be cut to reveal the articulation

Sternoclavicular Joint

- Articulation of the clavicle and the manubrium of the sternum
- Identify the following **(Figure 34-1)**:
  - **Sternoclavicular joint** — use a scalpel to scrape clean the joint capsule; use a scalpel to open the joint capsule
    - **Articular disc** — located between the manubrium, the clavicle, and rib 1
  - **Costoclavicular ligament** — attached to rib 1 and the inferior border of the clavicle

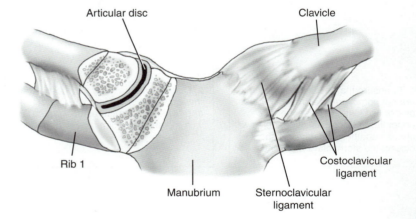

Figure 34-1 Sternoclavicular joint

Shoulder Joint

- Identify the following (when necessary cut and reflect overlying muscles) **(Figure 34-2)**:

  - **Coracoclavicular ligament** — consists of two ligaments:
    - **Conoid ligament** — courses between the conoid tubercle and superior aspect of the coracoid process
    - **Trapezoid ligament** — attached to the superior aspect of the coracoid process and the trapezoid line on the inferior aspect of the clavicle
  - **Acromioclavicular joint** — open with a scalpel
    - **Articular disc** — difficult to see; the disc separates the joint surfaces
  - **Coracoacromial ligament** — ligamentous attachment between the coracoid process and the anterior tip of the acromion
  - **Coracohumeral ligament** — a strong, ligamentous band that attaches the coracoid process to the anterior region of the greater tubercle of the humerus
  - **Transverse humeral ligament** — covers the intertubercular groove (between the greater and lesser tubercles); crosses anterior to the tendon of the long head of the biceps brachii m.
  - **Subscapular bursa** — deep to the subscapularis m.; attempt to identify the continuity of the subscapular bursa with the synovial membrane of the glenohumeral joint
  - **Rotator cuff** — observe the tendons of the supraspinatus, infraspinatus, teres minor, and subscapularis mm. where they insert into the glenohumeral joint capsule

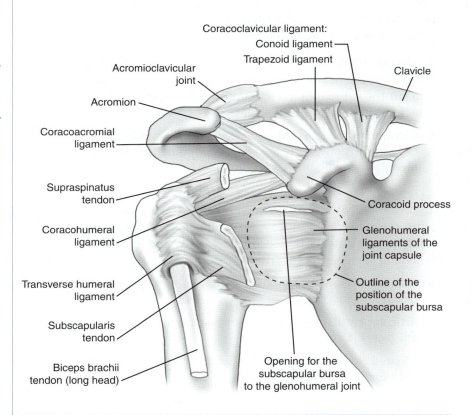

Figure 34-2 Anterior view of the right shoulder joint (expanded)

Glenohumeral Joint Capsule

- The glenohumeral joint capsule is attached from the periphery of the glenoid fossa of the scapula to the anatomic neck of the humerus

- To identify the ligaments of the glenohumeral joint capsule, cut the tendon of the supraspinatus m. from its attachment and cut the subscapularis tendon from its lesser tubercle attachment; reflect both muscles

  - **Glenohumeral ligaments** — intrinsic thickenings in the joint capsule anteriorly; there are **superior, middle,** and **inferior glenohumeral ligaments (Figure 34-3A)**, and there is one posterior glenohumeral ligament

- To better study the structures composing the glenohumeral joint, use a scalpel to make a vertical incision through the joint capsule anteriorly (see Figure 34-3A) and identify the following (see Figure 34-3B):

  - **Glenoid labrum** — fibrocartilaginous ring that adds depth to the glenoid fossa

  - **Articular cartilage** — hyaline cartilage covering the articular surfaces

  - **Glenoid cavity** — shallow fossa, which articulates with the head of the humerus

  - **Long head of the biceps brachii m.** — trace the tendon of this muscle to its attachment on the supraglenoid tubercle of the scapula; also trace the tendon of the long head of the triceps brachii m. to the infraglenoid tubercle of the scapula

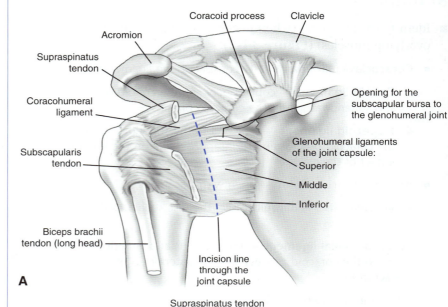

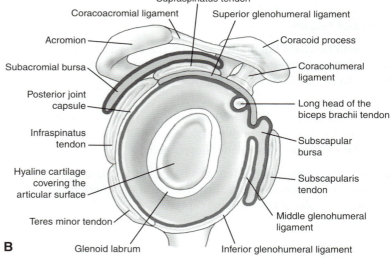

Figure 34-3 Right shoulder joint. **A,** Anterior view of the joint capsule. **B,** Lateral view of the opened joint capsule

Elbow Joint

- Palpate the olecranon process of the ulna and the medial and lateral epicondyles of the humerus; use a scalpel, forceps, and scissors to remove the muscles, arteries, veins, and nerves from the anterior, medial, and lateral surfaces of one elbow joint

- Use a sharp scalpel to scrape clean the underlying capsule of the elbow joint

- Identify the following ligaments **(Figure 34-4)**:

  - **Ulnar collateral ligament**
    - Anterior portion — between the medial epicondyle of the humerus and coronoid process of the ulna
    - Posterior portion — between the medial epicondyle of the humerus and olecranon process of the ulna

  - **Radial collateral ligament** — between the lateral epicondyle of the humerus and neck of the radius

  - **Annular ligament** — courses around the head of the radius; attaches to the anterior and posterior margins of the radial notch of the ulna; this ligament and its associated capsule form the proximal radioulnar joint

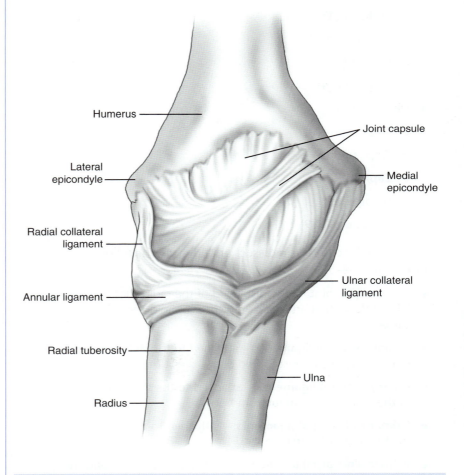

Figure 34-4 Right elbow joint

Wrist Joint

- If you desire to dissect the wrist joint, you will need to remove all muscles, arteries, veins, and nerves from the anterior region of one wrist and hand

- Using a skeleton, identify the carpal bones **(Figure 34-5A)**:

  - Proximal row
    - **Pisiform (1)**
    - **Triquetrum (2)**
    - **Lunate (3)**
    - **Scaphoid (4)**
  - Distal row
    - **Trapezium (5)**
    - **Trapezoid (6)**
    - **Capitate (7)**
    - **Hamate (8)**
    - **Metacarpals (9)**

- Return to the cadaver to dissect and identify the following (see Figure 34-5B):

  - **Radiocarpal joint** — the distal end of the radius has two joint surfaces that articulate with the scaphoid and lunate carpal bones
  - **Radial collateral ligament** — attached to the styloid process of the radius and the scaphoid bone
  - **Ulnar collateral ligament** — attached to the styloid process of the ulna and the triquetrum bone
  - **Palmar radiocarpal ligaments** — attached to the radius and the two rows of carpal bones
  - **Palmar ulnocarpal ligament** — attached to the ulna and the two rows of carpal bones

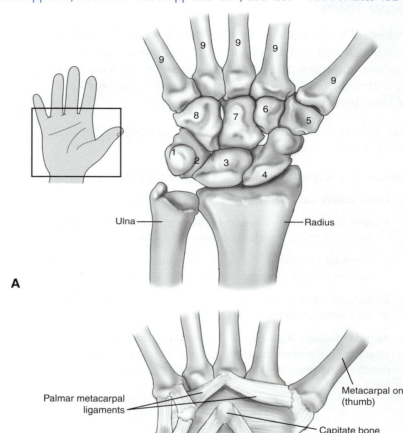

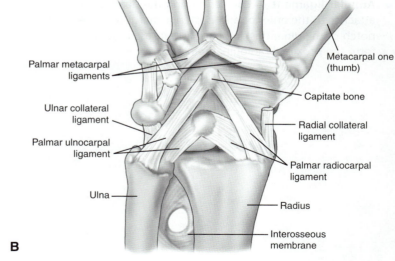

Figure 34-5 Carpal bone joints of the right hand. **A**, Osteology. **B**, Ligaments

Hand and Digit Joints

- Remove muscles and tendons to observe the joint capsules of the thumb and one digit

- Identify the following **(Figure 34-6)**:

  - **Carpometacarpal ligaments** — attached to the distal row of carpal bones and the base of the metacarpal bones

  - **Saddle joint** — articulation of the trapezium and base of the first metacarpal bones (thumb only)

  - **Hinge joints** — the interphalangeal joints of the thumb and digits 2–5

  - **Joint capsule** — each metacarpophalangeal (MP) and interphalangeal (IP) joint is surrounded by its own joint capsule

  - **Medial** and **lateral collateral digital ligaments** — medial and lateral thickenings of the joint capsule

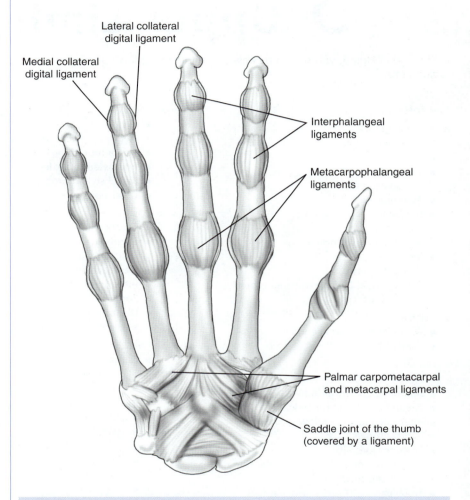

Figure 34-6 Joints of the right hand

Unit 5 Upper Limb Overview

At the end of Unit 5, you should be able to identify the following structures on cadavers, skeletons, and/or radiographs:

Osteology

- Scapula
  - Subscapular fossa
  - Spine
  - Supraspinous fossa
  - Infraspinous fossa
  - Acromion
  - Medial and lateral borders
  - Superior angle
    - Suprascapular notch
  - Inferior angle
  - Glenoid cavity
  - Supraglenoid and infraglenoid tubercles
  - Coracoid process
- Clavicle
  - Acromial and sternal ends
  - Conoid tubercle
- Humerus
  - Head
  - Anatomic and surgical necks
  - Greater and lesser tubercles
  - Intertubercular (bicipital) groove
  - Radial groove
  - Deltoid tuberosity
  - Lateral and medial supracondylar ridges
  - Lateral and medial epicondyles
  - Trochlea
  - Capitulum
  - Coronoid fossa
  - Olecranon fossa
- Radius
  - Head
  - Neck
  - Radial tuberosity
  - Interosseous border
  - Radial styloid process
  - Ulnar notch
- Ulna
  - Olecranon
  - Coronoid process
    - Radial notch
  - Trochlear notch
  - Interosseous border
  - Supinator crest
  - Ulnar head
    - Ulnar styloid process
- Hand
  - Carpal bones (8)
    - Scaphoid
    - Lunate
    - Triquetrum
    - Pisiform
    - Hamate
      - Hook of the hamate
    - Capitate
    - Trapezoid
    - Trapezium
  - Metacarpal bones (5)
  - Phalanges (14)
  - Proximal, middle, and distal phalanges

Muscles

- Shoulder
  - Deltoid m.
  - Trapezius m.
  - Levator scapulae m.
  - Serratus anterior m.
  - Pectoralis minor m.
  - Rhomboid major m.
  - Rhomboid minor m.
  - Subclavius m.
  - Rotator cuff muscles
    - Supraspinatus m.
    - Infraspinatus m.
    - Teres minor m.
    - Subscapularis m.
  - Teres major m.
  - Pectoralis major m.
  - Latissimus dorsi m.
- Arm
  - Coracobrachialis m.
  - Biceps brachii m.
    - Long head
    - Short head
  - Brachialis m.
  - Triceps brachii m.
    - Long head
    - Lateral head
    - Medial head
- Anterior compartment of the forearm

- Pronator teres m.
- Flexor carpi radialis m.
- Flexor carpi ulnaris m.
- Palmaris longus m.
- Flexor digitorum superficialis m.
- Flexor digitorum profundus m.
- Flexor pollicis longus m.
- Pronator quadratus m.
- Posterior compartment of the forearm
  - Brachioradialis m.
  - Extensor carpi radialis longus m.
  - Extensor carpi radialis brevis m.
  - Extensor digitorum m.
  - Extensor digiti minimi m.
  - Extensor carpi ulnaris m.
  - Extensor indicis m.
  - Extensor pollicis longus and brevis mm.
  - Abductor pollicis longus m.
  - Anconeus m.
  - Supinator m.
- Hand
  - Palmaris brevis m.
  - Thenar mm.
    - Abductor pollicis brevis, opponens pollicis, and flexor pollicis brevis mm.
  - Adductor pollicis m.
  - Hypothenar mm.
    - Abductor digiti minimi, opponens digiti minimi, and flexor digiti minimi mm.
  - Lumbrical mm.
  - Dorsal interossei mm.
  - Palmar interossei mm.

Arteries

- Aorta
  - Subclavian a.
    - Thyrocervical trunk
      - Transverse cervical a.
        - Superficial branch
        - Deep branch (dorsal scapular a.)
      - Suprascapular a.
  - Axillary a.
    - Superior thoracic a.
    - Thoracoacromial a.
      - Acromial, deltoid, pectoral, and clavicular branches
    - Lateral thoracic a.
    - Subscapular a.
      - Circumflex scapular a.
      - Thoracodorsal a.
    - Anterior humeral circumflex a.
    - Posterior humeral circumflex a.
  - Brachial a.
    - Deep a. of the arm
      - Radial collateral a.
      - Middle collateral a.
    - Superior ulnar collateral a.
    - Inferior ulnar collateral a.
  - Radial a.
    - Radial recurrent a.
    - Palmar carpal branch
    - Superficial palmar arch
    - Dorsal metacarpal aa.
    - Dorsal digital aa.
    - Princeps pollicis a.
    - Deep palmar arch
      - Palmar metacarpal aa.
- Ulnar a.
  - Anterior ulnar recurrent a.
  - Posterior ulnar recurrent a.
  - Common interosseous a.
    - Anterior interosseous a.
    - Posterior interosseous a.
      - Interosseous recurrent a.
  - Palmar carpal branch
  - Deep palmar branch
  - Superficial palmar arch
  - Common palmar digital aa.
    - Proper palmar digital aa.

Veins

- Axillary v.
  - Subscapular v.
  - Circumflex scapular v.
    - Thoracodorsal v.
    - Posterior circumflex humeral v.
    - Anterior circumflex humeral v.
  - Lateral thoracic v.
- Superficial veins of the upper limb
  - Cephalic v.
    - Thoracoacromial v.
  - Basilic v.
  - Median cubital v.
  - Dorsal venous network of the hand
- Deep veins of the upper limb
  - Brachial v.
  - Ulnar v.
  - Radial v.

Lymphatics

- Axillary lymph nodes

Nerves

- *Five Roots (C5, C6, C7, C8, T1)*
  - Dorsal scapular n. and long thoracic n.
- *Three Trunks*
  - Superior
    - Suprascapular n.
    - N. to the subclavius m.
  - Middle
  - Inferior
- *Six Divisions*
  - Three anterior and three posterior
- *Three Cords*
  - Lateral
    - Lateral pectoral n.
  - Medial

Continued

Nerves—cont'd
- *Three Cords*—cont'd
  - Medial—cont'd
    - Medial pectoral n.
    - Medial cutaneous n. of the arm
    - Medial cutaneous n. of the forearm
  - Posterior
    - Upper subscapular n.
    - Thoracodorsal n.
    - Lower subscapular n.
- *Five Terminal Branches*
  - Musculocutaneous n.
    - Muscular branches
    - Lateral cutaneous n. of the forearm
  - Median n.
    - Muscular branches
    - Palmar branch
    - Recurrent branch of the median n.
    - Digital branches of the median n. (common and proper palmar digital nn.)
  - Ulnar n.
    - Muscular branches
    - Superficial branch of the ulnar n.
    - Deep branch of the ulnar n.
    - Digital branches of the ulnar n. (common and proper palmar digital nn.)
  - Radial n.
    - Muscular branches
    - Posterior cutaneous nn. of the arm and forearm
    - Inferior lateral cutaneous n. of the arm
    - Deep branch (posterior interosseous n.)
    - Superficial branch
  - Axillary n.
    - Muscular branches
    - Superior lateral cutaneous n. of the arm

Joints
- Shoulder
  - Sternoclavicular joint
    - Articular disc
  - Costoclavicular joint
  - Acromioclavicular joint
  - Coracoclavicular ligaments
    - Conoid ligament
    - Trapezoid ligament
  - Glenohumeral capsule
    - Posterior region of the joint capsule
    - Superior glenohumeral ligament
    - Middle glenohumeral ligament
    - Inferior glenohumeral ligament
  - Subscapular bursa
  - Coracohumeral ligament
  - Transverse humeral ligament
  - Glenoid labrum
  - Articular cartilage
  - Tendon of the long head of the biceps brachii m.
- Elbow
  - Joint capsule
  - Radial collateral ligament of the elbow
  - Ulnar collateral ligament of the elbow
  - Annular ligament
- Wrist
  - Radial collateral ligament of the wrist
  - Ulnar collateral ligament of the wrist
  - Intercarpal ligaments
- Digits
  - Metacarpophalangeal joints
  - Interphalangeal joints
  - Lateral collateral digital ligaments
  - Medial collateral digital ligaments

Fascia
- Supraspinous fascia
- Infraspinous fascia
- Axillary fascia
- Suspensory ligament of the axilla
- Brachial fascia
- Medial intermuscular septum of the arm
- Lateral intermuscular septum of the arm
- Antebrachial fascia
- Flexor and extensor retinacula
- Carpal tunnel
- Fibrous digital sheaths
- Extensor expansion

Miscellaneous
- Deltopectoral triangle
- Anatomical snuff box

Unit 6
Lower Limb

Lab 35 Osteology of the Lower Limb   507

Lab 36 Superficial Structures of the Lower Limb and Gluteal Region   516

Lab 37 Thigh   524

Lab 38 Leg   537

Lab 39 Foot   546

Lab 40 Joints of the Lower Limb   554

Unit 6 Lower Limb Overview   562

Muscles of the Lower Limb

Muscle	Proximal Attachment	Distal Attachment	Action	Innervation
Iliopsoas				
• Psoas major	T12–L5 vertebrae	Lesser trochanter of the femur	Flexes the hip and vertebral column	Lumbar nn. (L1–L3)
• Psoas minor	T12–L1 vertebrae	Pectineal line of the femur	Acts as weak flexor of the pelvis	Lumbar n. (L1)
• Iliacus	Iliac fossa	Lesser trochanter of the femur	Flexes the hip	Femoral n. (L2–L3)
Muscles of the anterior region of the thigh				
Tensor fascia lata	Anterior superior iliac spine and anterior iliac crest	Iliotibial tract of the fascia lata to the lateral condyle of the tibia	Stabilizes the knee in extension	Superior gluteal n. (L4–S1)
Sartorius	Anterior superior iliac spine	Proximal and medial surfaces of the tibia	Flexes the hip and knee joint	Femoral n. (L2–L3)
Quadriceps femoris				
• Rectus femoris	Anterior inferior iliac spine	All four muscles of the quadriceps femoris form a common tendon that envelopes the patella and inserts on the tibial tuberosity	Flexes the hip; extends the knee	Femoral n. (L2–L4)
• Vastus medialis	Intertrochanteric line and linea aspera		Extend the knee	
• Vastus lateralis	Linea aspera			
• Vastus intermedius	Anterior and lateral surfaces of the femur			
Muscles of the medial region of the thigh				
Pectineus	Pectineal line of the superior pubic ramus	Pectineal line of the femur	Adducts and flexes the hip	Femoral n. (L2–L3); may receive a branch from the obturator n.

Muscles of the Lower Limb—cont'd

Muscle	Proximal Attachment	Distal Attachment	Action	Innervation
Muscles of the medial region of the thigh—cont'd				
Adductor longus	Pubis	Linea aspera (medial one third)	Adducts and medially rotates the hip	Obturator n. (L2–L4)
Adductor brevis	Inferior ramus of the pubis	Linea aspera (superior part)	Adducts the hip	Obturator n. (L2–L3)
Adductor magnus	Adductor division: ischiopubic ramus	Linea aspera	Adducts and medially rotates the hip	Obturator n. (L2–L4)
	Hamstring division: ischial tuberosity	Adductor tubercle		Tibial division of the sciatic n. (L2–L4)
Gracilis	Inferior ramus and body of the pubis	Proximal, medial surface of the tibia	Adducts the hip and flexes the knee	Obturator n. (L2–L3)
Obturator externus	Margins of the obturator foramen and obturator membrane	Trochanteric fossa of the femur	Rotates the hip laterally	Obturator n. (L3–L4)
Muscles of the gluteal region and posterior region of the thigh				
Gluteus maximus	Ilium and sacrum	Iliotibial tract and gluteal tuberosity	Acts as a powerful extensor of the flexed femur at the hip joint; laterally stabilizes the hip joint and knee joint	Inferior gluteal n. (L5–S2)
Gluteus medius	External surface of the ilium	Greater trochanter of the femur	Abduct the hip; hold the pelvis secure over the stance leg and prevent pelvic drop on the opposite, swing leg during walking	Superior gluteal n. (L4–S1)
Gluteus minimus				

Continued

Muscles of the Lower Limb—cont'd

Muscle	Proximal Attachment	Distal Attachment	Action	Innervation
Muscles of the gluteal region and posterior region of the thigh—cont'd				
Piriformis	Anterior surface of the sacrum	Greater trochanter of the femur	Laterally rotate the extended femur at the hip; abduct the flexed femur at the hip	Anterior rami L5–S2
Obturator internus	Pelvic surface of the obturator membrane			Nerve to the obturator internus (L5–S1)
Superior gemellus	Ischial spine			Nerve to the quadratus femoris (L5–S1)
Inferior gemellus	Ischial tuberosity			
Quadratus femoris		Intertrochanteric crest of the femur	Laterally rotates the hip	
Semitendinosus		Medial surface of the proximal tibia	Extends and medially rotates the hip; flexes the knee and medially rotates the tibia	Tibial n. (L5–S2)
Semimembranosus		Posterior medial surface of the condyle of the tibia	Extends and medially rotates the hip; flexes the knee and medially rotates the tibia	
Biceps femoris	Long head: ischial tuberosity Short head: lateral lip of the linea aspera of the femur	Head of the fibula	Long head: extends and laterally rotates the hip Long and short heads: flex the knee and laterally rotate the tibia	Long head: tibial n. (S1–S3) Short head: fibular n. (L5–S2)
Muscles of the anterior region of the leg				
Tibialis anterior	Lateral proximal surface of the tibia	Base of the first metatarsal bone	Dorsiflexes and inverts the foot at the ankle; dynamically supports the medial arch of the foot	Deep fibular n. (L4–L5)
Extensor digitorum longus	Lateral condyle of the tibia	Middle and distal phalanx of digits 2–5	Extends digits 2–5 and dorsiflexes the foot at the ankle	Deep fibular n. (L5–S1)
Extensor hallucis longus	Fibula	Distal phalanx of the great toe	Extends the great toe and dorsiflexes the foot at the ankle	
Fibularis tertius		Base of the fifth metatarsal bone	Dorsiflexes and everts the foot at the ankle	

Muscles of the Lower Limb—cont'd

Muscle	Proximal Attachment	Distal Attachment	Action	Innervation
Muscles of the lateral region of the leg				
Fibularis longus	Head and proximal surface of the fibula	Base of the first metatarsal and medial cuneiform bones	Evert and plantar flex the foot at the ankle	Superficial fibular n. (L5–S2)
Fibularis brevis	Distal two thirds of the lateral surface of the fibula	Posterior base of the fifth metatarsal bone		
Muscles of the posterior region of the leg				
Gastrocnemius	Medial and lateral condyles of the femur	Posterior surface of the calcaneus via the calcaneal tendon	Flexes the knee and plantar flexes the foot at the ankle	Tibial n. (S1–S2)
Soleus	Posterior aspect of the fibula and tibia		Plantar flexes the foot at the ankle	
Plantaris	Lateral supracondylar line of the femur		Assists the gastrocnemius; flexes the knee and plantar flexes the foot at the ankle	
Popliteus	Lateral condyle of the femur	Posterior surface of the proximal end of the tibia	Unlocks the knee joint (laterally rotates the femur on the fixed tibia)	Tibial n. (L4–S1)
Flexor hallucis longus	Posterior surface of the fibula and interosseous membrane	Base of the distal phalanx of the great toe	Flexes the great toe and plantar flexes the foot at the ankle	Tibial n. (S2–S3)
Flexor digitorum longus	Medial posterior surface of the tibia	Base of the distal phalanx of digits 2–5	Flexes digits 2–5 and plantar flexes the foot at the ankle	
Tibialis posterior	Posterior surface of the fibula, interosseous membrane, and tibia	Mainly to the tuberosity of the navicular and adjacent region of the medial cuneiform bones	Inverts and plantar flexes the foot at the ankle; supports the medial arch of the foot during walking	Tibial n. (L4–L5)
Extensor digitorum brevis	Superolateral surface of the calcaneus	Base of the proximal phalanx of the great toe and the lateral sides of digits 2–4	Flexes the metatarsophalangeal joint of the great toe and flexes digits 2–4	Deep fibular n. (S1–S2)

Continued

Muscles of the Lower Limb—cont'd

Muscle	Proximal Attachment	Distal Attachment	Action	Innervation
Plantar compartment of the foot (Layer 1)				
Abductor hallucis	Calcaneus bone	Proximal phalanx of the great toe (digit 1)	Abducts and flexes the great toe	Medial plantar n. (S2–S3)
Flexor digitorum brevis		Lateral surfaces of the middle phalanx of digits 2–5	Flexes digits 2–5	
Abductor digiti minimi		Lateral side of the base of the proximal phalanx for digit 5	Abducts and flexes digit 5	Lateral plantar n. (S2–S3)
Plantar compartment of the foot (Layer 2)				
Quadratus plantae	Calcaneus bone	Tendon of the flexor digitorum longus	Flexes digits 2–5	Lateral plantar n. (S1–S3)
Lumbricals	Tendons of the flexor digitorum longus	Expansion over digits 2–5	Flexes the proximal phalanges and extends the middle and distal phalanges of digits 2–5	Medial one: medial plantar n. (S2–S3) Lateral three: lateral plantar n. (S2–S3)
Plantar compartment of the foot (Layer 3)				
Flexor hallucis brevis	Cuboid and lateral cuneiform bones	Base of the proximal phalanx of the great toe	Flexes the great toe	Medial plantar n. (S1–S2)
Adductor hallucis	Oblique head: base of metatarsals 2–4 Transverse head: metatarsophalangeal joints	Proximal phalanx of the great toe	Adducts the great toe	Deep branch of the lateral plantar n. (S2–S3)
Flexor digiti minimi brevis	Base of the fifth metatarsal bone	Base of the proximal phalanx of digit 5	Flexes the proximal phalanx of digit 5	Superficial branch of the lateral plantar n. (S2–S3)
Plantar compartment of the foot (Layer 4)				
Plantar interossei (three muscles)	Base and medial side of metatarsals 3–5	Medial side of the base of the proximal phalanx of digits 3–5	Adducts digits 2–4 and flexes the metatarsophalangeal joints	Lateral plantar n. (S2–S3)
Dorsal interossei (four muscles)	Adjacent sides of metatarsals 1–5	First: medial side of the proximal phalanx of digit 2 Second to fourth: lateral side of digits 2–4	Abducts digits 2–4 and flexes the metatarsophalangeal joints	

Osteology of the Lower Limb

Lab 35

Prior to dissection, you should familiarize yourself with the following structures:

OSTEOLOGY

- Features of the os coxa
  - Acetabulum
  - Obturator foramen
  - Ischiopubic ramus
- Bones of the os coxae
  - Ilium
    - Ala (wing) of the ilium
    - Iliac crest
      - Anterior superior iliac spine
      - Anterior inferior iliac spine
      - Posterior superior iliac spine
      - Posterior inferior iliac spine
      - Iliac fossa
    - Anterior, posterior, and inferior gluteal lines
    - Auricular surface
  - Ischium
    - Ischial tuberosity, ramus, and spine
    - Greater sciatic notch
    - Lesser sciatic notch
  - Pubis
    - Pubic tubercle and crest
    - Superior pubic ramus
      - Pecten pubis (pectineal line)
    - Inferior pubic ramus
    - Obturator groove and crest
    - Pubic arch
- Pelvis
  - Pelvic cavity
  - Pubic symphysis
- Femur
  - Head
    - Fovea for the ligament of the head
  - Neck
    - Greater trochanter
      - Trochanteric fossa
    - Lesser trochanter
    - Intertrochanteric line and crest
  - Linea aspera
  - Pectineal line
  - Gluteal tuberosity
  - Medial condyle and epicondyle
    - Adductor tubercle
  - Lateral condyle and epicondyle
  - Popliteal and patellar surfaces
- Patella
  - Base and apex
  - Articular and anterior surfaces
- Tibia
  - Medial and lateral condyles
  - Intercondylar eminence
  - Tibial tuberosity
  - Soleal line
  - Interosseous border
  - Medial malleolus
  - Fibular notch
  - Inferior articular surface
- Fibula
  - Head and neck
  - Interosseous border
  - Lateral malleolus
- Foot
  - Tarsal bones (7)
    - Talus
    - Calcaneus — sustentaculum tali
    - Navicular
    - Medial cuneiform
    - Intermediate cuneiform
    - Lateral cuneiform
    - Cuboid
  - Metatarsal bones (5)
  - Phalanges (14)
    - Proximal, middle, and distal
  - Superficial fibular n.
  - Dorsal digital nn.

LYMPHATIC SYSTEM

- Femoral lymph nodes
- Inguinal lymph nodes

Lab 35 Dissection Overview

The purpose of this laboratory session is to learn the osteology of the lower limb through dissection. You will do so through the following suggested sequence:

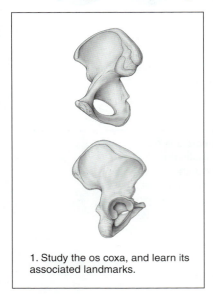

1. Study the os coxa, and learn its associated landmarks.

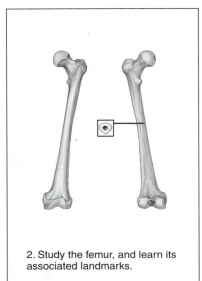

2. Study the femur, and learn its associated landmarks.

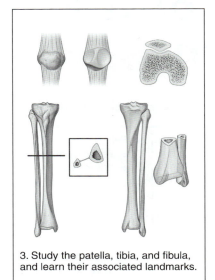

3. Study the patella, tibia, and fibula, and learn their associated landmarks.

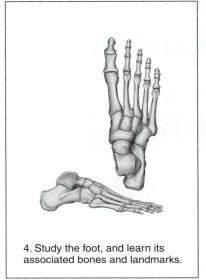

4. Study the foot, and learn its associated bones and landmarks.

Table 35-1 Osteology of the Lower Limb

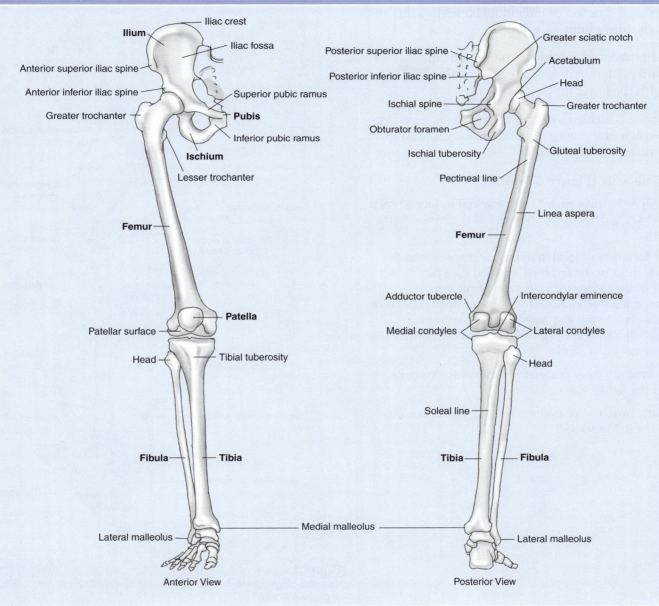

Lower Limb Osteology — Bony Pelvis

- Use an articulated skeleton or individual bones to study the osteology of the lower limb

- The external surfaces of the pelvic bones, sacrum, and coccyx are predominately the regions of the pelvis associated with the lower limb

- Each pelvic bone is formed by three bones (ilium, ischium, and pubis), which fuse during childhood along lines that intersect in the acetabular fossa

- Identify the following **(Figure 35-1)**:

  - **Acetabulum** — articular socket on the lateral surface of each **os coxa**, which, together with the head of the femur, forms the hip joint

  - **Obturator foramen** — located inferior and anterior to the acetabulum; most of the foramen is closed by a flat connective tissue membrane called the **obturator membrane**; a small obturator canal remains open superiorly between the membrane and adjacent bone, providing communication between the lower limb and the pelvic cavity for the obturator n., a., and v.

  - **Greater sciatic notch** — posterior margin of the os coxa, superior to the ischial spine

  - **Lesser sciatic notch** — posterior margin of the os coxa, inferior to the ischial spine

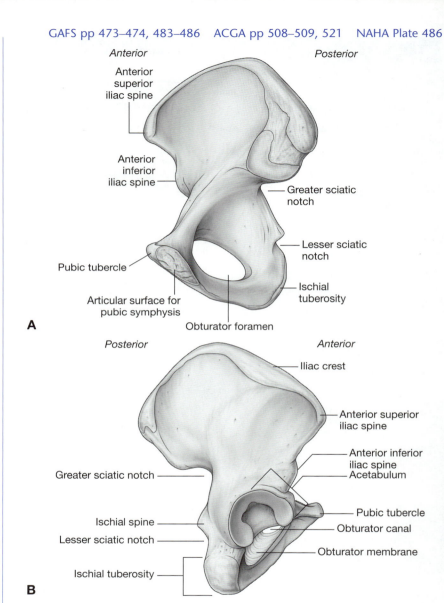

Figure 35-1 Os coxa, right side. **A**, Medial view. **B**, Lateral view. (Redrawn from Drake R, Vogl W, Mitchell A: Gray's Anatomy for Students. Philadelphia: Elsevier, 2005, Fig 5.19)

Lower Limb Osteology — Bony Pelvis—cont'd

- **Ilium** — the most superior of the os coxa bones; articulates with the sacrum **(Figure 35-2)**
  - **Iliac crest** — thickened, superior margin of the ilium that serves as an attachment for muscles and fascia
    - **Anterior superior iliac spine** — anterior termination of the iliac crest
    - **Anterior inferior iliac spine** — inferior to the anterior superior iliac spine
    - **Posterior superior iliac spine** — posterior termination of the iliac crest
    - **Posterior, anterior,** and **inferior gluteal lines** — rough, curved lines on the lateral surface of the ilium for the gluteal muscles to attach
- **Ischium** — the most inferior of the os coxa bones
  - **Ischial tuberosity** — the most prominent feature of the ischium, a large tuberosity on the posteroinferior aspect of the bone; an important site for lower limb muscle attachments and for supporting the body when sitting
  - **Ischial spine** — on the posterior margin of the ischium; that separates the lesser and greater sciatic notches
  - **Ischial ramus** — projects anteriorly and superiorly to join with the inferior ramus of the pubis; the ischial ramus and inferior pubic ramus are fused and therefore are often called the ischiopubic ramus or conjoint ramus
- **Pubis** — the most anterior of the os coxa bones
  - **Superior pubic ramus** — projects laterally and superiorly to join with the ilium; has notches for the external iliac a. and v., femoral n., and iliopsoas m./tendon
  - **Inferior pubic ramus** — a ramus that projects laterally and inferiorly to join with the ramus of the ischium; the inferior pubic ramus and ischial ramus are termed the **ischiopubic ramus**

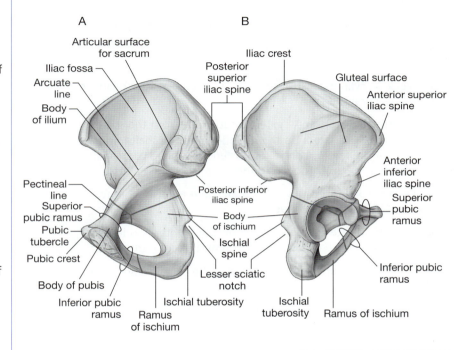

Figure 35-2 Components of the pelvic bone. **A,** Medial surface. **B,** Lateral surface. (Redrawn from Drake R, Vogl W, Mitchell A: Gray's Anatomy for Students. Philadelphia: Elsevier, 2005, Fig. 5.21)

Lower Limb Osteology — Femur

- **Femur** — bone of the thigh; the longest bone in the human body

- Identify the following **(Figure 35-3)**:
  - **Head** — proximal, spherical structure that articulates with the acetabulum
  - **Neck** — cylindrical strut of bone that connects the head to the femoral shaft
  - **Greater trochanter** — extends superiorly from the shaft of the femur just lateral to the region where the shaft joins the neck of the femur; continues posteriorly, where its medial surface is deeply grooved to form the trochanteric fossa
  - **Lesser trochanter** — smaller than the greater trochanter; has a blunt conical shape
  - **Intertrochanteric line** — between the greater and lesser trochanters on the anterior, proximal surface of the femur
  - **Intertrochanteric crest** — between the greater and lesser trochanters on the posterior, proximal surface of the femur
  - **Linea aspera** — vertical roughened crest along the posterior border; forms the medial and lateral supracondylar lines at the distal end of the femur
  - **Medial condyle** — articulates with the medial condyle of the tibia
  - **Medial epicondyle** — attachment for the medial collateral ligament of the knee; the adductor tubercle is a prominent pointed elevation on its superior aspect
  - **Lateral condyle** — articulates with the lateral condyle of the tibia
  - **Lateral epicondyle** — attachment for the lateral collateral ligament of the knee
  - **Intercondylar fossa** — the medial and lateral condyles are separated posteriorly by the intercondylar fossa and are joined anteriorly where they articulate with the patella (patellar surface)

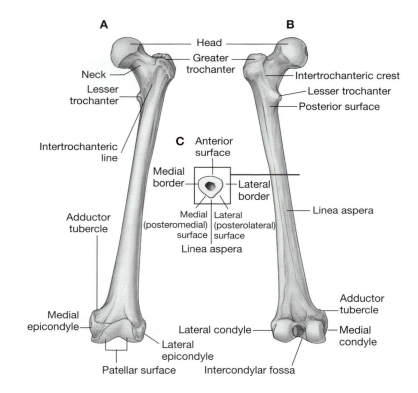

Figure 35-3 Left femur. **A**, Anterior view. **B**, Posterior view. **C**, Cross-section. (Redrawn from Drake R, Vogl W, Mitchell A: Gray's Anatomy for Students. Philadelphia: Elsevier, 2005, Fig. 6.51)

Lower Limb Osteology — Patella, Tibia, and Fibula

- **Patella** (knee cap) — largest sesamoid bone in the body; is located within the tendon of the quadriceps femoris m. as it crosses anterior to the knee joint to insert on the tibial tuberosity (patella not illustrated)

- **Tibia** — medial and larger of the two bones in the leg; articulates with the femur at the knee joint; identify the following **(Figure 35-4)**:
  - **Medial and lateral condyles** — the proximal end of the tibia is expanded on the transverse plane for weightbearing and consists of a medial and lateral condyle; separated by an intercondylar eminence, which serves as an attachment site for the cruciate ligaments and menisci
  - **Tibial tuberosity** — a palpable area on the anterior, proximal aspect of the tibia; site of attachment for the quadriceps femoris tendon
  - **Soleal line** — roughened oblique line on the posterior aspect of the tibia
  - **Medial malleolus** — a rectangular-shaped bony protuberance on the medial, distal end of the tibia
  - **Fibular notch** — a triangular notch on the distal, lateral surface of the tibia

- **Fibula** — lateral bone of the leg; does not take part in the formation of the knee joint or in weightbearing; identify the following:
  - **Head** — an oval-shaped expansion of the shaft of the fibula
  - **Neck** — separates the expanded head from the shaft; the common fibular nerve lies against its posterolateral aspect
  - **Lateral malleolus** — spear-shaped distal end of the fibula

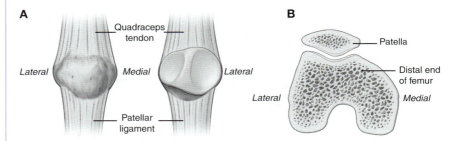

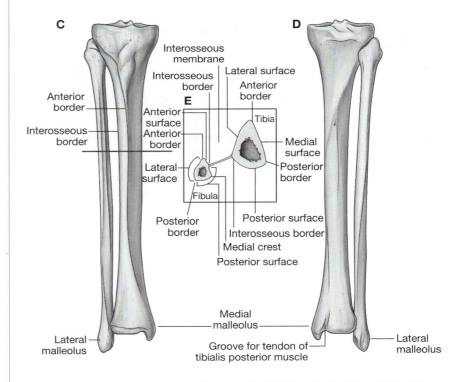

Figure 35-4 Patella: anterior view (**A**) and posterior view (**B**). Tibia and fibula: anterior view (**C**), posterior view (**D**), and cross-section (**E**). (Redrawn from Drake R, Vogl W, Mitchell A: Gray's Anatomy for Students. Philadelphia: Elsevier, 2005, Figs. 6.52, 6.80)

Lower Limb Osteology — Foot

- **Foot** — the region of the lower limb distal to the ankle joint; the bones of the foot are divided into the tarsal bones, the metatarsals, and the digits (phalanges)

- Identify the following seven tarsal bones and associated landmarks **(Figure 35-5)**:

  - **Talus** — most superior of the tarsal bones; sits on top of the calcaneus; articulates above with the tibia and fibula to form the ankle joint

  - **Calcaneus** — largest of the tarsal bones; forms the heel; sits under and supports the talus; its medial surface is concave, with a prominent upper margin called the **sustentaculum tali**

  - **Navicular** — boat-shaped bone on the medial side of the foot

  - **Cuboid** — articulates with the calcaneus (posteriorly) and the lateral two metatarsals (anteriorly)

  - **Cuneiforms** (medial, intermediate, and lateral) — Latin for *wedge*; articulate with the navicular and the three medial metatarsals

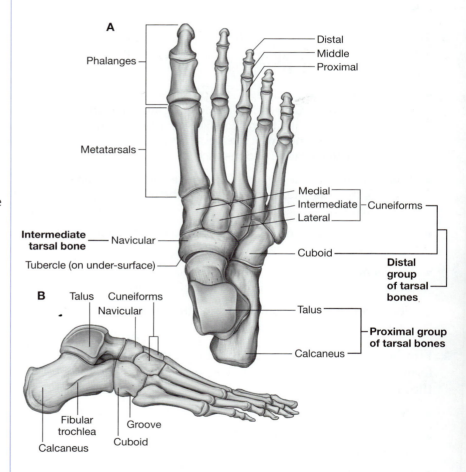

Figure 35-5 Bones of the foot. **A**, Dorsal view, left foot. **B**, Lateral view, left foot. (Redrawn from Drake R, Vogl W, Mitchell A: Gray's Anatomy for Students. Philadelphia: Elsevier, 2005, Fig. 6.91)

Lower Limb Osteology — Foot—cont'd

- **Metatarsals** — five metatarsals in the foot, numbered I to V from medial to lateral; each consists of a base, shaft, and head; all of the bases articulate with the tarsal bones and the heads each relate to one digit; identify the following **(Figure 35-5)**:

  - **Metatarsal I** — associated with the great toe; shortest and thickest
  - **Metatarsals II–V** — related to digits 2–5

- Identify the following regarding the digits:

  - **Great toe** — has two phalanges, a proximal and a distal phalanx
  - **Digits 2–5** — have three phalanges, a proximal, middle, and distal phalanx

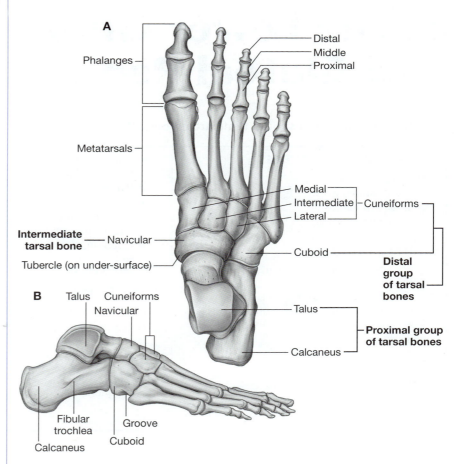

Figure 35-5 Bones of the foot. **A**, Dorsal view, left foot. **B**, Lateral view, left foot. (Redrawn from Drake R, Vogl W, Mitchell A: Gray's Anatomy for Students. Philadelphia: Elsevier, 2005, Fig. 6.91)

Lab 36

Superficial Structures of the Lower Limb and Gluteal Region

Prior to dissection, you should familiarize yourself with the following structures:

SUPERFICIAL STRUCTURES

- Superficial veins
  - Great saphenous v.
  - Small saphenous v.
  - Dorsal venous arch
- Superficial nerves
  - Lateral cutaneous n. of the thigh
  - Medial and intermediate cutaneous nn. of the thigh
  - Posterior cutaneous n. of the thigh
  - Cutaneous branch of the obturator n.
  - Medial and lateral sural cutaneous nn.
  - Saphenous n.

MUSCLES

- Gluteal region
  - Tensor fascia lata m.
  - Gluteus maximus m.
  - Gluteus medius m.
  - Gluteus minimus m.
  - Piriformis m.
  - Superior gemellus m.
  - Obturator internus m.
  - Inferior gemellus m.
  - Quadratus femoris m.

INNERVATION

Sacral Plexus

- Lumbosacral trunk (L4–L5)
- Nerve to the obturator internus m. (L5–S2)
- Nerve to the piriformis m. (S1–S2)
- Nerve to the quadratus femoris m. (L4–S1)
- Superior gluteal n. (L4–S1)
- Inferior gluteal n. (L5–S2)
- Posterior cutaneous n. of the thigh (S1–S3)
- Sciatic n. (L4–S3)

VASCULATURE

- Superior and inferior gluteal aa.

Lab 36 Dissection Overview

The purpose of this laboratory session is to learn the anatomy of the superficial structures of the lower limb and gluteal region through dissection. You will do so through the following suggested sequence:

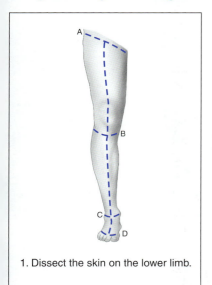

1. Dissect the skin on the lower limb.

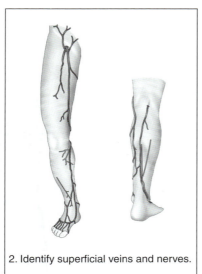

2. Identify superficial veins and nerves.

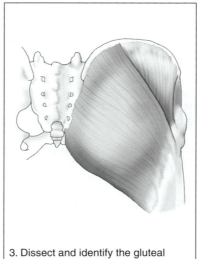

3. Dissect and identify the gluteal muscles and deep hip rotator muscles.

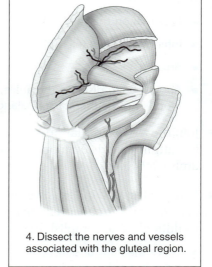

4. Dissect the nerves and vessels associated with the gluteal region.

Lower Limb — Skin Removal

- Use a scalpel to make the following circular incisions through the skin on the lower limb; do *not* cut the superficial nerves and veins in the superficial fascia **(Figure 36-1)**:
  - Proximal on the thigh *(A)*
  - Inferior to the patella *(B)*
  - Ankle *(C)*
  - About 10 cm distal to the ankle, on the dorsal surface of the foot along the metatarsophalangeal joints *(D)*

- Join the three circular and one semilunar incisions with a longitudinal incision along the anterior aspect of the lower limb *(A–D)*

- Remove the skin of the lower limb, leaving the superficial fascia, with the superficial nerves and veins intact (this may be difficult to accomplish in emaciated bodies)
  - Leave the flaps of skin between *C* and *D* attached at this time, but reflect the flaps from the dorsum of the foot

- Remove the skin and superficial fascia over the gluteal region if not done in a previous laboratory session; use the scraping technique and blunt dissection to remove the fat

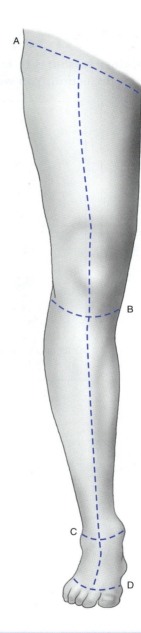

Figure 36-1 Right lower limb skin incisions

Lower Limb — Superficial Veins

- Use forceps to reveal and identify the following veins in the superficial fascia **(Figure 36-2)**:

  - **Dorsal venous arch** — identify the veins on the dorsal (superior) aspect of the foot; main tributary to the great saphenous v. (see Figure 36-2A)

  - **Great saphenous v.** — the longest vein in the body; begins at the medial side of the dorsal venous arch of the foot and ascends anterior to the medial malleolus, then ascends along the medial aspect of the leg

    - At the knee, the vein ascends posterior to the medial condyle of the femur, then courses along the anteromedial aspect of the thigh

    - Terminates in the thigh by passing through the deep fascia (saphenous opening), inferior to the inguinal ligament, as a tributary of the femoral v.

  - **Small saphenous v.** — begins on the lateral surface of the foot (see Figure 36-2B); ascends posterior to the lateral malleolus and penetrates the deep fascia in the popliteal fossa to terminate in the popliteal v., between the two heads of the gastrocnemius m.

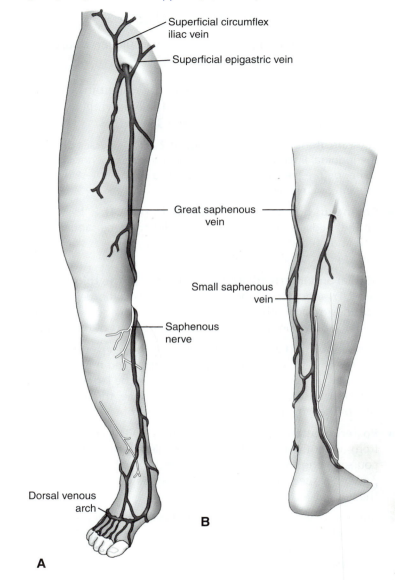

Figure 36-2 Superficial veins of the right lower limb. **A,** Anterior view. **B,** Posterior view

Lower Limb — Cutaneous Nerves

- In general, the main trunks of the cutaneous nerves are found just superficial to the deep fascia

- Use the scraping technique to remove the remaining fat and use forceps to reveal and identify the following superficial cutaneous nerves **(Figure 36-3)**:

  - **Lateral cutaneous n. of the thigh (L2–L3)** — passes deep to the inguinal ligament, inferior to the anterior superior iliac spine, before piercing the deep fascia to supply the skin over the anterolateral region of the thigh

  - **Cutaneous branch of the obturator n. (L2–L4)** — located on the medial surface of the thigh; inferior to the saphenous ring and medial to the great saphenous v.; supplies skin over the upper medial aspect of the thigh

  - **Medial and intermediate cutaneous nn. of the thigh (L2–L4)** — branches emerge along the medial border of the sartorius m. and course along the anteromedial surface of the thigh; supply skin over the anteromedial aspect of the thigh

  - **Saphenous n. (L2–L4)** — courses along the deep surface of the sartorius m. and pierces the fascia distal and medial to the knee; follows the great saphenous v. in the leg; supplies skin over the anteromedial region of the knee, the medial side of the leg, and the medial side of the foot

  - **Posterior cutaneous n. of the thigh (S1–S3)** — emerges from under the inferior border of the gluteus maximus m.; courses along the posterior surface of the thigh; supplies the posterior aspect of the thigh and upper posterior region of the leg

  - **Sural n.** — emerges from the deep fascia near the middle of the posterior aspect of the leg; follow this nerve inferiorly as it courses together with the small saphenous v., posterior to the lateral malleolus; supplies the posterior aspect of the leg

  - **Superficial fibular n.** — pierces the deep fascia in the lateral distal one third of the leg; follow it distally to the dorsum of the foot; supplies some skin over the dorsal surface of the foot

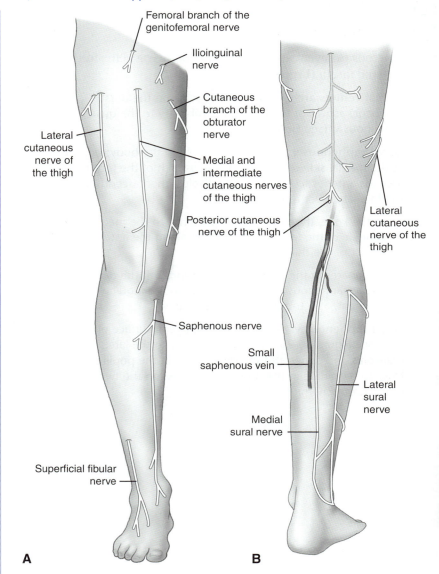

Figure 36-3 Cutaneous nerves of the right lower limb. **A,** Anterior view. **B,** Posterior view

Lower Limb — Superficial Lymph Nodes

■ Use forceps to reveal and identify the following lymph nodes of the thigh **(Figure 36-4)**:

- **Superficial inguinal lymph nodes**
  - **Horizontal group** — inferior to the inguinal ligament
  - **Vertical group** — bilaterally flank the great saphenous v. where the vein penetrates the deep fascia

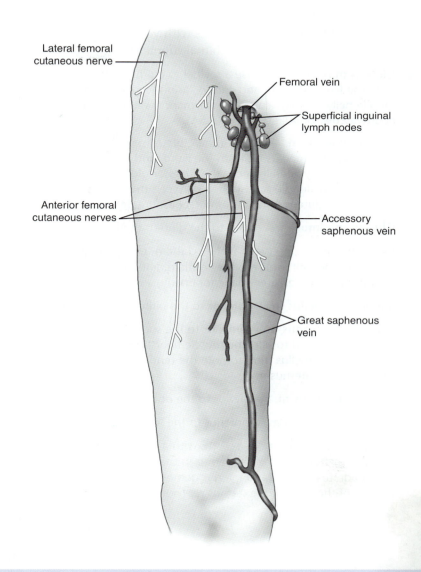

Figure 36-4 Superficial lymph nodes of the right thigh

Muscles of the Gluteal Region

- Turn the limb prone

- As you reveal the following muscles with your fingers or forceps, preserve the nerve and blood supplies:

  - **Gluteus maximus m.** — use a scalpel to cut its attachment from the ilium, sacrum, and coccyx, and then reflect the muscle belly laterally; cut and note/mark the inferior gluteal neurovascular bundle (**Figure 36-5A**)

  - **Gluteus medius m.** — deep to the gluteus maximus m.; cut the gluteus medius m. from the ilium, and then reflect the muscle belly laterally; note the superior gluteal neurovascular bundle sandwiched between the gluteal medius and gluteus minimus mm. (see Figure 36-5B)

  - **Gluteus minimus m.** — deep to the gluteus medius m.

  - **Piriformis m.** — observe that the **sciatic n.** exits the pelvis inferior to the piriformis m.; the sciatic n. and piriformis m. pass through the greater sciatic foramen

  - **Superior gemellus m.** — inferior to the piriformis m.

  - **Obturator internus m.** — inferior to the superior gemellus m.; you may need to part the muscle fibers of the superior and inferior gemellus mm. to note the tendinous portion of the obturator internus m.

  - **Inferior gemellus m.** — inferior to the obturator internus m.

  - **Quadratus femoris m.** — inferior to the inferior gemellus m.

  - **Obturator externus m.** — search, with a probe, deep near the greater trochanter of the femur in the interval between the quadratus femoris and inferior gemellus mm. to find the tendon of the obturator externus m. (not shown)

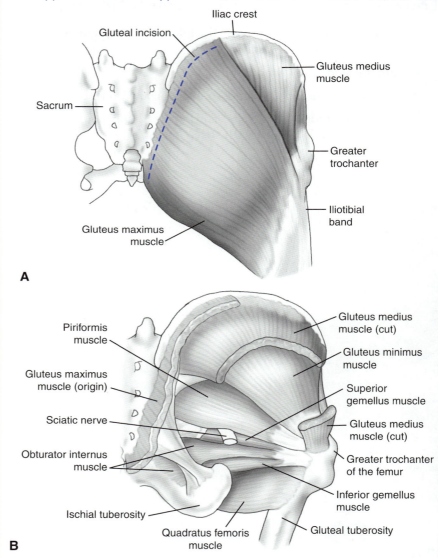

Figure 36-5 Muscles of the gluteal region. **A,** Posterior view. **B,** Posterior view with the gluteus maximus muscle removed and the gluteus medius muscle cut to show the gluteus minimus muscle

Nerves and Vessels of the Gluteal Region

- Veins (vena comitantes) are not shown but accompany each artery; ask your instructor if you may remove the veins

- Turn the lower limb prone; use forceps to reveal and identify the following by using blunt dissection and the scraping technique to remove the fat **(Figure 36-6)**:

  - **Superior gluteal a. and n.** — exit the pelvis through the greater sciatic foramen, superior to the piriformis m. (accompanied by the superior gluteal v.)
  - **Inferior gluteal a. and n.** — exit the pelvis through the greater sciatic foramen, inferior to the piriformis m. (accompanied by the inferior gluteal v.)
  - **Posterior cutaneous n. of the thigh** — exits the pelvis with the sciatic and inferior gluteal nn.
  - **Medial circumflex femoral a.** — courses between the proximal parts of the adductor magnus and quadratus femoris mm.
  - **Sciatic n.** — the largest nerve in the body; exits the pelvis with the inferior gluteal n., inferior to the piriformis m.; descends between the greater trochanter of the femur and ischial tuberosity, between the hamstring muscles
    - Identify tibial branches of the sciatic n. to the hamstring musculature and hamstring division of the adductor magnus m.

- Attempt to identify the nerves that supply the quadratus femoris, inferior gemellus, obturator internus, superior gemellus, and piriformis mm.; these nerves are small

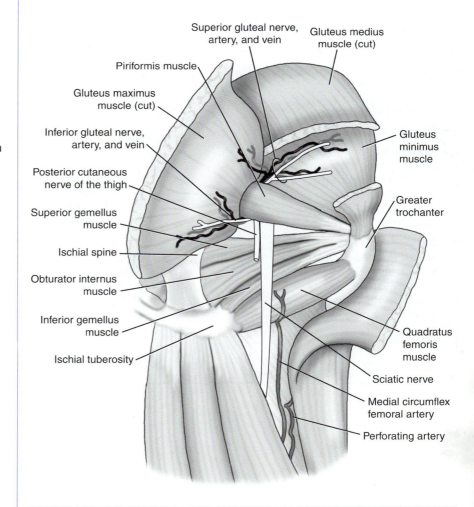

Figure 36-6 Posterior view of the nerves of the right gluteal region

Lab 37

Thigh

Prior to dissection, you should familiarize yourself with the following structures:

MUSCLES
- Iliopsoas m.
  - Iliacus m.
  - Psoas major m.
- Psoas minor m.
- Anterior muscles of the thigh
  - Quadriceps femoris m.
    - Rectus femoris m.
    - Vastus medialis m.
    - Vastus intermedius m.
    - Vastus lateralis m.
  - Sartorius m.
- Medial muscles of the thigh
  - Pectineus m.
  - Adductor brevis m.
  - Adductor longus m.
  - Adductor magnus m.
  - Gracilis m.
  - Obturator externus m.
- Posterior muscles of the thigh
  - Biceps femoris m.
  - Semitendinosus m.
  - Semimembranosus m.

INNERVATION

Lumbar Plexus
- Subcostal n. (T12)
- Ilioinguinal n. (L1)
- Genitofemoral n. (L1–L2)
  - Genital branch
  - Femoral branch
- Lateral cutaneous n. of the thigh (L2–L3)
- Obturator n. (L2–L4)
  - Anterior branch
    - Cutaneous branch
  - Posterior branch
- Accessory obturator n.
- Femoral n. (L2–L4)
  - Muscular branches
  - Medial cutaneous n. of the thigh (L2–L4)
  - Intermediate cutaneous n. of the thigh (L2–L4)
  - Saphenous n. (L2–L4)
- Lumbosacral trunk (L4–L5)

Sacral Plexus
- Lumbosacral trunk (L4–L5)
- Posterior cutaneous n. of the thigh (S1–S3)
- Sciatic n. (L4–S3)
  - Common fibular (peroneal) n. (L4–S3)
  - Tibial n. (L4–S3)

VASCULATURE
- Obturator a.
- Femoral a.
  - Deep a. of the thigh
  - Medial circumflex femoral a.
  - Lateral circumflex femoral a.
    - Ascending, transverse, and descending branches
  - Perforating branches

Lab 37 Dissection Overview

The purpose of this laboratory session is to learn the anatomy of the thigh through dissection. You will do so through the following suggested sequence:

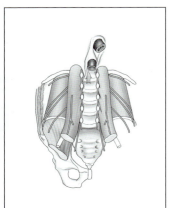

1. Review and identify the lumbar plexus of nerves in the posterior abdominal and lateral pelvic walls.

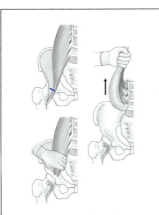

2. Dissect and reflect the psoas major muscle to better view the lumbar plexus of nerves.

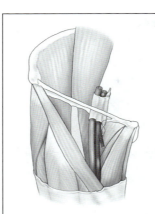

3. Dissect and identify the borders and contents of the femoral triangle and the contents of the femoral sheath.

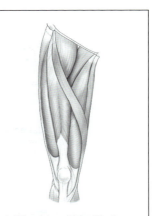

4. Dissect and identify the anterior musculature of the thigh.

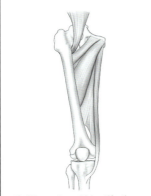

5. Dissect and identify the medial muscles of the thigh.

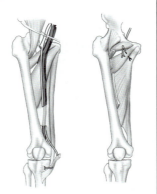

6. Dissect and identify the branches of the femoral and obturator nerves and femoral artery.

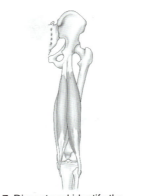

7. Dissect and identify the posterior musculature of the thigh and associated nerves and vessels.

Table 37-1 Lumbosacral plexus of nerves.

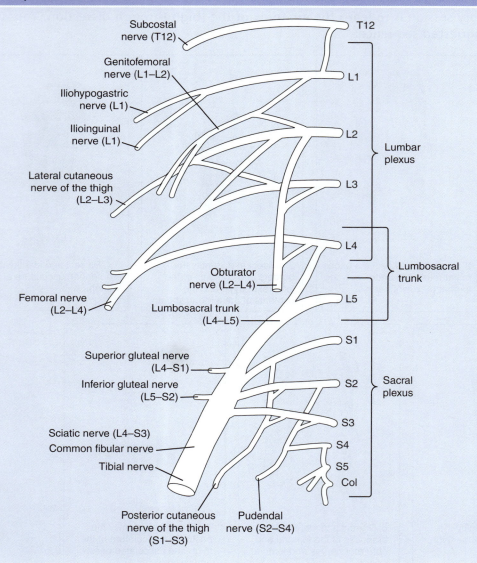

Lumbar Plexus — Posterior Abdominal Wall

Place the cadaver supine; expose the previously dissected posterior abdominal wall; use forceps to reveal and identify the following components of the lumbar plexus **(Figure 37-1)**:

- **Subcostal n.** — lateral to the psoas major m.; courses parallel to the inferior border of rib 12, in the same fashion as the intercostal nn.
- **Iliohypogastric n.** — emerges lateral to the psoas major m.; courses parallel to the iliac crest to reach the inguinal and pubic regions; supplies the skin in the pubic region
- **Ilioinguinal n.** — emerges lateral to the psoas major m.; courses through the inguinal canal and terminates as the anterior scrotal/labial branches; supplies the skin over the upper medial thigh and the skin over either the root of the penis and anterior scrotum or the mons pubis and labia majora
- **Genitofemoral n.** — descends on the anterior surface of the psoas major m.; divides into genital and femoral branches; the genital branch supplies the skin over the anterior scrotum or skin of the mons pubis and labia majora; the femoral branch supplies the skin of the upper anterior thigh
- **Lateral cutaneous n. of the thigh** — emerges lateral to the psoas major m.; courses obliquely toward the anterior superior iliac spine and then passes inferior to the inguinal ligament to supply skin on the lateral aspect of the thigh
- **Femoral n.** — lateral to the psoas major m.; arises from the anterior rami of L2, L3, and L4 lumbar nn.; exits the pelvis lateral to the femoral a. and v., inferior to the inguinal ligament; supplies the iliacus and pectineus mm. and muscles in the anterior compartment of the thigh, as well as the skin on the anterior thigh and medial surfaces of the leg
- **Obturator n.** — medial to the psoas major m.; also originates from the anterior rami of L2, L3, and L4; exits the pelvis through the obturator foramen and pierces the obturator internus and externus mm.; supplies the obturator externus m. and muscles of the medial compartment of the thigh, as well as the skin on the medial aspect of the thigh

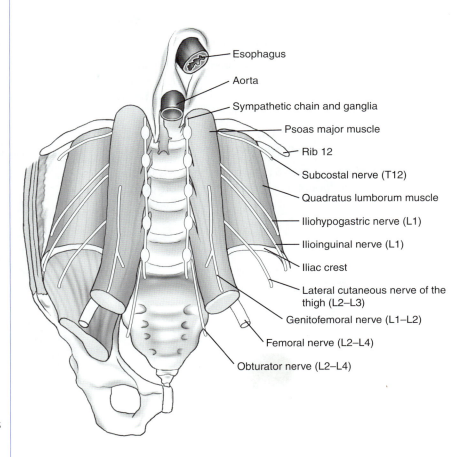

Figure 37-1 Posterior abdominal wall, demonstrating the lumbar plexus of nerves (the psoas major muscle is shown for orientation)

Lumbar and Sacral Plexuses — Pelvic Cavity

- Use forceps to reveal and identify the following nerves along the lateral wall of the pelvis **(Figure 37-2)**:

  - **Obturator n. (L2–L4)** — courses along the lateral wall of the pelvis en route to the obturator foramen

  - **Lumbosacral trunk (L4–L5)** — branches from anterior primary rami at the level of L4 and L5 join to become the lumbosacral trunk; the trunk descends into the pelvic cavity to contribute to the sacral plexus

  - **Superior gluteal n. (L4–L5)** — exits the pelvis through the greater sciatic foramen, superior to the piriformis m.

  - **Inferior gluteal n. (L5–S1)** — exits the pelvis through the greater sciatic foramen, inferior to the piriformis m.

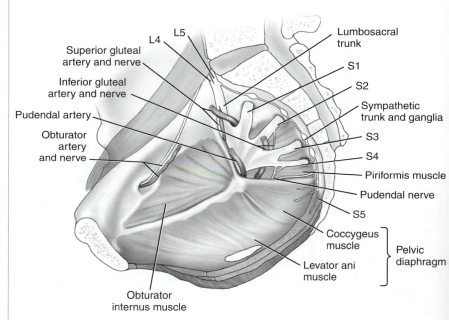

Figure 37-2 Medial view of a sagittal section through the right pelvis

Dissection of the Lumbar Plexus

- Verify with your instructor that you may cut and reflect the psoas major m.

- To study the anterior rami that contribute the nerves of the lumbar plexus, remove the psoas major m. from its attachments on one side of your cadaver in the following three steps **(Figure 37-3)**:

  - Isolate the obturator, genitofemoral, and femoral nn.; use a scalpel to transect the distal end of the belly of the psoas major m., without cutting the isolated nerves *(A)*

  - Grasp the proximal end of the transected psoas major m. firmly with your hand *(B)*

  - Pull anteriorly and superiorly, tearing the proximal attachment of the psoas major m. from the ilium and lumbar vertebrae to reveal the underlying lumbar plexus *(C)*; review the revealed nerves

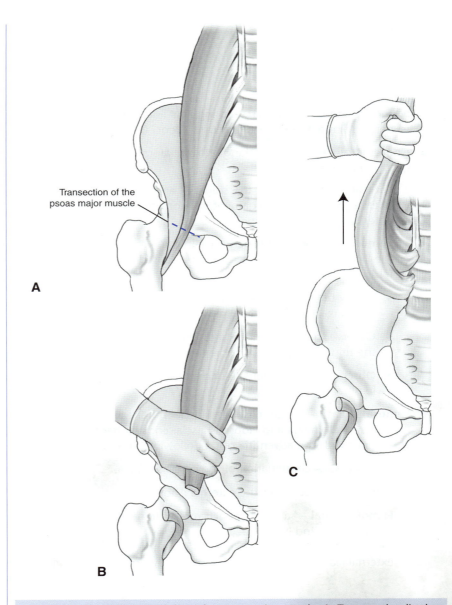

Figure 37-3 Reflection of the right psoas major muscle. **A,** Transect the distal end of the psoas major muscle. **B,** Grasp the proximal end of the cut psoas major muscle. **C,** Pull superiorly on the psoas major muscle to peel it from its attachments

Femoral Triangle

■ Turn the lower limb supine; use forceps to reveal and identify the following:

- **Borders of the femoral triangle** — sartorius m. (lateral), adductor longus m. (medial), and inguinal ligament (superior); iliopsoas and pectineus mm. (floor) **(Figure 37-4A)**

- **Contents of the femoral triangle** (from lateral to medial) (see Figure 37-4B):

  - **Lateral cutaneous n. of the thigh** — enters the thigh inferior to the inguinal ligament, inferomedial to the anterior superior iliac spine

  - **Femoral n.** — located superficially in the furrow between the iliopsoas and pectineus mm.; not housed in the femoral sheath

    ◆ Follow branches of the femoral n. to the pectineus, sartorius, and quadriceps mm.

    ◆ Observe the intermediate and medial cutaneous nn. of the thigh branching from the femoral n.

    ◆ Observe the saphenous n. originating from the femoral n.

- **Femoral sheath** — a funnel-shaped fascial tube; extension of the transversalis fascia and iliopsoas fascia; ends by becoming continuous with the adventitia of the following structures:

  - **Femoral a.** — continuation of the external iliac a.

  - **Femoral v.** — becomes the external iliac v.

  - **Femoral canal** — a closed pouch medial to the femoral v.; lymph nodes and lymphatic vessels occupy the femoral canal (potential space for hernias) and connect to the external iliac lymph nodes and lymphatic vessels

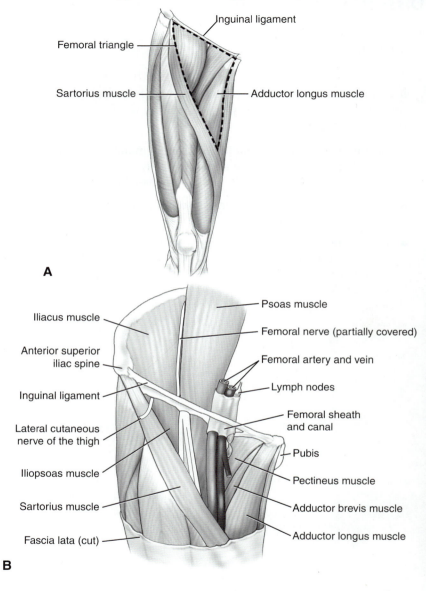

Figure 37-4 Right femoral triangle. **A,** Borders. **B,** Contents

Muscles of the Anteromedial Region of the Thigh

- If possible, flex the thigh at the hip joint to reduce tension on the muscles; if necessary, to separate one muscle from another, use a scalpel to incise the deep fascia at the border of two adjoining muscles, then slide your fingers up and down the adjoining borders to free one muscle from another; keep in mind that many neurovascular bundles run between adjoining muscle bellies

- Use your fingers or forceps to separate and identify the following **(Figure 37-5)**:

  - **Sartorius m.** — longest muscle in the body; crosses two joints (hip and knee)
  - **Quadriceps femoris mm.** (four heads) — inferolateral to the sartorius m.
    - **Rectus femoris m.** — the most superficial and medial muscle of the quadriceps femoris group
    - **Vastus lateralis m.** — lateral to the rectus femoris m.
    - **Vastus medialis m.** — medial to the rectus femoris m.
    - **Vastus intermedius m.** — deep to the rectus femoris m.
  - **Tensor fascia lata m.** — most lateral of the thigh muscles; its tendon becomes the iliotibial tract
  - **Iliopsoas m.** — union of the iliacus and psoas major mm.; posterolateral to the **femoral sheath** and **femoral n.**
  - **Pectineus m.** — posteromedial to the femoral sheath and femoral n.

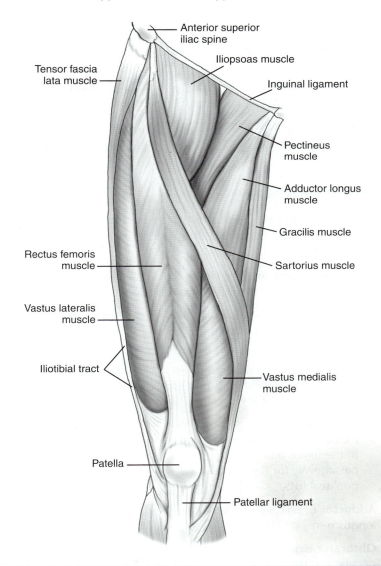

Figure 37-5 Muscles of the anterior region of the thigh

Muscles of the Anteromedial Region of the Thigh Continued

Muscles of the Anteromedial Region of the Thigh—cont'd

- Flex the thigh at the hip joint to reduce tension; if the hip joint cannot be flexed, use a scalpel to transect the sartorius and rectus femoris mm. near the proximal attachment, then reflect to identify the following **(Figure 37-6A)**:

- **Gracilis m.** — the most medial muscle in the medial compartment of the thigh; courses vertically between the pubis and tibia

- **Pectineus m.** — posteromedial to the femoral sheath

- **Adductor longus m.** — inferior to the pectineus m.; use a scalpel to bisect the adductor longus m. to see the deeper muscles

  - **Adductor magnus m.** (see Figure 37-6B) — deep to the adductor longus m. and inferior to the adductor brevis m.

    - **Adductor canal** — muscular channel that transmits the femoral a. and v. from the femoral sheath to the adductor hiatus

      - **Boundaries** — sartorius m. (roof), vastus medialis m. (lateral wall and floor), and adductor magnus m. (medial wall and floor)

    - **Adductor hiatus** — an opening in the adductor magnus m. between the adductor tubercle on the medial condyle of the femur and the linea aspera; provides a deep passageway for the femoral a. and v. to reach the popliteal fossa

  - **Adductor brevis m.** — deep to the pectineus and adductor longus mm.

  - **Obturator externus m.** — deep to the iliopsoas and pectineus mm.; you may cut the iliopsoas and pectineus mm. on one lower limb of the cadaver to better identify the obturator externus m.

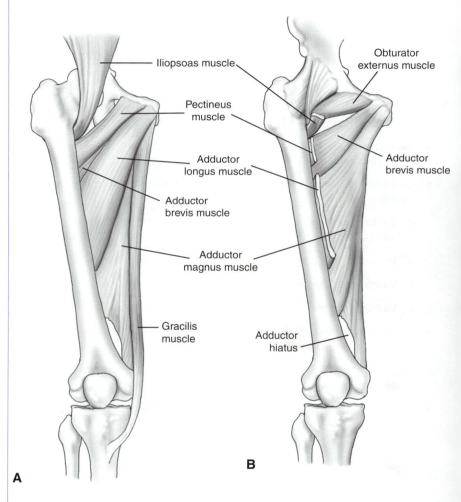

Figure 37-6 Muscles of the medial region of the right thigh. **A,** Intermediate layer. **B,** Deep layer

Nerves of the Anteromedial Region of the Thigh

■ Use forceps to reveal and identify the following:

- **Saphenous n. (Figure 37-7A)** — a branch from the femoral n.; note the following:

  - Accompanies the femoral vessels distally through the **adductor canal**

  - Does not traverse the **adductor hiatus**; instead, it curves anterior to the adductor magnus tendon toward the medial aspect of the knee

  - Find the saphenous n. where it emerges from the deep fascia inferior to the knee, proximal to the attachment of the gracilis and sartorius mm.; use forceps to reveal the nerve proximally to the adductor canal

- **Obturator n.** (see Figure 37-7B) — exits the pelvis through the obturator foramen, by coursing through an opening in the obturator internus m., then an opening in the obturator membrane, and finally through the obturator externus m.; identify the following divisions:

  - **Anterior division of the obturator n.** — superficial to the adductor brevis

  - **Posterior division of the obturator n.** — deep to the adductor brevis m.

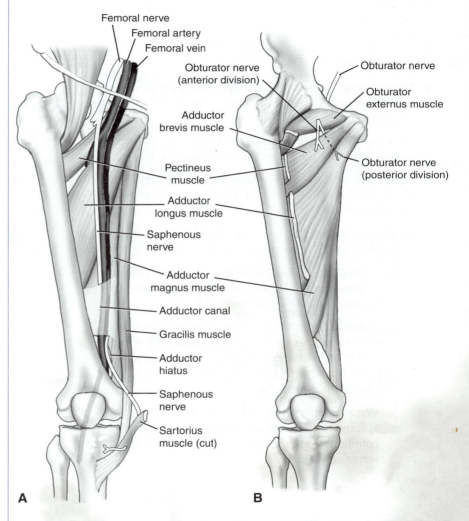

Figure 37-7 Nerves of the anterior and medial regions of the right thigh. **A,** Femoral and saphenous nerves. **B,** Obturator nerve.

Vessels of the Anteromedial Region of the Thigh

- Turn the lower limb supine; identify the **femoral triangle** bordered by the sartorius m., adductor longus m., and inguinal ligament

- Use forceps to reveal and identify the following structures **(Figure 37-8)**:

  - **Obturator a.** — emerges through the obturator canal (accompanied by the obturator n.) and divides into anterior and posterior divisions

  - **Femoral sheath** — surrounds the femoral a., v., and lymph nodes; note that the femoral n. is outside the femoral sheath

  - **Femoral a. and v.** — use scissors to open the anterior wall of the femoral sheath by making a vertical cut to expose the femoral a. and v.

    - **Deep a. of the thigh** — arises from the lateral surface of the femoral a.; gives rise to two proximal circumflex aa.

      - **Medial circumflex femoral a.** — passes between the iliopsoas and pectineus mm.; courses around the posterior aspect of the femoral neck

      - **Lateral circumflex femoral a.** — passes superficial to the iliopsoas tendon; courses around the anterior aspect of the femoral neck; attempt to identify its three branches: **ascending, transverse,** and **descending branches**

      - **Venae comitantes** — observe that the femoral a. is accompanied by smaller paired veins called venae comitantes; ask your instructor if you may remove the venae comitantes

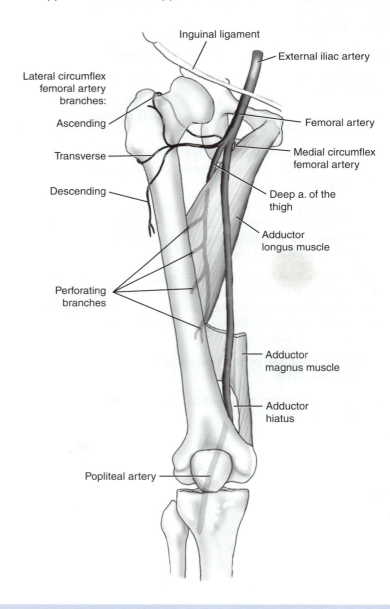

Figure 37-8   Right femoral artery and its branches

Vessels of the Anteromedial Region of the Thigh—cont'd

- Use forceps to reveal and identify the following structures **(Figure 37-9)**:

  - **Femoral a.**

    - **Deep a. of the thigh**

      - **Perforating branches** — trace the deep a. of the thigh distally, as it passes posterior to the adductor longus m.; identify the perforating branches of the deep a. of the thigh that pierce the adductor mm.; the perforating branches terminate in the posterior compartment of the thigh

  - **Adductor canal** — a fascial tunnel that courses from the apex of the femoral triangle to the adductor hiatus; the canal lies deep to the sartorius m. (see Figure 37-9A)

    - Use forceps to follow the femoral a. and v. and the saphenous n. as they descend through the adductor canal

  - **Adductor hiatus** — an opening through the distal end of the adductor magnus m., through which pass the femoral a. and v. to enter the popliteal fossa

    - The saphenous n. does not course through the adductor hiatus (see Figure 37-9A)

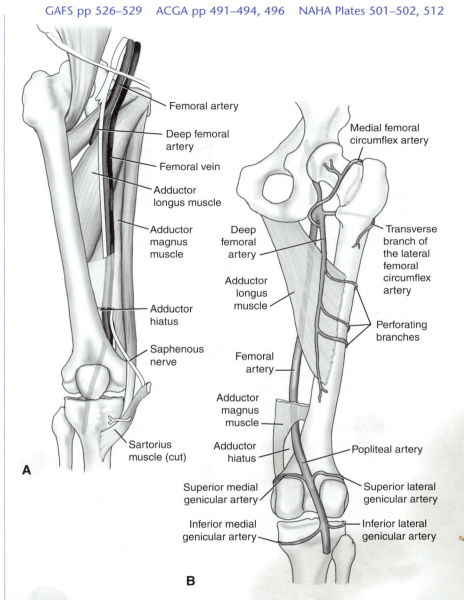

Figure 37-9 Vasculature of the right thigh. **A,** Anterior view. **B,** Posterior view (some veins are not shown).

Posterior Muscles of the Thigh

- Turn the lower limb in prone position

- Use your fingers or forceps to separate and identify the following; try to flex the leg at the knee to reduce tension on the muscles that cross the posterior surface of the knee joint **(Figure 37-10)**:

  - **Hamstrings** — a group of muscles that attach proximally to the ischial tuberosity, span both the hip and knee joints, and are innervated by the tibial division of the sciatic n.; observe the tibial n. coursing inferior to the piriformis m., along the adductor magnus m. and crossed by the biceps femoris m.; proximal to the knee the sciatic n. separates into its two terminal branches: the tibial n. and the common fibular n.

    - **Biceps femoris m. (long head only)** — the most lateral of the three hamstring muscles; attached distally to the fibular head

    - **Semitendinosus m.** — middle of the three hamstring muscles; attached distally to the same region as the sartorius and gracilis mm., medial to the tibial tuberosity

    - **Semimembranosus m.** — most medial of the three hamstring muscles; attached distally to the medial condyle of the tibia

  - **Biceps femoris m. (short head)** — on the lateral side of the thigh (linea aspera) and deep to the long head of the biceps femoris m.

    - Because the short head of the biceps femoris m. does not originate on the ischial tuberosity, span two joints, or have the same innervation as the hamstring muscles, it is not considered a hamstring muscle

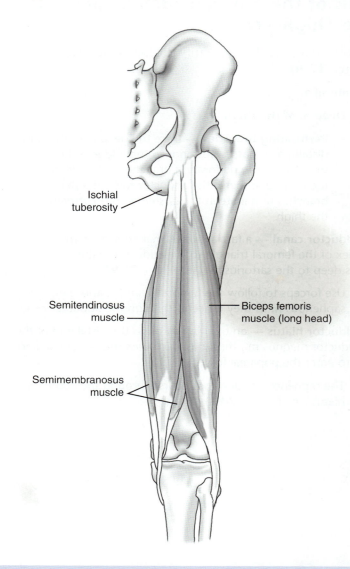

Figure 37-10 Hamstring muscles of the posterior region of the right thigh

Lab 38

Leg

Prior to dissection, you should familiarize yourself with the following structures:

MUSCLES
- Lateral muscles of the leg
  - Fibularis (peroneus) longus m.
  - Fibularis (peroneus) brevis m.
- Anterior muscles of the leg
  - Tibialis anterior m.
  - Extensor digitorum longus m.
  - Fibularis (peroneus) tertius m.
  - Extensor hallucis longus m.
- Posterior muscles of the leg
  - Superficial layer
    - Gastrocnemius m.
    - Plantaris m.
    - Soleus m.
  - Deep layer
    - Tibialis posterior m.
    - Flexor hallucis longus m.
    - Flexor digitorum longus m.
    - Popliteus m.

VASCULATURE
- Popliteal a.
  - Superior medial genicular a.
  - Superior lateral genicular a.
  - Inferior medial genicular a.
  - Inferior lateral genicular a.
- Anterior tibial a.
  - Dorsalis pedis a.
- Posterior tibial a.
  - Fibular a.

Note: Deep veins are named the same as the arteries they accompany. Vasculature of the foot will be dissected in another laboratory session.

INNERVATION
- Sciatic n. (L4–S3)
  - Common fibular (peroneal) n. (L4–S3)
    - Lateral sural cutaneous n.
    - Superficial fibular (peroneal) n.
    - Deep fibular (peroneal) n.
  - Tibial n. (L4–S3)
    - Interosseous n.
    - Medial sural cutaneous n.
    - Medial plantar n.
      - Common plantar digital nn.
        - Proper plantar digital nn.
    - Lateral plantar n.
      - Common plantar digital nn.
        - Proper plantar digital nn.

Lab 38 Dissection Overview

The purpose of this laboratory session is to learn the anatomy of the leg through dissection. You will do so through the following suggested sequence:

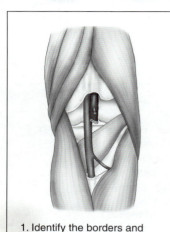

1. Identify the borders and contents of the popliteal fossa.

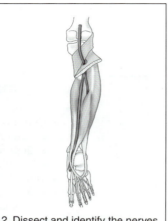

2. Dissect and identify the nerves and vessels associated with the popliteal fossa.

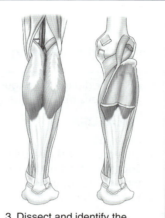

3. Dissect and identify the gastrocnemius and soleus muscles on the posterior aspect of the leg.

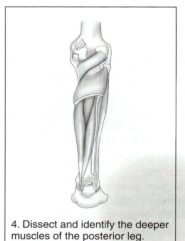

4. Dissect and identify the deeper muscles of the posterior leg.

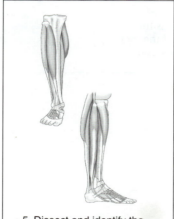

5. Dissect and identify the muscles of the anterior and lateral regions of the leg.

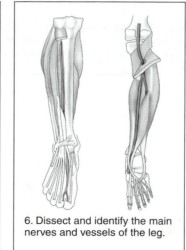

6. Dissect and identify the main nerves and vessels of the leg.

Muscles of the Popliteal Fossa

- Turn the lower limb prone to reveal the posterior surface of the knee

- Greater access to the popliteal fossa may be gained by flexing the leg at the knee joint to ease the tension of the deep fascia and tendons; keep vessels and nerves intact

- Use your fingers or forceps to separate and identify the following **(Figure 38-1)**:

  - **Popliteal fossa** — a diamond-shaped region on the posterior aspect of the knee
    - Boundaries — superior angle
      - Lateral border — biceps femoris tendon
      - Medial border — semimembranosus and semitendinosus tendons
    - Boundaries — inferior angle
      - Both heads of the gastrocnemius m.
  - **Tibial n.** — pull the two heads of the gastrocnemius m. apart at the popliteal fossa to observe the tibial n.

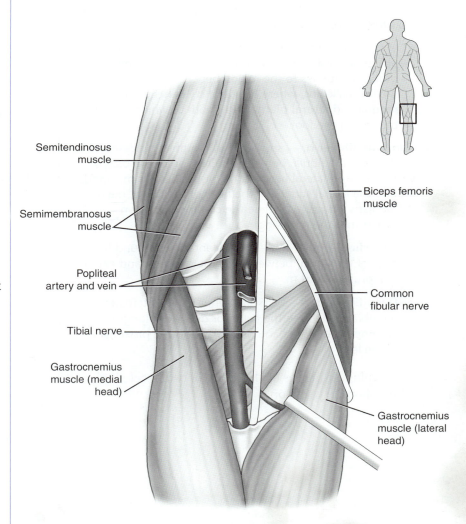

Figure 38-1 Muscles of the popliteal fossa (posterior aspect of the knee)

Nerves of the Popliteal Fossa and Leg

- Use forceps to reveal and identify the following **(Figure 38-2)**:

  - **Tibial n.** — courses through the middle of the popliteal fossa, next to the popliteal a. and v.

    - In the leg, the tibial n. descends in company with the posterior tibial vessels between the superficial and deep group of muscles to the region between the heel and medial malleolus, where the tibial n. branches into the **medial** and **lateral plantar nn.**, both of which course to the sole of the foot

  - **Common fibular n.** — smaller than the tibial n.; descends to the head of the fibula, between the tendon of the biceps femoris m. and lateral head of the gastrocnemius m.; winds around the lateral surface of the neck of the fibula, deep to the fibularis longus m., where the common fibular n. bifurcates into the following:

    - **Superficial fibular n.** — courses anteriorly around the neck of the fibula, between the fibularis mm. and extensor digitorum longus m.

    - **Deep fibular n.** — courses anterior to the interosseous membrane, deep to the extensor digitorum longus m., accompanied by the anterior tibial a. in the proximal part of the leg

- *Note:* The plantar nerves of the foot will be dissected in another laboratory session

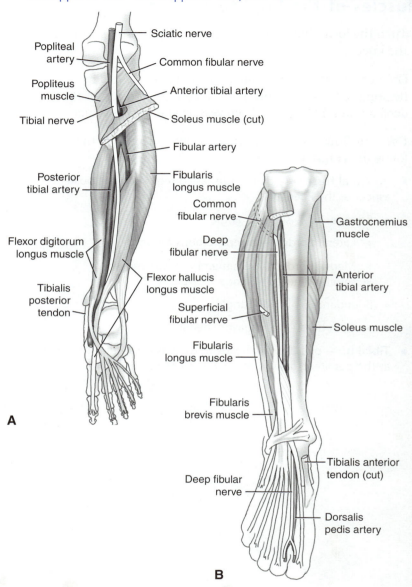

Figure 38-2 The right popliteal fossa and leg. **A,** Posterior view. **B,** Anterior view

Vessels of the Popliteal Fossa

- Use forceps to reveal and identify the following (**Figure 38-3**):

  - **Popliteal a.** — trace the femoral a. and v. distally through the adductor hiatus, at which location their names change to the popliteal a. and v.

    - Ask your instructor if you may remove the popliteal v. and its tributaries, which accompany the following arteries

  - Identify the following anastomotic branches of the popliteal a.:

    - **Superior medial genicular a.** — passes superior to the medial condyle of the femur and anterior to the semitendinosus and semimembranosus mm.

    - **Superior lateral genicular a.** — passes superior to the lateral condyle of the femur and anterior to the biceps femoris tendon

    - **Inferior lateral genicular a.** — emerges deep to the lateral head of the gastrocnemius m.

    - **Inferior medial genicular a.** — emerges deep to the medial head of the gastrocnemius m.

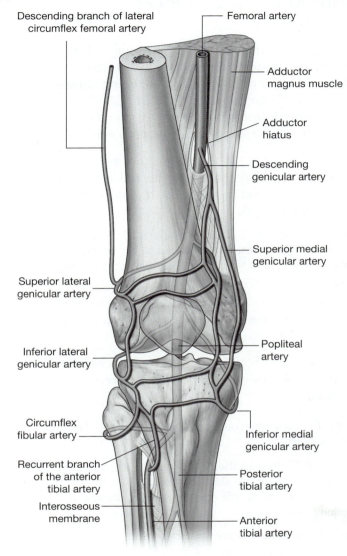

Figure 38-3 Genicular arteries of the right knee. (Redrawn from Drake R, Vogl W, Mitchell A: Gray's Anatomy for Students. Philadelphia: Elsevier, 2005, Fig. 6.74)

Posterior Muscles of the Leg — Superficial Layer

- Observe the sural nn. and small saphenous v.; if necessary, to separate one muscle from another, use a scalpel to incise the deep fascia at the border of two adjoining muscles, and then slide your fingers up and down the adjoining borders to free one muscle from another; keep in mind that many neurovascular bundles run between adjoining muscle bellies

- Use your fingers or forceps to separate and identify the following muscles that converge on the calcaneal (Achilles) tendon **(Figure 38-4)**:

  - **Gastrocnemius m.** — the most superficial muscle in the posterior region of the leg; attached to the condyles of the femur and the calcaneus; thus, this muscle spans two joints (knee and ankle joints)
  - **Plantaris m.** — the smallest of the three muscles in the superficial layer; the muscle and its tendon also span the same two joints

- Use a scalpel to cut both heads of the gastrocnemius m., where the two heads unite into one belly; keep vessels and nerves intact

- As you reflect the gastrocnemius m. inferiorly, identify the following:

  - **Soleus m.** — deep to the gastrocnemius m.; attached to the posterior aspect of the tibia and fibula; inserted with the gastrocnemius m. on the calcaneus; thus, the soleus m. spans one joint (ankle joint)
  - **Plantaris tendon** — sometimes referred to as the "freshman's nerve" because it looks like a nerve

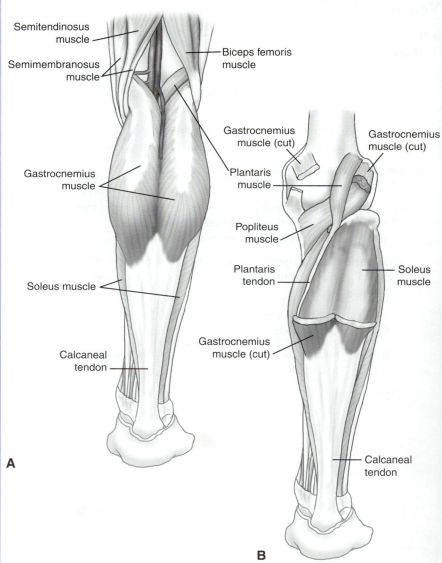

Figure 38-4 Posterior muscles of the right leg. **A,** Superficial muscles. **B,** Deep muscles

Posterior Muscles of the Leg — Deep Layer

- To better identify the deep muscles in the posterior aspect of the leg, use scissors or a scalpel to transect the soleus m. (in a similar fashion to the gastrocnemius m.), and then reflect the two cut ends of both muscles superiorly and inferiorly
  - Keep vessels and nerves intact during the reflection

- Use your fingers or forceps to separate and identify the following **(Figure 38-5)**:
  - **Popliteus m.** — deepest muscle in the popliteal fossa; passes obliquely downward and medially from the femur to the tibia
  - **Tibialis posterior m.** — thick, flat muscle between the flexor hallucis longus and flexor digitorum longus mm.
  - **Flexor digitorum longus m.** — medial to and partially overlies the tibialis posterior m.
  - **Flexor hallucis longus m.** — its muscle belly is lateral to the flexor digitorum longus m.; its tendon crosses the medial side of the ankle joint
  - **Flexor retinaculum** — fibrous band that tethers tendons that cross the ankle joint on its medial side; spans the interval between the medial malleolus and the medial surface of the calcaneus; secures the tendons of the tibialis posterior, flexor digitorum longus, and flexor hallucis longus mm.
    - The plantar attachments will be studied in a future laboratory session
  - A helpful way to remember the three deep muscle tendons on the medial side of the ankle is *Tom*, *Dick*, and *Harry* (from anterior to posterior at the medial malleolus):
    - *T*ibialis posterior, flexor *D*igitorum longus, flexor *H*allucis longus mm.

GAFS pp 548–550   ACGA p 556   NAHA Plate 518

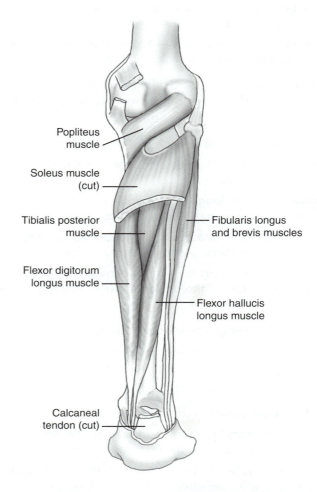

Figure 38-5 Deep view of the posterior muscles of the right leg

Anterolateral Muscles of the Leg

- Turn the lower limb so that it is supine

- Use forceps to reveal and identify the following structures at the ankle **(Figure 38-6)**:
  - **Superior extensor retinaculum** — courses between the anterior borders of the distal ends of the tibia and fibula above the ankle joint
  - **Inferior extensor retinaculum** — Y-shaped structure; attached to the calcaneus, medial malleolus, and plantar fascia

- Cut both of the retinacula vertically to free the underlying tendons; dorsiflex the foot to relieve some tension from the tendons; keep vessels and nerves intact

- **Anterior compartment muscles of the leg**
  - **Tibialis anterior m.** — located along the lateral border of the anterior surface of the tibia
  - **Extensor digitorum longus m.** — visible inferior and lateral to the tibialis anterior m.; follow the tendon to digits 2–5
  - **Fibularis tertius m.** — attached to the fibula; inserts on the base of the fifth metatarsal bone; your cadaver may not have this muscle
  - **Extensor hallucis longus m.** — deep between the tibialis anterior and extensor digitorum longus mm.; follow the tendon to digit 1

- **Lateral compartment muscles of the leg**
  - **Fibularis longus m.** — the most superficial muscle on the lateral aspect of the fibula
  - **Fibularis brevis m.** — deep to the fibularis longus m.

- **Intrinsic dorsal muscles of the foot**
  - **Extensor digitorum brevis m.** — located on the dorsal surface of the foot, deep to the extensor digitorum longus m.
  - **Extensor hallucis brevis m.** — located on the dorsal surface of the foot, deep to the extensor digitorum longus m.

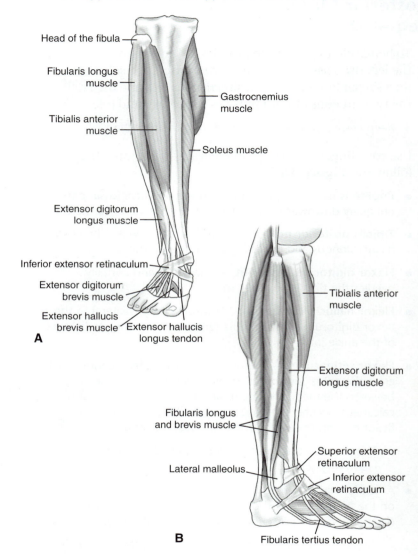

Figure 38-6 Superficial view of the anterior and lateral muscles of the right leg. **A**, Anterior view. **B**, Lateral view

Arteries of the Leg

- Use forceps to reveal and identify the following; veins accompany each artery; ask your instructor if you may remove them to clear up the dissection field (**Figure 38-7**):

  - **Posterior tibial a.** — trace the popliteal a. distally to where it crosses the soleus m.; at this location, the name of the artery changes to the posterior tibial a.

  - **Anterior tibial a.** — pierces the belly of the tibialis posterior m. and the interosseus membrane to enter the anterior compartment of the leg

  - **Fibular a.** — branch of the posterior tibial a. that courses to the lateral compartment of the leg

  - **Dorsalis pedis a.** — follow the anterior tibial a. distally to the foot, where the name of the artery changes to the dorsalis pedis a. on the dorsal surface of the foot; located between the tendons of the extensor hallucis longus and extensor digitorum longus mm.; used to assess the peripheral arterial pulse

    - Attempt to locate the **arcuate a., dorsal metatarsal aa., and dorsal digital aa.**; they are small

- Plantar vessels of the foot will be dissected in another laboratory session

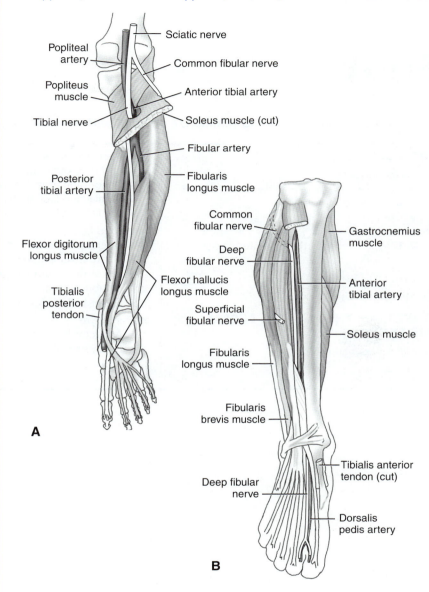

Figure 38-7 Vessels of the right leg. **A**, Posterior view. **B**, Anterior view

Foot

Lab 39

Prior to dissection, you should familiarize yourself with the following structures:

OSTEOLOGY
- Tarsal bones (7)
  - Calcaneus
    - Sustentaculum tali
  - Cuboid
  - Navicular
  - Cuneiform bones (lateral, intermediate, medial)
- Metatarsal bones (5)
- Phalanges (14)

LAYERS OF THE PLANTAR SURFACE OF THE FOOT
- Plantar aponeurosis
- First layer
  - Abductor hallucis m.
  - Abductor digiti minimi m.
  - Flexor digitorum brevis m.
  - Medial and lateral plantar nn.
  - Medial and lateral plantar aa.
- Second layer
  - Lateral plantar n.
  - Quadratus plantae m.
  - Flexor digitorum longus tendon
  - Lumbrical mm. (4)
  - Flexor hallucis longus tendon
- Third layer
  - Adductor hallucis m. (oblique and transverse heads)
  - Flexor hallucis brevis m.
  - Common plantar digital nn.
  - Proper plantar digital nn.
  - Flexor digiti minimi brevis m.
  - Deep plantar arch
  - Plantar metatarsal aa.
  - Common plantar digital aa.
- Fourth layer
  - Dorsal interosseous mm. (4)
  - Plantar interosseous mm. (3)
  - Tibialis posterior tendon
  - Fibularis longus tendon
  - Medial and lateral plantar aa.

Lab 39 Dissection Overview

The purpose of this laboratory session is to learn the anatomy of the foot through dissection. You will do so through the following suggested sequence:

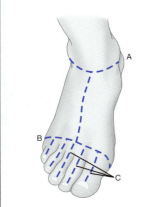

1. Dissect and remove the skin of the foot.

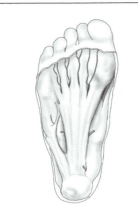

2. Using a sharp scalpel, reflect the plantar aponeurosis. You will dissect the plantar surface of the foot in four layers.

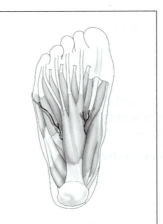

3. Dissect and identify muscles, nerves, and vessels of the first layer.

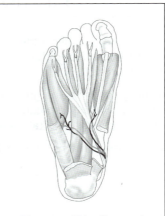

4. Dissect and identify muscles, nerves, and vessels of the second layer.

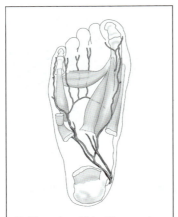

5. Dissect and identify muscles, nerves, and vessels of the third layer.

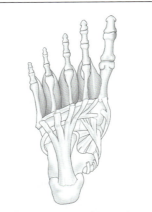

6. Dissect and identify muscles, nerves, and vessels of the fourth layer.

Skin Removal — Foot

- Use a scalpel with a new blade to make the following skin incisions **(Figure 39-1)**:

  - Remove the flaps between *A* and *B* from the ankle and dorsal and plantar surfaces of the foot

  - Make longitudinal incisions *(C)* along the dorsal and plantar surfaces of the great toe and along the top of the other digits connected to the incision at *B*

  - Remove the remaining skin from the great toe and at least one other digit; expect difficulty separating the skin from the plantar aponeurosis; be patient, and take your time

    - Ask your instructor about the number of toes to dissect

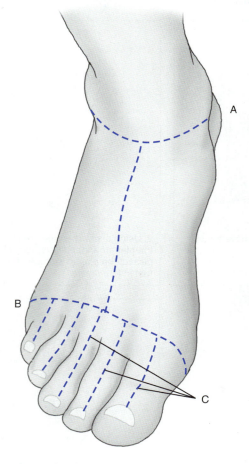

Figure 39-1   Skin incisions of the right foot

Dissection of the Plantar Surface of the Foot

- Use a scalpel handle (with the blade off) to scrape the remaining superficial fascia from the plantar aponeurosis **(Figure 39-2)**

- Identify digital bands of the plantar aponeurosis that extend to each toe; look for **proper digital n., a.,** and **v.** lateral and medial to each band

- Use a scalpel or scissors to cut the digital bands from the plantar aponeurosis proximally to the base of the toes distally; do not damage the underlying neurovascular bundles

- Use a scalpel or scissors to make a longitudinal incision through the plantar aponeurosis, from the **calcaneus** to the base of the toes

- Plantar structures are customarily grouped into four layers:
  - First layer
  - Second layer
  - Third layer
  - Fourth layer

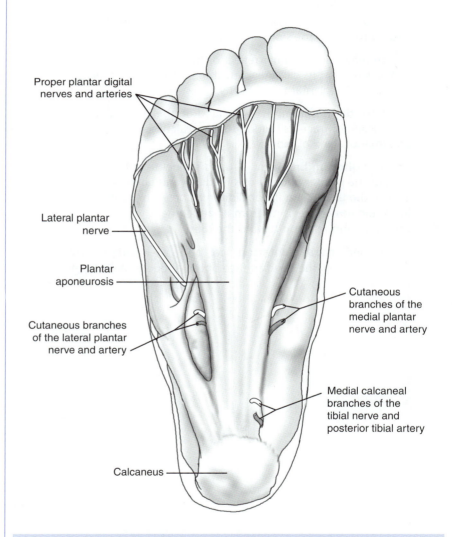

Figure 39-2 Plantar surface of the right foot (veins not shown)

Plantar Surface of the Foot — First Layer

- Use forceps to reveal and identify the following (Figure 39-3):

  - **Abductor hallucis m.** — located on the medial surface of the calcaneus; trace the muscle's tendon to its attachment on the base of the great toe's proximal phalanx

    - You may want to either reflect or transect the abductor hallucis m. at its calcaneal attachment to see the course of the medial plantar n., a., and v.

  - **Abductor digiti minimi m.** — located on the lateral side of the calcaneus; trace its tendon to the attachment on the proximal phalanx of digit 5

  - **Flexor digitorum brevis m.** — use a scalpel to reflect the flaps of the plantar aponeurosis medially and laterally to expose the underlying flexor digitorum brevis m.; cut the flexor digitorum brevis m. from its attachment to the calcaneus and reflect it toward the toes

  - **Medial** and **lateral plantar nn., aa.,** and **vv.** — enter the sole of the foot from the deep surface of the abductor hallucis m.

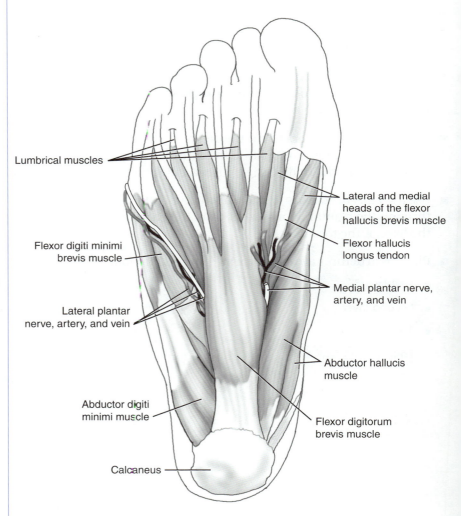

Figure 39-3 First layer of the plantar surface of the right foot

Plantar Surface of the Foot — Second Layer

■ Use forceps to reveal and identify the following **(Figure 39-4)**:

- **Quadratus plantae m.** — arises by two heads from the calcaneus and inserts into the tendon of the flexor digitorum longus m.

- **Flexor digitorum longus tendons** — trace the tendons distally to digits 2–5; note that these tendons pass deep to the tendons of the flexor digitorum brevis m.

- **Lumbrical mm.** — the four lumbrical mm. arise from the tendons of the flexor digitorum longus m.

- **Flexor hallucis longus tendon** — trace the tendon as it crosses deep to the tendon of the flexor digitorum longus m. to attach to digit 1

- **Tibial n.** and **posterior tibial a.** and **v.** — before entering the plantar surface of the foot, the nerve and vessels branch into the following:

  - **Medial plantar n., a., and v.** — course between the abductor hallucis and flexor digitorum brevis mm.

  - **Lateral plantar n., a., and v.** — course laterally across the sole of the foot between the quadratus plantae m. and the reflected flexor digitorum brevis m.

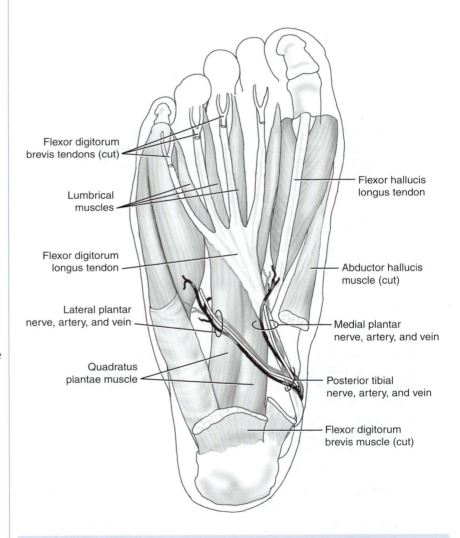

Figure 39-4 Second layer of the plantar surface of the right foot

Plantar Surface of the Foot — Third Layer

■ To see the structures in the third layer, use a scalpel to make the following transections:
- The quadratus plantae m. from the calcaneus; reflect the muscle toward the toes
- The tendon of the flexor digitorum longus m., inferior to the tendon of the flexor hallucis longus m.; reflect the cut muscle toward the toes

■ Use forceps to reveal and identify the following (**Figure 39-5**):
- **Flexor hallucis brevis m.** — two heads, one on each side of the flexor hallucis longus tendon; note that sesamoid bones may be within the tendon
  - Detach the lateral head of the flexor hallucis brevis m. from its origin on the bases of metatarsals 2–4 and reflect the muscle medially
- **Adductor hallucis m.** — lateral to the flexor hallucis brevis m.; has oblique and transverse heads
  - Reflect the oblique head of the adductor hallucis m. toward the great toe
- **Flexor digiti minimi m.** — medial to the abductor digiti minimi m.
- **Deep plantar arterial arch** — at the interface between the third and fourth layers; observe that the medial and lateral plantar aa. anastomose to form the deep plantar arterial arch, deep to the flexor hallucis brevis m. and oblique head of the adductor hallucis m.
  - **Plantar metatarsal aa.** — the deep plantar arterial arch gives rise to four plantar metatarsal aa. located in the region of the metatarsal bones
    - **Plantar digital aa. proper** — supply the digits
  - **Deep plantar a.** — joins the deep plantar arterial arch with the dorsalis pedis a. by piercing interosseous space 1
- **Lateral** and **medial plantar nn.** — branches of the posterior tibial n.
  - **Common plantar digital nn.**
  - **Proper plantar digital nn.**

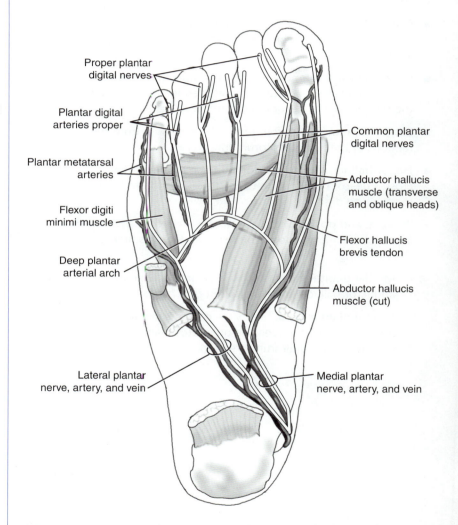

Figure 39-5 Third layer of the plantar surface of the right foot

Plantar Surface of the Foot — Fourth Layer

■ Use forceps to reveal and identify the following (**Figure 39-6**):

- **Plantar interosseous mm.** (3) — located on the medial side of the metatarsals for digits 3–5; *add*uct digits 3–5
- **Dorsal interosseous mm.** (4) — located on the lateral side of the metatarsals for digits 3 and 4 and both sides of the metatarsals for digit 2; *abd*uct digits 2–4
- **Tibialis posterior tendon** — trace the tendon of the tibialis posterior m. to its multiple insertions on the tarsal bones
- **Tibialis anterior tendon** — note its attachment on metatarsal 1
- **Fibularis longus tendon** — follow the tendon of the fibularis longus m. across the deep plantar surface of the foot to the base of metatarsal 1 and the medial cuneiform bone
- **Long plantar ligament** — courses from the plantar surface of the calcaneus to the cuboid and base of the metatarsals; a tunnel is formed deep to the ligament for the tendon of the fibularis longus m.; helps maintain the arches of the foot
- **Plantar calcaneonavicular ("spring") ligament** — courses from the sustentaculum tali to the posterior and inferior surface of the navicular bone; helps maintain the longitudinal arch of the foot

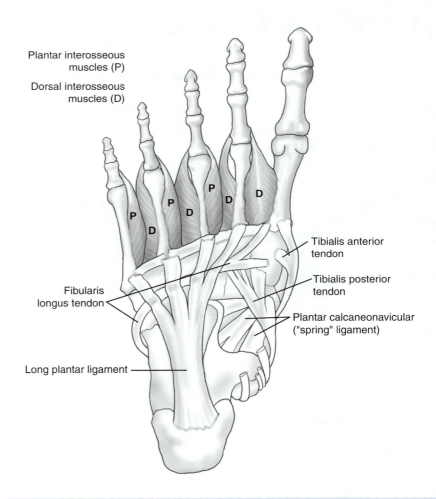

Figure 39-6 Fourth layer of the plantar surface of the right foot

Joints of the Lower Limb

Lab 40

Prior to dissection, you should familiarize yourself with the following structures:

HIP
- Iliofemoral ligament
- Pubofemoral ligament
- Ischiofemoral ligament
- Round ligament of the femur
- Acetabular ligament
- Articular cartilage
- Transverse acetabular ligament

KNEE
- Fibular (lateral) collateral ligament
- Tibial (medial) collateral ligament
- Medial meniscus
- Lateral meniscus
- Anterior cruciate ligament
- Posterior cruciate ligament

ANKLE
- Medial deltoid ligament
- Anterior talofibular ligament
- Posterior talofibular ligament
- Calcaneofibular ligament
- Plantar calcaneonavicular ("spring") ligament
- Long plantar ligament

FOOT AND DIGITS
- Plantar metatarsal ligaments
- Plantar ligaments
- Metatarsophalangeal joints
- Interphalangeal joints
- Joint capsule
- Medial and lateral collateral digital ligaments

Lab 40 Dissection Overview

The purpose of this laboratory session is to learn the anatomy of the joints of the lower limb through dissection. You will do so through the following suggested sequence:

1. To ensure that the limb dissections are not completely destroyed, choose only one or two joints to dissect on the lower limb. Other dissection tables will choose other limb joints.

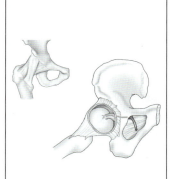

2. Dissect and cut away the muscles that cross the hip joint. Dissect and reveal the structures associated with the hip joint.

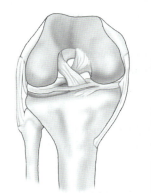

3. Dissect and cut away the muscles that cross the knee joint. Dissect and reveal the structures associated with the knee joint.

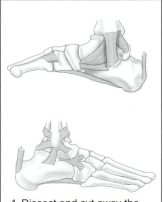

4. Dissect and cut away the muscles that cross the ankle joints. Dissect and reveal the structures associated with the ankle joints.

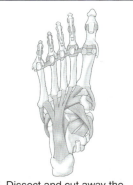

5. Dissect and cut away the muscles that cross the metatarsophalangeal and interphalangeal joints. Dissect and reveal the structures associated with these joints.

LOWER LIMB — JOINT DISSECTION

- Select one lower limb on which to dissect the joints; use a scalpel and forceps to perform the dissection in the following steps:
  - First, muscles that surround each joint will be removed from the joint to reveal the joint capsule
  - Second, the joint capsule and tendons that traverse the capsule will be cut to reveal the articulation

Hip Joint

- The joint capsule extends from the acetabular rim to the neck of the femur at the intertrochanteric line and root of the greater trochanter
- Thick parts of the joint capsule form the ligaments of the hip joint, which pass in a spiral fashion from the os coxae to the femur
- To identify the three capsular ligaments, cut all muscles that cross the hip joint; leave the joint capsule intact:
  - **Iliofemoral ligament** — attached to the anterior inferior iliac spine and the acetabular rim and courses inferiorly to the intertrochanteric line of the femur; reinforces the anterior aspect of the hip joint capsule **(Figure 40-1)**
  - **Pubofemoral ligament** — attached to the obturator crest of the pubis and courses laterally and inferiorly to the femur; reinforces the inferior and anterior aspects of the hip joint capsule (see Figure 40-1A)
  - **Ischiofemoral ligament** — attached to the ischial part of the acetabular rim; spirals superior and lateral to the neck of the femur and base of the greater trochanter; reinforces the posterior aspect of the hip joint capsule (see Figure 40-1B)

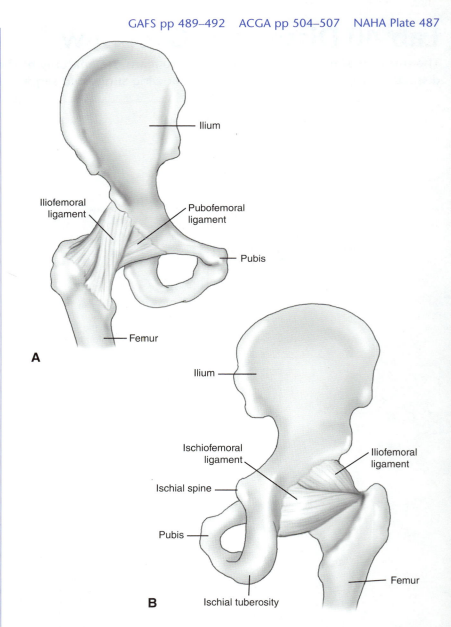

Figure 40-1 Right hip joint. **A,** Anterior view. **B,** Posterior view

Hip Joint—cont'd

- Identify the following:

  - Use a scalpel to cut the ligaments of the capsule of the dissected joint around its circumference **(Figure 40-2A)**
  - Open the hip joint to disconnect the round ligament of the femur, either by twisting the femur or cutting the round ligament with a scalpel
  - Identify the following (see Figure 40-2B and 40-2C):

    - **Round ligament of the femur** — attached to the margins of the acetabular notch, the transverse acetabular ligament, and the fovea in the head of the femur; provides little support to the hip joint but is accompanied by an important artery:

      - **The a. to the head of the femur** — a branch of the obturator a.

    - **Acetabular labrum** — a fibrocartilaginous rim that is attached to the acetabulum and the transverse acetabular ligament; increases the depth of the acetabulum

    - **Transverse acetabular ligament** — forms part of the acetabular labrum; crosses the notch, forming a foramen through which vessels and nerves enter the joint

    - **Articular cartilage** — hyaline cartilage that converges with the head of the femur and fills the acetabulum, except for the fovea, for attachment of the round ligament of the femoral head

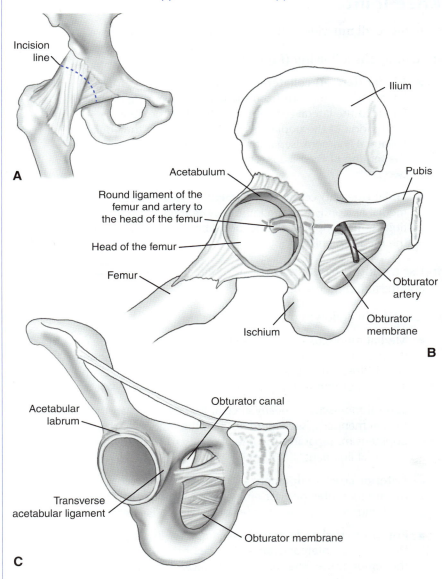

GAFS pp 489–492   ACGA pp 504–507   NAHA Plate 487

Figure 40-2   Right hip joint. **A**, Capsule incision. **B**, Capsule open. **C**, Hip joint

Knee Joint

- Remove all muscles that cross one knee joint

- Identify the following (**Figure 40-3A** and **40-3B**):

  - **Fibular (lateral) collateral ligament** — round, cordlike ligament that extends from the lateral epicondyle of the femur to the lateral surface of the head of the fibula; the tendon of the popliteus m. passes deep to the fibular collateral ligament, separating it from the lateral meniscus; the tendon of the biceps femoris splits the ligament into two parts

  - **Tibial (medial) collateral ligament** — extends from the medial epicondyle of the femur to the medial surface of the tibia; at its midpoint, the deepest fibers are firmly attached to the medial meniscus

- Use a scalpel to cut away the joint capsule, but leave the collateral ligaments intact

- Identify the following:

  - **Medial meniscus** — C-shaped fibrocartilaginous wedge on the medial aspect of the tibia (see Figure 40-3C); its anterior end is attached to the anterior cruciate ligament (ACL) and its posterior end to the posterior cruciate ligament (PCL)

  - **Lateral meniscus** — nearly circular and smaller than the medial meniscus (see Figure 40-3C); the tendon of the popliteus m. separates the lateral meniscus from the fibular collateral ligament

  - **Anterior cruciate ligament** — named for its attachment to the anterior intercondylar eminence of the tibia; attached to the femur at the posterior, medial surface of its lateral condyle

  - **Posterior cruciate ligament** — named for its attachment to the posterior intercondylar eminence of the tibia; attached to the femur at the anterior, lateral surface of its medial condyle

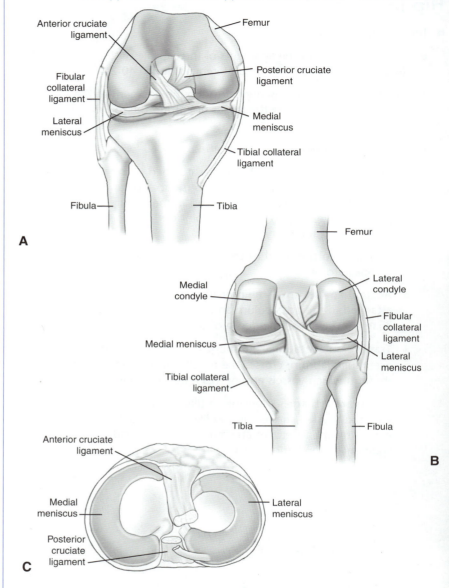

Figure 40-3 Right knee joint. **A**, Anterior view (flexed). **B**, Posterior view (extended). **C**, Superior view of the tibia

Ankle and Foot Joints

- Remove all muscles, arteries, veins, nerves, and tendons that cross the ankle joint of one lower limb to identify the following:

  - **Tibiotalar joint** — allows dorsal and plantar flexion

    - **Collateral ligaments** — medial side of the ankle (Figure 40-4A)

      ◆ **Deltoid ligament** — attached to the medial malleolus of the tibia; consists of four parts that attach to the navicular, calcaneus, and two parts of the talus

    - **Collateral ligaments** — lateral side of the ankle (see Figure 40-4B)

      ◆ **Posterior** and **anterior** *talo*fibular ligaments — attached between the talus and the lateral malleolus of the fibula

      ◆ **Calcaneofibular ligament** — attached at the calcaneus and the apex of the lateral malleolus of the fibula

    - **Posterior** and **anterior** *tibio*fibular ligaments — hold the tibia and fibula together, along with the interosseous membrane

  - **Talocalcaneonavicular joint** — allows inversion and eversion

    - **Plantar calcaneonavicular ("spring") ligament** — attached from the calcaneus to the navicular bone

  - **Long plantar ligament** — courses from the plantar surface of the calcaneus to the cuboid and base of the metatarsals

GAFS pp 562–569   ACGA pp 564–566, 568–569   NAHA Plates 527–528

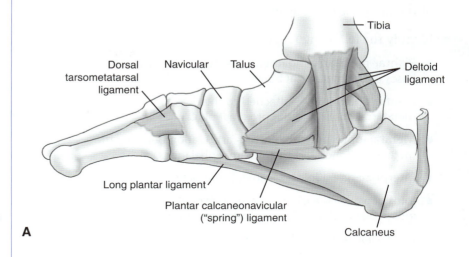

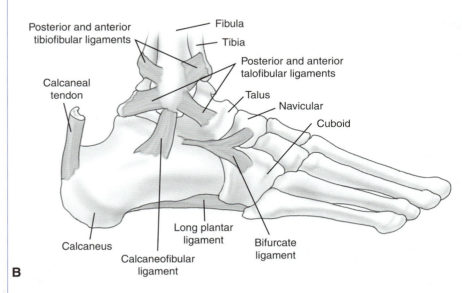

Figure 40-4   Right ankle and foot joints. **A,** Medial view. **B,** Lateral view

Foot and Digit Joints

- Remove muscles and tendons to observe the joint capsules of the great toe and one other digit
- Identify the following **(Figure 40-5)**:
  - **Plantar metatarsal ligaments** — attached between the bases of the metatarsal bones
  - **Plantar ligaments** — attached to the distal end of the metatarsal bones and the proximal phalanges
  - **Metatarsophalangeal joints** — articulation between the metatarsal bones and the proximal phalanges
  - **Interphalangeal joints** — articulation between the phalanges
  - **Joint capsule** — each metatarsophalangeal and interphalangeal joint is surrounded by its own joint capsule
    - **Medial** and **lateral collateral digital ligaments** — medial and lateral thickenings of the joint capsule

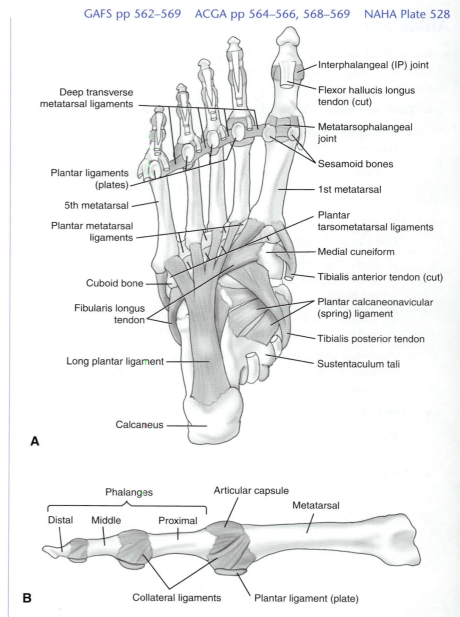

Figure 40-5 Right foot and digit joints. **A,** Plantar view. **B,** Lateral view.

Arches of the Foot

- Identify the following **(Figure 40-6)**:
  - **Arches of the foot** — the tarsal and metatarsal bones are arranged in longitudinal and transverse arches that enable the weightbearing capabilities and movements of the foot
    - **Longitudinal arch of the foot** — composed of both the medial and lateral longitudinal arches
      - **Medial longitudinal arch** — higher than the lateral arch; composed of the calcaneus, talus, navicular, three cuneiforms, and three metatarsal bones; the talar head is the keystone of the medial longitudinal arch
      - **Lateral longitudinal arch** — flatter than the medial longitudinal arch; composed of the calcaneus, cuboid, and lateral two metatarsals
    - **Transverse arch of the foot** — courses from side to side; formed by the cuboid, cuneiforms, and bases of the metatarsals

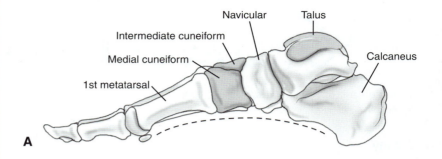

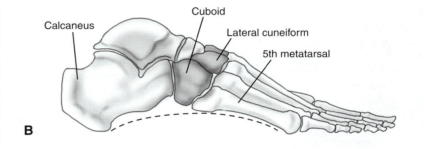

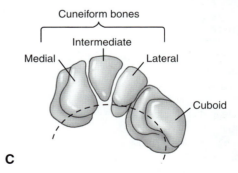

Figure 40-6 Arches of the foot. **A,** Medial longitudinal arch. **B,** Lateral longitudinal arch. **C,** Anterior view of the transverse arch

Unit 6 Lower Limb Overview

At the end of Unit 6, you should be able to identify the following structures on cadavers, skeletons, and/or radiographs:

Osteology

- Features of the os coxae
  - Acetabulum
  - Obturator foramen
  - Ischiopubic ramus
- Bones of the os coxae
  - Ilium
    - Ala (wing) of the ilium
    - Iliac crest
      - Anterior superior iliac spine
      - Anterior inferior iliac spine
      - Posterior superior iliac spine
      - Posterior inferior iliac spine
    - Iliac fossa
    - Anterior, posterior, and inferior gluteal lines
    - Auricular surface
  - Ischium
    - Ischial tuberosity, ramus, and spine
    - Greater sciatic notch
    - Lesser sciatic notch
  - Pubis
    - Pubic tubercle and crest
    - Superior pubic ramus
      - Pecten pubis (pectineal line)
    - Inferior pubic ramus
    - Obturator groove and crest
    - Pubic arch
- Pelvis
  - Pelvic cavity
  - Pubic symphysis
- Femur
  - Head
    - Fovea for the ligament of the head
  - Neck
    - Greater trochanter
      - Trochanteric fossa
    - Lesser trochanter
    - Intertrochanteric line and crest
  - Linea aspera
  - Pectineal line
  - Gluteal tuberosity
  - Medial condyle and epicondyle
    - Adductor tubercle
  - Lateral condyle and epicondyle
  - Popliteal and patellar surfaces
- Patella
  - Base and apex
  - Articular and anterior surfaces
- Tibia
  - Medial and lateral condyles
  - Intercondylar eminence
  - Tibial tuberosity
  - Soleal line
  - Interosseous border
  - Medial malleolus
  - Fibular notch
  - Inferior articular surface
- Fibula
  - Head and neck
  - Interosseous border
  - Lateral malleolus
- Foot
  - Tarsal bones (7)
    - Talus
    - Calcaneus — sustentaculum tali
    - Navicular
    - Medial cuneiform
    - Intermediate cuneiform
    - Lateral cuneiform
    - Cuboid
  - Metatarsal bones (5)
    - Phalanges (14)
      - Proximal, middle, and distal

Muscles

- Gluteal region
  - Tensor fascia lata m.
  - Gluteus maximus m.
  - Gluteus medius m.
  - Gluteus minimus m.
  - Piriformis m.
  - Superior gemellus m.
  - Obturator internus m.
  - Inferior gemellus m.
  - Quadratus femoris m.
- Iliopsoas m.
  - Iliacus m.
  - Psoas major m.
- Psoas minor m.
- Anterior muscles of the thigh
  - Quadratus femoris m.

- Rectus femoris m.
- Vastus medialis m.
- Vastus intermedius m.
- Vastus lateralis m.
- Sartorius m.
- Medial muscles of the thigh
  - Pectineus m.
  - Adductor brevis m.
  - Adductor longus m.
  - Adductor magnus m. (adductor hiatus)
  - Gracilis m.
  - Obturator externus m.
- Posterior muscles of the thigh
  - Biceps femoris m.
  - Semitendinosus m.
  - Semimembranosus m.
- Anterior muscles of the leg
  - Tibialis anterior m.
  - Extensor digitorum longus m.
  - Extensor hallucis longus m.
  - Fibularis (peroneus) tertius m.
- Lateral muscles of the leg
  - Fibularis (peroneus) longus m.
  - Fibularis (peroneus) brevis m.
- Posterior muscles of the leg
  - Superficial layer
    - Gastrocnemius m.
    - Plantaris m.
    - Soleus m.
  - Deep layer
    - Tibialis posterior m.
    - Flexor hallucis longus m.
    - Flexor digitorum longus m.
    - Popliteus m.
- Dorsal muscles of the foot
  - Extensor digitorum brevis m.
  - Extensor hallucis brevis m.
- Plantar aponeurosis

- Plantar muscles of the foot
  - First layer
    - Abductor hallucis m.
    - Flexor digitorum brevis m.
    - Abductor digiti minimi m.
  - Second layer
    - Quadratus plantae m.
    - Lumbrical mm. (4)
  - Third layer
    - Flexor hallucis brevis m.
    - Adductor hallucis m.
      - Oblique head
      - Transverse head
    - Flexor digiti minimi brevis m.
  - Fourth layer
    - Plantar interossei mm. (3)
    - Dorsal interossei mm. (4)

Nerves

Lumbar Plexus
- Subcostal n. (T12)
- Iliohypogastric n. (L1)
- Ilioinguinal n. (L1)
- Genitofemoral n. (L1–L2)
  - Genital branch
  - Femoral branch
- Lateral cutaneous n. of the thigh (L2–L3)
- Obturator n. (L2–L4)
  - Anterior branch
    - Cutaneous branch
  - Posterior branch
- Accessory obturator n.
- Femoral n. (L2–L4)
  - Muscular branches
  - Medial cutaneous n. of the thigh (L2–L4)
  - Intermediate cutaneous n. of the thigh (L2–L4)
  - Saphenous n. (L2–L4)
- Lumbosacral trunk (L4–L5)

Sacral Plexus
- Lumbosacral trunk (L4–L5)
- Nerve to the obturator internus m. (L5–S2)
- Nerve to the piriformis m. (S1–S2)
- Nerve to the quadratus femoris m. (L4–S1)
- Superior gluteal n. (L4–S1)
- Inferior gluteal n. (L5–S2)
- Posterior cutaneous n. of the thigh (S1–S3)
- Sciatic n. (L4–S3)
  - Common fibular (peroneal) n. (L4–S3)
    - Lateral sural cutaneous n.
    - Superficial fibular (peroneal) n.
    - Deep fibular (peroneal) n.
  - Tibial n. (L4–S3)
    - Interosseous n.
    - Medial sural cutaneous n.
    - Medial plantar n.
      - Common plantar digital nn.
        - Proper plantar digital nn.
    - Lateral plantar n.
      - Common plantar digital nn.
        - Proper plantar digital nn.

Arteries
- Internal iliac a.
  - Superior gluteal a.
  - Inferior gluteal a.
  - Obturator a.
- External iliac a.
  - Femoral a.
    - Deep a. of the thigh
      - Medial circumflex femoral a.
      - Lateral circumflex femoral a.
        - Ascending, transverse, and descending branches
      - Perforating branches
  - Popliteal a.

Continued

Arteries—cont'd

- External iliac a.—cont'd
  - Popliteal a.—cont'd
    - Superior medial genicular a.
    - Superior lateral genicular a.
    - Inferior medial genicular a.
    - Inferior lateral genicular a.
  - Anterior tibial a.
    - Dorsalis pedis a.
  - Posterior tibial a.
    - Fibular a.
    - Medial plantar a.
      - Deep branch
      - Superficial branch
    - Lateral plantar a.
      - Deep plantar arch
      - Plantar metatarsal aa.
      - Common plantar digital aa.
      - Plantar digital aa. proper

Veins

- Internal iliac v.
  - Superior gluteal v.
  - Inferior gluteal v.
  - Obturator v.
- External iliac v.
  - Great saphenous v.
  - Small saphenous v.
    - Dorsal venous arch of the foot
    - Plantar venous arch
    - Dorsal metatarsal vv.
    - Plantar metatarsal vv.
    - Plantar digital vv.
  - Femoral v.
    - Deep femoral v. of the thigh
      - Medial and lateral circumflex femoral vv.
      - Perforating vv.
  - Popliteal v.
    - Sural v.
    - Genicular vv.
    - Anterior tibial v.
    - Posterior tibial v.
    - Fibular v.

Lymphatics

- Femoral lymph nodes
- Inguinal lymph nodes

Joints

Hip

- Iliofemoral ligament
- Pubofemoral ligament
- Ischiofemoral ligament
- Round ligament of the femur
- Acetabular ligament
- Articular cartilage
- Transverse acetabular ligament

Knee

- Fibular (lateral) collateral ligament
- Tibial (medial) collateral ligament
- Medial meniscus
- Lateral meniscus
- Anterior cruciate ligament
- Posterior cruciate ligament

Ankle

- Medial deltoid ligament
- Anterior talofibular ligament
- Posterior talofibular ligament
- Calcaneofibular ligament
- Plantar calcaneonavicular ("spring") ligament
- Long plantar ligament

Foot and Digits

- Plantar metatarsal ligaments
- Plantar ligaments
- Metatarsophalangeal joints
- Interphalangeal joints
- Joint capsule
- Medial and lateral collateral ligaments

Miscellaneous

- Flexor and extensor retinacula
- Iliotibial band of fascia
- Femoral triangle, sheath, and canal
- Fibrous digital sheaths

Index

A

Abdomen
  arteries of, 246
  ligaments of, 248
  lymphatics of, 247
  muscles of, 245–246
  nerves of, 247
    cutaneous, 136
  orientation of, 133
  osteology of, 117–119, 245
  overview of, 245–249
  skin incisions of, 134
  surface anatomy of, 133
  veins of, 246–247
Abdominal aorta, 183, 186, 187, 238
  branches of, 157
Abdominal viscera, 248
  adrenal glands, 153
  cecum, 153
  colon, 153
  duodenojejunal junction, 163
  duodenum, 153, 162
  gallbladder, 153
  ileocecal junction, 153
  ileum, 153
  jejunum, 153
  kidneys, 153
  liver, 153, 165–168
  overview of, 153
  pancreas, 153
  spleen, 153, 164
  stomach, 153, 156
  vasculature of, 147, 157–161, 169
  vermiform appendix, 153
Abdominal wall
  anterior, 129–144, 247
    dissection overview of, 130
    incisions of, 139
    layers of, 129, 132, 140, 247
    muscles of, 129, 131, 137

Abdominal wall *(Continued)*
    nerves of, 129
    osteology of, 129
    rectus sheath of, 141–142
    superficial fascia of, 135
    superficial inguinal ring of, 129, 138
    vessels of, 129
  layers of, 132, 206
  osteology of, 118
  posterior, 183–195
    abdominal aorta, 183, 186, 187
    adrenal glands, 189, 191
    arteries of, 183
    diaphragm, 183, 186, 192
    dissection overview of, 184
    inferior vena cava, 183, 186, 188
    kidneys, 183, 186, 189–190
    lymphatics of, 183
    muscles of, 183, 185, 193
    nerves of, 183, 194–195
    overview of, 186
    veins of, 183
Abducens nerve, 312, 323, 324, 328, 333, 334
Abductor digiti minimi muscle, 424, 485, 506, 540
Abductor hallucis muscle, 506, 550, 551
Abductor pollicis brevis muscle, 423, 484
Abductor pollicis longus muscle, 471, 472, 488
Abductor pollicis muscle, 423
Accessory hemiazygos vein, 106–108
Accessory meningeal artery, 367
Accessory meningeal branch, of mandibular division of trigeminal nerve, 322
Accessory pancreatic duct, 172
Accessory saphenous vein, 521
Acetabular labrum, 557
Acetabular ligament, transverse, 557
Acetabulum, 119, 122, 123, 509, 510

Acoustic canal, external, 405, 408
  opening of, 406
Acoustic meatus, internal, 262, 322, 326, 327, 408
Acromial artery, 452
Acromial branch, 67, 68
Acromioclavicular joint, 54, 58, 61, 493
Acromion, of scapula, 13, 54, 58, 61, 272, 427, 429, 493
Acute marginal artery, 92, 93
Adam's apple, 272
Adductor brevis muscle, 502, 530, 532, 533
Adductor canal, 532, 533, 535
Adductor compartment, of hand, 479, 487
Adductor hallucis muscle, 506, 552
Adductor hiatus, 532, 533–535, 541
Adductor longus muscle, 502, 530–535
Adductor magnus muscle, 503, 532, 534, 535, 541
Adductor pollicis muscle, 423, 487
Adductor tubercle, 508, 512
Adenoids, 371
Adrenal arteries
  inferior, 187, 191
  middle, 187, 191
  superior, 187, 191
Adrenal glands, 153, 186, 189, 191
Adrenal veins
  left, 188
  right, 188
Air cells, 332
Ala, of sacrum, 120, 127
Alar branch, of lateral nasal artery, 383
Alar ligaments, 345
Alveolar arch, 261
Alveolar artery
  inferior, 365–367
  superior
    anterior, 387
    middle, 387
    posterior, 387

Alveolar foramina, posterior superior, 265
Alveolar nerve
  inferior, 364–367
  superior
    anterior, 387
    middle, 387
    posterior, 367, 377, 387
Alveolar process, 258
Alveolar vein
  inferior, 365–367
  superior
    anterior, 387
    middle, 387
    posterior, 387
Anal canal, 155
Anal sphincter
  external, 201, 202, 215, 216, 223, 224
  internal, 201, 202
Anal triangle, 211, 218
Anatomical snuff box, 472, 488
Anconeus muscle, 421, 463, 471
Ankle joint, 554, 559, 564
Annular ligament, 495
Anococcygeal ligament, 201, 202
Ansa cervicalis, 270, 282, 288
Anterior abdominal wall, 129–144, 247
  dissection overview of, 130
  incisions of, 139
  internal surface of, 144
  layers of, 129, 132, 140, 247
  muscles of, 129, 131, 137
  nerves of, 129
  osteology of, 129
  rectus sheath of, 141–142
  superficial fascia of, 135
  superficial inguinal ring of, 129, 137, 138
  vessels of, 129
Anterior cardiac veins, 94
Anterior chamber, of eye, 337

Anterior chest wall, 55–72
  arteries and veins of, 55
  breasts in, 55, 60
  deltopectoral triangle of, 63, 64, 66–68
  dissection overview of, 56
  examination of removed, 72
  intercostal structures of, 69
  miscellaneous terms and structures of, 55
  muscles of, 55, 57, 63–65
  nerves of, 55
  orientation and incisions for
    female, 58–59
    male, 61–62
  osteology of, 55
  removal of, 70–71
  superficial fascia of, 63
Anterior circumflex humeral artery, 452
Anterior clinoid process, 262, 321, 322
Anterior communicating artery, 314, 315
Anterior cranial fossa, 262, 317, 320, 321
Anterior cruciate ligament, 558
Anterior cutaneous nerves, of abdomen, 136
Anterior cutaneous neurovascular bundles, 63
Anterior ethmoidal air cells, 382
Anterior ethmoidal artery, 334, 380, 383, 384
  septal branch of, 383
Anterior ethmoidal nerve, 334, 380
  external nasal branch of, 351
Anterior femoral cutaneous nerves, 521
Anterior gluteal line, 511
Anterior inferior cerebellar arteries, 314, 315
Anterior inferior iliac spine, 124–126, 508, 510, 511
Anterior inferior pancreaticoduodenal artery, 177
Anterior intercostal artery, 112
Anterior interosseous artery, 462, 473, 474
Anterior interosseous nerve, 475
Anterior interventricular artery, 91–93, 100
Anterior interventricular groove, 91
Anterior jugular vein, 285
Anterior labial artery, 225
Anterior labial nerve, 225
Anterior labial vein, 225
Anterior mediastinum, 84, 102
Anterior nasal spine, 258
Anterior papillary muscle, 98, 100
Anterior perforating branches, 112
Anterior primary rami, 55, 63
Anterior roots, spinal, 42
Anterior sacral foramina, 127
Anterior sacrococcygeal ligament, 231, 232

Anterior scalene muscle, 276, 277, 343, 348
Anterior scrotal artery, 217
Anterior scrotal nerves, 208
Anterior scrotal vein, 217
Anterior scrotal vessels, 208
Anterior spinal artery, 314, 315
Anterior superior alveolar artery, 387
Anterior superior alveolar nerve, 387
Anterior superior alveolar vein, 387
Anterior superior iliac spine, 119, 121, 122, 124, 133, 509–511
Anterior superior pancreaticoduodenal arteries, 160, 169, 177
Anterior talofibular ligament, 559
Anterior tibial artery, 540, 541, 545
  recurrent branch of, 541
Anterior tympanic artery, 367
Anterior ulnar recurrent artery, 461, 462, 473, 474
Anterior vagal trunk, 104
Anterolateral abdominal wall, layers of, 129, 247
Antihelix, of ear, 406
Antitragus, 406
Anus, 153, 176, 215, 219
Aorta, 86, 100, 111, 112, 170
  abdominal, 183, 186, 187, 238
    branches of, 157
  ascending, 88–93
  descending, 102, 104, 111, 112
  thoracic, 55, 111, 112
Aortic arch, 100, 102, 110
Aortic hiatus, 192
Aortic impression, 81
Aortic valve, 100, 101
Apex
  of heart, 91
  of lung
    left, 80, 81
    right, 82, 83
Appendicular artery, 178, 179
Appendicular lymph nodes, 179
Appendix(ices)
  omental (epiploic), 176
  vermiform, 153, 175
Arachnoid granulations, 307, 308
  indentations caused by, 305
Arachnoid mater
  cranial, 307, 308
  spinal, 42
Arachnoid trabeculae, 307, 308
Arcuate artery, 545
Arcuate eminence, 263

Arcuate ligament(s)
  lateral, 192, 193
  medial, 192, 193
  median, 192, 193
Arcuate line, 120, 124–126, 142–144, 511
Areola, 58, 60, 61
Arm, 454–465
  arteries of, 454
    brachial, 461
    deep, 444, 445, 465
    posterior region, 465
    proximal portions of radial and ulnar, 462
  brachial plexus in
    posterior branches in shoulder of, 464
    terminal branches of, 454, 456, 459–460
  dissection overview of, 455–456
  muscles of, 454, 498
    anterior, 457–458
    posterior, 463
  nerves of, 454
    inferior lateral cutaneous, 441
    medial cutaneous, 440, 451, 459, 475
    posterior cutaneous, 441
    superior lateral cutaneous, 441
  veins of, 454
    deep, 461
Arterial arcades, 178
Articular cartilage, 494, 557
Articular disc, 492, 493
Articular facet, of sacrum, 127
Articular process
  inferior, 6
    thoracic, 51, 53
  superior, 6
    of sacrum, 127
    thoracic, 51, 53
Articular surface, of ilium, 124
Articular tubercle, 261
Aryepiglottic fold, 399, 401
Aryepiglotticus muscles, 400, 402
Arytenoid cartilages, 397, 401
Arytenoid muscle
  oblique, 395, 400, 420
  transverse, 395, 400, 402
Ascending cervical artery, 297
Ascending pharyngeal artery, 290
Asterion, 259
Atlanto-occipital joint, 7, 345
Atlanto-occipital membrane, 306
Atlas, 5, 7, 345
  transverse ligament of, 345
  transverse process of, 348

Atrial artery, 92, 93
Atrial branch, of right coronary artery, 92
Atrioventricular (AV) node, 96
Atrioventricular (AV) valve
  left, 99–101
  right, 96, 98, 101
Atrium
  cardiac
    left, 84, 92, 93, 99, 114
      auricle of, 91
    right, 84, 91–94, 98, 114
      incisions of, 95
      internal structures of, 96
  nasal, 381
Auditory tube, 388, 399, 405
  dissection of, 410
  groove for, 261
  opening of, 371, 379, 382
Auricle
  of ear, 406
  of heart. See Atrium.
Auricular artery
  deep, 367
  posterior, 290
Auricular nerve
  greater, 270, 275, 282
  superficial, 355
Auricular vein, posterior, 285
Auricularis muscles, 356
Auriculotemporal nerve, 353, 367
Autonomic nerves, of abdomen and pelvis, 247
AV (atrioventricular) node, 96
AV (atrioventricular) valve
  left, 99–101
  right, 96, 98, 101
Axilla, suspensory ligament of, 66
Axillary artery, 448, 449, 453, 461
  branches of, 68, 452
Axillary nerve, 444, 453, 460, 464
Axillary sheath, 448
Axillary veins, 439, 448, 449
Axis, 5, 7, 345
Azygos veins, 106–108

B

Back
  osteology of, 3–9, 44
  overview of, 44–45
  superficial, 10–22
    muscles of, 10, 11, 12, 17–22
    orientation and surface anatomy of, 13

Back (Continued)
  osteology of, 10
  overview of dissection of, 11
  skin incisions of, 11, 14
  skin reflection of, 11, 15
  vessels and nerves of, 10, 11, 16
Back muscles, 44
  deep (intrinsic), 10, 23–32, 44
  intermediate, 10, 22, 44
  superficial (extrinsic), 10, 12, 17–21, 44
Basilar artery, 314, 315
Basilar venous plexus, 323
Basilic vein, 439, 440
Biceps aponeurosis, 458
Biceps brachii muscle, 421, 457
  long head of, 493
Biceps brachii tendons, 457, 493, 494
Biceps femoris muscle, 504, 536, 539, 542
Bicipital aponeurosis, 468
Bicipital groove, 430
Bicuspid valve, 99–101
Bifurcate ligament, 559
Bile duct, common, 159, 168, 172
Bladder, 154, 228, 248
  female, 236
  male, 234
Bony labyrinth, of ear, 405, 408
Bony pelvis, 510–511
Brachial artery, 448, 461, 462, 474
  deep, 445
Brachial plexus, 277, 296, 456
  branches of
    forearm, 475–476
    posterior, of shoulder region, 464
    terminal, 454, 456, 459–460
  cords of, 450, 454
    lateral, 450
      branches from, 451
    medial, 450
      branches from, 451
    posterior, 450
      branches from, 453
  divisions of, 450
  roots of, 447, 450
  trunks of, 449, 450
Brachialis muscle, 421, 457
Brachiocephalic trunk, 110, 111, 297
Brachiocephalic veins, 110
  left, 106
  right, 106
Brachioradialis muscle, 422, 468, 471
Brain, 301, 416
  arterial supply of, 300, 314–315
  dissection overview of, 302

Brain (Continued)
  examination of removed, 313
  exposure of, 306
  innervation of, 301
  removal of, 311–312
  venous drainage of, 300
  ventricular system of, 301, 316
Breasts, 55, 60, 113
Broad ligament, 155, 229, 230
Bronchial arteries, 111, 112
  left, 80, 81
  right, 82, 83
Bronchopulmonary lymph nodes
  left, 80
  right, 82
Bronchus(i)
  left, 80, 81
  primary, 105, 111
  right, 82, 83
  secondary, 105
  tertiary, 105
Buccal artery, 367
Buccal branches, of facial nerve, 355
Buccal fat pad, 354
Buccal nerve, 353, 365, 367
Buccinator muscle, 341, 354, 356, 357
Buccopharyngeal fascia, 346
Bulbospongiosus muscle
  female, 223
  male, 215
Bulbourethral gland, 214, 216, 234, 235

C

C7, spinous process of, 13
Calcaneal tendon, 542, 543, 559
Calcaneonavicular ligament, plantar, 553, 559, 560
Calcaneus, 514, 549, 559–561
Calvarium
  dissection overview of, 302
  internal surface of, 305
  osteology of, 300
  removal of, 304
Calyx (calyces)
  major, 190
  minor, 190
Camper's fascia, 133, 135
Capitate, 433, 434, 496
Capitulum, 430
Cardia, 156

Cardiac impression
  left, 81
  right, 83
Cardiac notch, 80, 81
Cardiac plexus, 104, 110
Cardiac sphincter, 156
Cardiac vein(s), 94
  anterior, 94
  great, 94, 100
  middle, 94
  small, 94
Cardinal ligament, 237
Carina, 105
Carotid artery
  common, 288–291
    left, 110, 111, 297
    right, 110, 111
  external, 289, 365, 367
    branches of, 290
  internal, 288–290, 312, 315, 323
Carotid canal, 261
  opening of, 263
Carotid sheath, 271, 288, 346, 362, 370
Carotid sinus, 289, 290
Carotid triangle, 278, 286–291
  borders of, 286
Carpal arch, 433, 434
Carpal bones, 427, 433, 434
Carpal ligament, palmar, 481
Carpal tunnel, 481
Carpometacarpal ligaments, 497
Cauda equina, 43
Cavernous sinuses, 310, 323
  lumen of, 323
Cecal lymph nodes, 179
Cecum, 153, 163, 175
Celiac ganglia, 159
Celiac trunk, 147, 157–158, 187
  branches of, 158
    common hepatic artery as, 158, 160
    left gastric artery as, 158, 161
    splenic artery as, 158, 161
  location of, 157
  review of, 169
  topography of, 157
Central artery, of retina, 334, 337
Central compartment, of palm of hand, 479, 486
Central sulcus, 313
Central tendon, of diaphragm, 192, 193
Central vein, of retina, 337
Cephalic vein, 66, 68, 439, 440

Cerebellar arteries
  inferior
    anterior, 314, 315
    posterior, 314, 315
  superior, 314, 315
Cerebellar fossa, 306
Cerebellum, 313
Cerebral aqueduct, 316
Cerebral arterial circle, 314, 315
Cerebral arteries
  anterior, 314, 315
  middle, 314, 315
  posterior, 314, 315
Cerebral cortex, 307, 308
Cerebral vein, great, 310
Cerebrum
  lobes of, 313
  poles of, 313
Cervical artery
  ascending, 297
  transverse, 276, 277, 290, 297
    deep branch of, 21, 276, 445
    superficial branch of, 19, 276
Cervical branches, of facial nerve, 355
Cervical canal, 236
Cervical fascia, 267, 271
  deep, 271
  superficial, 271
Cervical ganglia
  inferior, 370
  middle, 370
  superior, 370
Cervical ligament, transverse, 237
Cervical lymph nodes
  deep, 285, 289
  superficial, 285, 289
Cervical nerve, transverse, 270, 275, 282
Cervical parietal pleura, 75, 76
Cervical plexus, 270, 282
Cervical spinal enlargement, 43
Cervical sympathetic trunks, 370
Cervical vertebrae, 5, 7, 346
Cervix, 236
  external os of, 236
  internal os of, 236
Chest wall, anterior. See Anterior chest wall.
Chiasmatic sulcus, 263
Choana, 261, 371, 379
Chorda tympani nerve, 367, 390, 405
Chordae tendineae, 98, 100
Choroid, 337
Ciliary artery
  long, 334
  short, 333

Ciliary body, 337
Ciliary ganglion, 333, 334
Ciliary nerve
   long, 334
   short, 333, 334
Ciliary vein
   long, 334
   short, 333
Circle of Willis, 314, 315
Circular folds
   of duodenum, 172
   of ileum, 174
   of jejunum, 174
Circumflex artery, 92, 93, 100
Circumflex fibular artery, 541
Circumflex iliac vein, superficial, 136
Circumflex scapular artery, 445, 452
Cisterna chyli, 108, 186
Cisterna magna, 316
Clavicle, 54, 272, 425, 427, 428
   acromial end of, 428
   overview of, 498
   sternal end of, 428
Clavicular artery, 452
Clavicular branch, 67, 68
Clavicular head, 446
Clavipectoral fascia, 66
Clinoid process
   anterior, 262, 321, 322
   middle, 263
   posterior, 263, 322
Clitoral fascia
   deep, 222
   superficial, 222
Clitoris, 155, 219, 223, 249
   crus of, 221
   shaft of, 222
Clivus, 262, 326, 347
Coccygeus muscle, 231, 232
Coccyx, 5, 8, 119, 122, 127
Cochlea, 405, 408
Colic artery
   left, 180
   middle, 178, 179
   right, 178, 179
Colic flexure
   left, 162
   right, 162, 175
Collateral artery
   middle, 461, 462, 465, 473
   radial, 461, 462, 465, 473
   ulnar
      inferior, 461, 462, 473
      superior, 461, 462, 465, 473

Collateral intercostal nerve, 69
Collateral intercostal vessels, 69
Collateral ligaments, of ankle, 559
Colon
   ascending, 149, 153, 162, 175
   descending, 153, 162, 176
   sigmoid, 153, 176
   transverse, 153, 162, 175, 176
Common bile duct, 159, 168, 172
Common carotid artery, 288–291
   left, 110, 111, 297
   right, 110, 111
Common digital arteries, 480, 482
Common digital nerves, 480
Common digital veins, 480
Common facial vein, 285
Common fibular nerve, 526, 539, 540, 545
Common hepatic artery, 158–160, 168, 169, 177
Common hepatic duct, 168
Common iliac artery, 187, 228, 238–242
Common iliac lymph nodes, 186, 238
Common iliac vein, 188, 226, 228
Common iliac vessels, 154, 155, 229
Common interosseous artery, 462, 473, 474
Common palmar digital arteries, 482
Common palmar digital nerves, 483
Common plantar digital nerves, 552
Communicating artery
   anterior, 314, 315
   posterior, 314, 315
Concha
   of ear, 406
   nasal
      inferior, 381, 383
      middle, 381, 383
      superior, 381, 383
Condylar process, 259
Condyle
   lateral, 508, 512, 513, 558
   medial, 508, 512, 513, 558
Conjoint ramus, 126, 511
Conjoint tendon, 145, 146
Conjunctiva, 335, 337
Conoid ligament, 493
Conoid tubercle, 428
Contact impressions, of lung
   left, 81
   right, 83
Conus arteriosus, 98
Conus medullaris, 43
Coracoacromial ligament, 493, 494
Coracobrachialis muscle, 421, 457
Coracoclavicular ligament, 493

Coracohumeral ligament, 493, 494
Coracoid process, 54, 427, 429, 493
Cornea, 337
Corniculate cartilages, 397, 401
Corniculate tubercle, 401
Coronal suture, 259, 305
Coronary arteries, 84, 114
   left, 92, 93, 100, 101, 114
   right, 92, 93, 101, 114
Coronary ligaments, 165, 166
Coronary sinus, 94, 96
Coronary sulcus, 91
Coronary veins, 84, 114
Coronoid fossa, 427, 430
Coronoid process
   of mandible, 259, 364
   of ulna, 427, 432, 457
Corpora cavernosa
   female, 222, 223
   male, 213, 215
Corpus spongiosum, 213, 215
Corrugator supercilii muscle, 341, 356
Costal arch, 54
Costal cartilage, 53, 54
Costal facet, thoracic
   inferior, 51, 53
   superior, 51, 53
   transverse, 51, 53
Costal groove, 52
Costal margin, 119, 133
Costal parietal pleura, 75–77, 107, 109
Costocervical artery, 297
Costocervical trunk, 112, 297
Costoclavicular ligament, 492
Costodiaphragmatic recess, 76
Costomediastinal recess, 77
Cranial cavity, venous plexus of, 327
Cranial fossae, 254, 320–327
   anterior, 262, 320, 321
   middle, 263, 312, 320, 322–325
   posterior, 262, 320, 326–327
Cranial nerves, 312, 318, 323, 328
Craniovertebral joints, 345
Cranium. *See* Skull.
Cremasteric fascia, 208
Cremasteric fibers, 208
Cribriform plates, 262, 312, 321
   foramina of, 262
Cricoarytenoid muscle
   lateral, 395, 402
   posterior, 395, 400, 402
Cricoid cartilage, 284, 298, 397–402
Cricothyroid joint, 402
Cricothyroid membrane, 298, 396, 397

Cricothyroid muscle, 291, 292, 370, 395, 396
Crista galli, 262, 321
Crista terminalis, 96
Cruciate ligament, 345
   anterior, 558
   posterior, 558
Crus (crura)
   of clitoris, 221, 223
   left, 192
   of penis, 214–216
   right, 192
Cubital fossa, 458
Cubital vein, median, 439, 440
Cuboid bone, 514, 515, 559–561
Cuneiform bones, 514, 515, 561
   intermediate, 561
   lateral, 561
   medial, 560, 561
Cuneiform cartilage, 401
Cutaneous nerves, 440
   of abdomen, 136
      anterior, 136
      lateral, 136
   of arm
      lateral, 459
         inferior, 441
         superior, 441
      medial, 440, 451, 459, 475
      posterior, 441
   of forearm
      lateral, 440, 457, 475
      medial, 440, 441, 451, 459
      posterior, 441
   of lower limb, 520
      intermediate, 520
      lateral, 520, 526, 527, 530
      medial, 520
      posterior, 520, 523, 526
Cutaneous neurovascular bundles
   anterior, 63
   lateral, 63
   posterior, 10, 16
Cutaneous veins, 439
Cystic artery, 160
Cystic duct, 167, 168

D

Dartos fascia, 132, 208, 209
Deep artery
   of arm, 444, 445, 465
   of clitoris, 222, 225

Deep artery (Continued)
 of penis, 213, 217
 of thigh, 534, 535
Deep auricular artery, 367
Deep brachial artery, 445
Deep cervical fascia, 271
Deep cervical lymph nodes, 285, 289
Deep clitoral fascia, 222
Deep dorsal vein
 female, 222
 male, 213, 234, 235
Deep femoral artery, 535
Deep fibular nerve, 540, 545
Deep inguinal ring, 144, 146, 154, 228
Deep lingual artery, 390
Deep palmar arch, 487
Deep penile fascia, 213
Deep perineal nerve, 217, 225
Deep perineal space
 female, 203, 205, 221, 224, 236
 male, 203, 205, 214, 215, 234, 235
Deep plantar arterial arch, 552
Deep plantar artery, 552
Deep radial nerve, 475, 476
Deep temporal arteries, 365, 367
Deep temporal nerves, 365, 367
Deep transverse metatarsal ligaments, 560
Deep transverse perineal muscle
 female, 224
 male, 216
Deep vein, of arm, 461
Deltoid artery, 452
Deltoid branch, 67, 68
Deltoid ligament, 559
Deltoid muscle, 64, 420, 442, 446
Deltoid tuberosity, 427, 430
Deltopectoral triangle, 63, 64, 66–68
Dens, 7
Denticulate ligaments, 42
Depressor anguli oris muscle, 341, 356
Depressor labii inferioris muscle, 341, 356
Descending artery, posterior, 92
Diaphragm, 183, 186, 192
 central tendon of, 192, 193
 lumbar part of, 159
 pelvic, 201, 202, 214, 226, 231–232
 urogenital
  female, 221, 223, 224
  male, 214–216, 234–235
Diaphragmatic parietal pleura, 75, 76
Diaphragmatic surface
 of heart, 91
 of liver, 165

Digastric muscle, 281, 286, 290, 295
 anterior belly of, 293, 294
 posterior belly of, 294, 369
Digit(s)
 extensor expansion of, 489
 joints of
  lower limb, 554, 560, 564
  upper limb, 490–492, 497, 500
Digital arteries
 dorsal, 545
 of foot
  dorsal, 545
  proper, 549
 of hand
  common, 480
  proper, 480
 palmar
  common, 482
  proper, 482
 plantar, proper, 552
Digital ligaments
 of foot
  lateral collateral, 560
  medial collateral, 560
 of hand
  lateral collateral, 497
  medial collateral, 497
Digital nerves
 of foot
  common, 552
  dorsal, 476
  proper, 549, 552
 of hand
  common, 480
  proper, 480
 palmar
  common, 483
  proper, 483
 plantar
  common, 552
  proper, 552
Digital veins
 of foot, proper, 549
 of hand
  common, 480
  proper, 480
Diploic bone, 303, 304
Dorsal artery
 of clitoris, 222, 224, 225
 of penis, 213, 217
Dorsal digital arteries, 545
Dorsal digital nerves, 476, 488
Dorsal hood, 489

Dorsal interosseous muscles, 424, 488, 506, 553
Dorsal metatarsal arteries, 545
Dorsal muscles, intrinsic, of foot, 544
Dorsal nerve
 of clitoris, 222, 224, 225
 of penis, 213, 216, 217
Dorsal scapular artery, 21, 444, 449
Dorsal scapular nerve, 21, 444, 447, 449
Dorsal tarsometatarsal ligament, 559
Dorsal vein
 of clitoris, 225
  deep, 222
  superficial, 222
 of penis, 217
  deep, 213, 234, 235
  superficial, 213
Dorsal venous arch, 439, 441, 519
Dorsalis pedis artery, 540, 545
Dorsum sellae, 263
Ductus deferens, 144, 154, 208–210, 228, 234
Duodenal fossa, 163
Duodenal papilla
 major, 172
 minor, 172
Duodenal sphincter, 172
Duodenojejunal junction, 163, 173
 transection of, 182
Duodenum, 162, 170, 172
 circulatory folds of, 172
 nerves of, 159
 suspensory ligaments of, 163, 192
Dura mater
 cranial, 306–308, 311
  endosteal layer of, 307, 308
  meningeal layer of, 307, 308
  separation of calvarium from, 304
 spinal, 42
Dural folds, cranial, 309
Dural sinuses
 occipital, groove for, 306
 transverse, grooves for, 306
Dural venous sinuses, cranial, 300, 307, 310, 318, 323–325
 confluence of, 306, 310

E

Ear, 403–410, 416–417
 dissection overview of, 404–405
 external, 403, 405, 406
 inner, 403, 405
 middle, 403, 405, 407–410

Ear lobe, 406
Efferent ductules, 210
Ejaculatory ducts, 234, 235
Elbow joint, 490–492, 495, 500
Emissary vein, 310
Endocardium, 87
Endothoracic fascia, 71, 77
Epicondyle
 of femur
  lateral, 512
  medial, 512
 of humerus
  lateral, 427, 430, 431, 495
  medial, 427, 430, 431, 444, 495
Epididymis, 208–210
 sinus of, 210
Epidural fat, spinal, 42
Epigastric artery
 inferior, 132, 187, 229
 superior, 72, 112
Epigastric vein
 inferior, 188, 229
 superficial, 136, 519
Epigastric vessels
 inferior, 140, 143, 144
 in rectus abdominis muscle, 143
 superior, 143
Epiglottic cartilage, 397, 401
Epiglottis, 371, 392, 397, 399–401
Epiploic appendages, 162
Epiploic appendices, 176
Epiploic foramen, 151, 152, 166
Epitympanic recess, 405, 408
Erector spinae muscles, 22, 25, 28
Esophageal arteries, 111, 112, 161
Esophageal hiatus, 192
Esophageal plexus, 104
Esophageal vein, 181
Esophagus, 104, 156, 371
Ethmoid bone, 253–254, 256, 262, 264, 321
 cribriform plates of, 262, 312, 321
  foramina of, 262
 perpendicular plate of, 379
Ethmoid sinuses, lining of, 332
Ethmoidal air cells, 378
 anterior, 382
 middle, 382
 posterior, 382
Ethmoidal artery
 anterior, 334, 380, 383, 384
  septal branch of, 383
 posterior, 334, 383
  septal branch of, 383

Ethmoidal bulla, 382
Ethmoidal foramina, 264
Ethmoidal nerve
　anterior, 334, 380
　　external nasal branch of, 351
　posterior, 334, 380
Ethmoidal vein, posterior, 334
Eustachian tube, 388, 399, 405
　dissection of, 410
　groove for, 261
　opening of, 371, 379, 382
Extensor carpi radialis brevis muscle, 422, 471, 473
Extensor carpi radialis longus muscle, 422, 471
Extensor carpi ulnaris muscle, 422, 471
Extensor digiti minimi muscle, 422, 471
Extensor digitorum brevis muscle, 505, 544
Extensor digitorum longus muscle, 504, 544
Extensor digitorum muscle, 422, 471, 488
Extensor expansion, of digits, 489
Extensor hallucis brevis muscle, 544
Extensor hallucis longus muscle, 504, 544
Extensor hallucis longus tendon, 544
Extensor indicis muscle, 423, 472
Extensor pollicis brevis muscle, 423, 471, 472
Extensor pollicis brevis tendon, 488
Extensor pollicis longus muscle, 423, 471, 472
Extensor pollicis longus tendon, 488
Extensor retinaculum, 472, 488
　inferior, 544
　superior, 544
External acoustic canal, 405, 408
　opening of, 406
External anal sphincter, 201, 202, 215, 216, 223, 224
External carotid artery, 289, 365, 367
　branches of, 290
External ear, 403, 405, 406
External genitalia
　female, 203, 219, 222, 249
　male, 203, 207–213, 249
External iliac artery, 225, 238
External iliac lymph nodes, 186, 238
External iliac vein, 188, 226
External iliac vessels, 143, 154, 228
External intercostal muscles, 57, 63, 69, 72
External jugular vein, 275, 285, 286, 294
External laryngeal nerve, 291, 298, 370, 396
External nasal artery, 383
External nasal nerve, 334, 351

External oblique aponeurosis, 137
External oblique fascia, 145, 146
External oblique muscle, 17, 131, 133, 137, 138, 140
External occipital crest, 260, 261
External occipital protuberance, 9, 13, 17, 260, 261
External pudendal artery
　female, 225
　male, 217
External pudendal vein
　female, 225
　male, 217
External spermatic fascia, 208
External urethral orifice, 219
Extrahepatic portal triad, 168
Extraperitoneal fat, 133, 140–142
Eye(s). See Orbit.
Eyeball, 329, 336–337

F

Face
　deep, 358–368
　　arch of ramus of mandible of, 364
　　dissection overview of, 359
　　infratemporal fossa of, 358, 362, 365, 367
　　muscles of, 358, 360
　　　masseter, 363
　　　removal of lateral pterygoid, 366
　　nerves of, 358
　　osteology of, 358
　　parotid gland of, 363
　　temporomandibular joint of, 368
　　vessels of, 358
　　zygomatic arch of, 364
　superficial, 338–357
　　arteries of, 339
　　bisection of head and neck for, 344, 349
　　dissection of craniovertebral joints for, 345
　　dissection of retropharyngeal space for, 346
　　dissection overview of, 340
　　fascia of, 338
　　ligaments of, 338
　　muscles of, 338, 341–343, 356–357
　　nerves of, 338, 351–353, 355
　　osteology of, 338
　　parotid region of, 339, 354–355

Face (Continued)
　　prevertebral region of, 343, 348
　　removal of head and neck viscera from vertebral column for, 347
　　skin removal from, 350
　　veins of, 339
Facial artery, 290, 294, 295, 354
　transverse, 354
Facial expression, muscles of, 341, 356
Facial nerve, 312, 325, 328, 386
　geniculate ganglion of, 386, 409
　in parotid region, 355
Facial vein, 285, 294, 295, 310, 354
　common, 285
　transverse, 354
Falciform ligament, 144, 149, 165, 166
False vocal cords, 398
Falx cerebelli, 309, 310
Falx cerebri, 307–310
Fascia lata, 530
Femoral artery, 238, 530, 533, 534, 541
　deep, 535
　lateral circumflex, 534, 535, 541
　medial circumflex, 522, 523, 534, 535
Femoral branch, of genitofemoral nerve, 194, 520
Femoral canal, 530
Femoral cutaneous nerves
　anterior, 521
　lateral, 194, 195, 521
Femoral nerve, 194, 195, 526, 527, 530
Femoral sheath, 530, 531, 534
Femoral triangle, 530, 534
Femoral vein, 521, 530, 533–535
Femur, 507, 508, 512, 562
　head of, 508, 512
　　artery to, 557
　neck of, 512
　round ligament of, 557
Fibrous capsule, of kidney, 190
Fibrous digital sheaths, 480, 486
Fibula, 507, 508, 513, 562
　head of, 508, 513, 544
　neck of, 513
Fibular artery, 540, 545
　circumflex, 541
Fibular collateral ligament, 558
Fibular nerve
　common, 526, 539, 540, 545
　deep, 540, 545
　superficial, 520, 540, 545
Fibular notch, 513
Fibular trochlea, 514, 515
Fibularis brevis muscle, 505, 540, 543–545

Fibularis longus muscle, 505, 540, 543–545
Fibularis longus tendon, 553, 560
Fibularis tertius muscle, 504, 544
Filiform papillae, 392
Filum terminale, 43
Fimbriae, 236
First dorsal interosseus muscle, 488
Flexor carpi radialis muscle, 421, 468, 471
Flexor carpi ulnaris muscle, 422, 468
Flexor digiti minimi brevis muscle, 424, 506, 550
Flexor digiti minimi muscle, 485, 552
Flexor digitorum brevis muscle, 506, 540, 551
Flexor digitorum brevis tendons, 551
Flexor digitorum longus muscle, 505, 540, 543, 545
Flexor digitorum longus tendons, 551
Flexor digitorum profundus muscle, 422, 470, 481, 489
Flexor digitorum profundus tendon, 486
Flexor digitorum superficialis muscle, 422, 468, 469, 481, 489
Flexor digitorum superficialis tendon, 486
Flexor digitorum tendons, 486
Flexor hallucis brevis muscle, 506, 550, 552
Flexor hallucis brevis tendon, 552
Flexor hallucis longus muscle, 505, 540, 543
Flexor hallucis longus tendon, 550, 551, 560
Flexor pollicis brevis muscle, 423, 484
Flexor pollicis longus muscle, 422, 469, 470, 481
Flexor retinaculum, 481–485, 543
Floating ribs, 54
Foot, 546–553
　arches of, 561
　dissection overview of, 547
　joints of, 554, 559–560, 564
　muscles of
　　intrinsic dorsal, 544
　　plantar compartment, 506
　osteology of, 507, 514–515, 546, 562
　plantar surface of, 549–553
　　layers of, 546, 550–553
　skin removal from, 548
Foramen cecum, 262, 321, 392
Foramen lacerum, 261, 263, 322
Foramen magnum, 261, 262, 306, 326, 327
Foramen ovale, 261, 263, 322, 324
Foramen rotundum, 263, 322, 324
Foramen spinosum, 261, 263, 322, 324

Foramina
    of cribriform plate, 262
    of skull, 256–257
Forearm, 466–476
    brachial plexus branches in, 475–476
    dissection overview of, 467
    fascia of, 466
    muscles of, 466
        anterior, 468–470, 498–499
        posterior, 471–472, 499
    nerves of, 466
        lateral cutaneous, 440, 457, 475
        medial cutaneous, 440, 441, 451, 459
        posterior cutaneous, 441
    radial and ulnar arteries of, 473–474
    vasculature of, 466
Foregut
    dissection overview of, 148
    duodenojejunal junction in, 163
    duodenum in, 162
    stomach in, 156
    vasculature of, 147, 157–161
Fossa ovalis, 96
Fourth ventricle, 316
Frenulum
    lingual, 390
    of upper lip, 372
"Freshman's nerve," 542
Frontal bone, 253, 256, 258, 259
    in anterior cranial fossa, 262, 321
    in calvarium, 305
    orbital part of, 262, 264
    zygomatic process of, 258
Frontal crest, 262
Frontal lobe, 313
Frontal nerve, 332
Frontal pole, 313
Frontal process, of maxilla, 258
Frontal sinus, 332, 378, 379
Frontalis muscle, 303
Fundiform ligament, 135, 136
Fundus, of stomach, 156
Fungiform papillae, 392

G

Galea aponeurotica, 303
Gallbladder, 153
Gastric arteries
    left, 158, 159, 161, 168, 169
    right, 158–160, 169
    short, 158, 161, 169

Gastric canal, 156
Gastric rugae, 156
Gastric vein
    left, 181
    right, 181
Gastric vessels, short, 164
Gastrocnemius muscle, 505, 542, 544
    medial head of, 539
Gastrocolic ligament, 150
Gastroduodenal artery, 159, 177
Gastrointestinal (GI) tract, removal of, 182
Gastro-omental artery
    left, 158, 159, 161, 164, 169
    right, 158, 160, 169
Gastro-omental veins, 181
    left, 159, 164
Gastrosplenic ligament, 150, 163
Gemellus muscle
    inferior, 504, 522, 523
    superior, 504, 522, 523
Gender difference, in pelvis, 128
Genicular artery
    descending, 541
    inferior
        lateral, 535, 541
        medial, 535, 541
    superior
        lateral, 535, 541
        medial, 535, 541
Geniculate ganglion, 386, 409
Genioglossus muscle, 376, 389–391
Geniohyoid muscle, 281, 389, 391
    innervation of, 270, 282
Genital branch, of genitofemoral nerve, 145, 146, 194, 209
Genitofemoral nerve, 194, 195, 209, 526, 527
    femoral branch of, 194, 520
    genital branch of, 145, 146, 194, 209
GI (gastrointestinal) tract, removal of, 182
Glabella, 258
Glans penis, 212
Glenohumeral joint capsule, 494
Glenohumeral ligaments, 493, 494
Glenoid cavity, 427, 429, 494
Glenoid labrum, 494
Globe, 329, 336–337
Glossoepiglottic folds
    lateral, 392
    medial, 392
Glossopharyngeal nerve, 312, 327, 328, 370, 372
Glottis, 398

Gluteal artery
    inferior, 225, 239–243, 523, 528
    superior, 225, 239–243, 523, 528
Gluteal lines, 511
Gluteal nerve
    inferior, 200, 243, 523, 526, 528
    superior, 243, 523, 526, 528
Gluteal region, 196–200
    dissection overview of, 197, 517
    ligaments of, 196
    muscles of, 196, 503, 516, 522
    nerves and vessels of, 516, 523
    osteology of, 196
    skin incisions of, 198
Gluteal tuberosity, 508, 522
Gluteal vein
    inferior, 200, 523
    superior, 523
Gluteus maximus muscle, 199–202, 503, 522, 523
Gluteus medius muscle, 503, 522, 523
Gluteus minimus muscle, 503, 522, 523
Gonadal arteries, 187, 229
    left, 189
    right, 189
Gonadal vein
    left, 188, 189, 229
    right, 188, 189, 229
Gracilis muscle, 503, 531, 532, 533
Gray rami communicantes, 107, 109
Great cardiac vein, 94, 100
Great cerebral vein, 310
Great saphenous vein, 519, 521
Great toe, 515
Greater auricular nerve, 270, 275, 282
Greater curvature, of stomach, 150, 156
Greater occipital nerve, 33, 34, 36, 275
Greater omentum, 147, 149–150, 159, 161, 162
Greater palatine artery, 383–385
    terminal part of, 383
Greater palatine foramen, 261
Greater palatine nerve, 377, 384–386
Greater palatine vein, 385
Greater petrosal nerve, 325, 386, 408, 409
    groove and hiatus for, 263, 322
Greater sac, 149, 150
Greater scapular notch, 429
Greater sciatic foramen, 121
Greater sciatic notch, 121, 123, 508, 510
Greater splanchnic nerves, 107, 109
Greater trochanter, 508, 512, 523
Greater tubercle, 427, 430

Greater vestibular glands, 222, 223
Gubernaculum testis, 210

H

Hamate, 433, 434, 496
Hamstring muscles, 536
Hand, 477–489
    carpal tunnel of, 481
    dissection overview of, 478
    dorsal hood of, 489
    dorsal surface of, 488
    extensor expansion of digits of, 489
    fibrous digital sheaths of, 480
    joints of, 490–492, 497
    muscles of, 477, 499
    nerves of, 477
    osteology of, 433–434, 477, 498
    palm of
        adductor compartment of, 479, 487
        central compartment of, 479, 486
        hypothenar compartment of, 479, 485
        nerves of, 483
        thenar compartment of, 479, 484
        vessels of, 482
    palmar aponeurosis of, 480
    skin removal from, 479
    tendons of, 477
    vasculature of, 477
Hard palate, 261, 372, 379, 380
Haustra, 162, 176
Head
    arteries of, 414–415
    dissection overview of, 255
    fascia/membranes of, 417
    glands of, 415–416
    joints of, 412
    ligaments of, 412
    lymphatics of, 415
    muscles of, 412–413
    nerves of, 413–414
    osteology of, 253–254, 256–266, 411–412
    veins of, 415
Heart, 84–101, 114
    dissection overview of, 85
    inspection of removed, 91
    left atrium of, 84, 99
    left ventricle of, 84, 100
    orientation to, 86
    in pericardial sac, 86
    removal from middle mediastinum of, 89–90
    right atrium of, 84

Index 571

Heart (Continued)
  incisions of, 95
  internal structures of, 96
  right ventricle of, 84
Heart valve(s), 101
  aortic semilunar, 100, 101
  bicuspid (left AV, mitral), 99–101
  pulmonary semilunar, 98, 101
  tricuspid (right AV), 96, 98, 101
Helix, of ear, 406
Hemiazygos vein, 106, 108
  accessory, 106–108
Hepatic artery, 167
  common, 158–160, 168, 169, 177
  left, 160
  proper, 158, 160, 168, 169
  right, 160
Hepatic duct
  common, 168
  left, 168
  right, 168
Hepatic flexure, right, 175
Hepatic vein(s), 181, 188
  proper, 159
Hepatoduodenal ligament, 151, 168
Hepatogastric ligament, 151
Hiatus semilunaris, 382
Hilum, 164
  left, 80
  right, 82
Hindgut, 170
  dissection overview of, 171
  inferior mesenteric artery to, 180
  large intestine in, 176
Hinge joints, 497
Hip joint, 554, 556–557, 564
Horizontal fissure, of right lung, 82, 83
Humeral artery
  anterior circumflex, 452
  posterior circumflex, 445, 452, 465
Humeral ligament, transverse, 457, 493
Humerus, 54, 425, 427, 430–431
  head of, 427, 430
  neck of
    anatomical, 430
    surgical, 430
  overview of, 498
Hyoglossus muscle, 376
Hyoid bone, 284, 295, 397
  greater horns of, 369, 399
Hypogastric plexus
  inferior, 244
  superior, 244
Hypoglossal canal, 261, 262, 326, 327

Hypoglossal nerve, 270, 282, 288, 295, 327, 328, 390
Hypoglossus muscle, 390, 391
Hypophysial fossa, 263
Hypothenar compartment, of hand, 479, 485
Hypothenar eminence, 480
Hypothenar muscles, 424, 480, 482, 483, 485

I

Ileal artery, 178, 179
Ileocecal junction, 153, 175
Ileocecal valve, 173
Ileocolic artery, 179
Ileocolic lymph nodes, 179
Ileum, 153, 162, 173–174
Iliac artery
  common, 187, 228, 238–242
  external, 225, 238
  internal, 225, 238–242
Iliac crest, 13, 17, 119, 124, 133, 186, 507, 511
Iliac fossa, 119, 124–126, 508, 511
Iliac lymph nodes
  common, 186, 238
  external, 186, 238
  internal, 186, 238
Iliac spine
  anterior
    inferior, 124–126, 508, 510, 511
    superior, 119, 121, 122, 124, 133, 509–511
  posterior
    inferior, 124–126, 508, 511
    superior, 124–126, 508, 511
Iliac tuberosity, 124–126, 511
Iliac vein
  common, 188, 226, 228
  external, 188, 226
  internal, 188, 226
  superficial circumflex, 136, 519
Iliac vessels
  common, 154, 155, 229
  external, 143, 154, 228
Iliacus muscle, 185, 193, 520, 530
Iliococcygeus muscle, 231, 232, 244
Iliocostalis cervicis muscle, 25, 28
Iliocostalis lumborum muscle, 25, 28
Iliocostalis muscle, 25, 28
Iliocostalis thoracis muscle, 25, 28
Iliofemoral ligament, 556

Iliohypogastric nerve, 136, 194, 195, 526, 527
Ilioinguinal nerve, 136, 194, 195, 225, 520, 526, 527
Iliolumbar artery, 239–242
Iliolumbar ligament, 119, 193
Iliopsoas muscle, 193, 502, 530–532
Iliotibial band, 522
Iliotibial tract, 531
Ilium, 117, 123, 124, 507, 511, 556
Incisive canal, 380
Incisive foramen, 386
Incisive fossa, 261
Incus, 405, 408
Inferior adrenal artery, 187, 191
Inferior alveolar artery, 365–367
Inferior alveolar nerve, 364–367
Inferior alveolar vein, 365–367
Inferior articular process, 6
  thoracic, 51, 53
Inferior cervical ganglia, 370
Inferior concha, 381, 383
Inferior costal facet, thoracic, 51, 53
Inferior epigastric artery, 132, 187, 229
Inferior epigastric vein, 188, 229
Inferior epigastric vessels, 140, 143, 144
Inferior extensor retinaculum, 544
Inferior gemellus muscle, 504, 522, 523
Inferior gluteal artery, 225, 239–243, 523, 528
Inferior gluteal line, 511
Inferior gluteal nerve, 200, 243, 523, 526, 528
Inferior gluteal vein, 200, 523
Inferior horn, of thyroid cartilage, 397
Inferior hypogastric plexus, 244
Inferior lateral cutaneous nerve, of arm, 441
Inferior lateral genicular artery, 535, 541
Inferior lobe, of lung
  left, 80, 81
  right, 82, 83
Inferior longitudinal ligament, 345
Inferior meatus, 378, 381
Inferior medial genicular artery, 535, 541
Inferior mesenteric artery, 157, 180, 187
Inferior mesenteric lymph nodes, 180
Inferior mesenteric vein, 181
Inferior nasal concha, 258, 378
Inferior nuchal line, 260, 261
Inferior oblique muscle, 335
Inferior orbital fissure, 264
Inferior pancreaticoduodenal artery, 178
Inferior pelvic aperture, 122

Inferior petrosal sinuses, 310, 323, 327
  groove for, 262
Inferior pharyngeal constrictor muscle, 361, 369, 370
Inferior phrenic arteries, 187, 191
Inferior phrenic vein, 188
Inferior pubic ramus, 124–126, 508, 511
Inferior rectal artery, 201, 202, 217, 225
Inferior rectal nerve, 201, 202, 217, 225
Inferior rectal vein, 201, 202
  female, 225
  male, 217
Inferior rectus muscle, 335
Inferior sagittal sinus, 310
Inferior subscapular nerve, 461
Inferior suprarenal arteries, 187, 191
Inferior thyroid artery, 290, 297, 298
Inferior thyroid vein, 298
Inferior ulnar collateral artery, 461, 462, 473
Inferior vagal ganglion, 370
Inferior vena cava (IVC), 89, 92, 93, 186, 188, 189
Inferior vertebral notch, 6
Inferior vesical artery, 239, 240
Infraglenoid tubercle, 427, 429
Infrahyoid muscles, 281, 292
Infraorbital artery, 335, 367, 384, 387
Infraorbital canal, 387
Infraorbital fissure, 265, 266
Infraorbital foramen, 258, 265, 351
Infraorbital nerve, 335, 352, 377, 384, 387
Infraorbital vein, 310, 335, 387
Infraspinatus muscle, 421, 443–445, 463, 464
Infraspinatus tendon, 494
Infraspinous fossa, 427, 429
Infratemporal fossa, 362
  contents of, 358
    deep, 367
    superficial, 365
  overview of, 362
Infratrochlear nerve, 334, 351
Inguinal canal, 145–146
Inguinal ligament, 119, 138, 193, 238, 530
Inguinal lymph nodes, superficial, 521
Inguinal ring
  deep, 144, 146, 154, 228
  superficial, 129, 137, 138, 145, 146
Inguinal triangle, 144
Inion, 260
Inner ear, 403, 405
Innermost intercostal muscles, 57, 63, 69, 72

Interatrial septum, 96
Intercavernous sinus, 323
Intercondylar eminence, 508
Intercondylar fossa, 512
Intercostal arteries, 69, 72, 107, 109
   anterior, 112
   collateral, 69
   posterior, 16, 111, 112
Intercostal muscles, 60
   external, 57, 63, 69, 72
   innermost, 57, 63, 69, 72
   internal, 57, 63, 69, 72
Intercostal nerve, 69, 72, 107, 109
   collateral, 69
Intercostal neurovascular bundles, 63, 109
Intercostal structures, 69
Intercostal veins, 69, 72
   collateral, 69
   left, 107
   posterior, 108
   right, 106
Intercostal vessels, 16
Intercostobrachial nerve, 440
Intercrural fibers, of superficial inguinal ring, 138
Intermediate cuneiform, 561
Intermediate cutaneous nerve, of thigh, 520
Internal acoustic meatus, 262, 322, 326, 327, 408
Internal anal sphincter, 201, 202
Internal carotid artery, 288–290, 312, 315, 323
Internal genitalia
   female, 226, 236–237, 248–249
   male, 226, 234–235, 249
Internal iliac artery, 225, 238–242
Internal iliac lymph nodes, 186, 238
Internal iliac vein, 188, 226
Internal intercostal muscles, 57, 63, 69, 72
Internal jugular vein, 288, 289, 310
   left, 108
Internal laryngeal nerve, 291, 298, 370, 396, 399
Internal oblique muscle, 131, 133, 140
Internal occipital crest, 262
Internal occipital protuberance, 262, 326
Internal pudendal artery, 201, 202, 243
   female, 225, 241, 242
   male, 217, 239, 240
Internal pudendal vein, 201, 202
   female, 225
   male, 217

Internal spermatic fascia, 208
Internal thoracic artery, 112, 143, 297
Internal thoracic vein, 136
Internal thoracic vessels, 70, 72
Interossei muscles, palmar, 424, 487
Interosseous artery, 461
   anterior, 462, 473, 474
   common, 462, 473, 474
   posterior, 462, 473
Interosseous border, 513
Interosseous crest, 432
Interosseous membrane, 462, 473, 496, 513, 541
Interosseous muscles, 489
   dorsal, 424, 488, 506, 553
   plantar, 506, 553
Interosseous nerve, anterior, 475
Interosseous recurrent artery, 462, 465, 473
Interphalangeal (IP) joint(s)
   of foot, 560
   of hand, 489
Interphalangeal (IP) joint capsules
   of foot, 560
   of hand, 497
Interphalangeal ligaments, 497
Interscalene triangle, 277
Interspinalis muscles, 26
Interspinous ligaments, 39
Intertransversarii muscles, 26, 32
Intertransverse ligaments, 39
Intertrochanteric crest, 512
Intertrochanteric line, 512
Intertubercular groove, 430, 446, 457
Intertubercular sulcus, 430
Interventricular artery
   anterior, 91–93, 100
   posterior, 92, 93
Interventricular foramen, 316
Interventricular groove
   anterior, 91
   posterior, 91
Interventricular septum, 100
Intervertebral discs, 6
   thoracic, 53
Intervertebral foramina, 6
   thoracic, 51
Intestine(s)
   large, 147, 175–176, 248
   small, 147, 162, 248
Intrahepatic portal triads, 167
Intrahepatic veins, 167
Intrinsic dorsal muscles, of foot, 544
Intrinsic muscles, of tongue, 389

Investing fascia, 271, 275
IP (interphalangeal) joint(s)
   of foot, 560
   of hand, 489
IP (interphalangeal) joint capsules
   of foot, 560
   of hand, 497
Iris, 335, 337
Ischial body, 126
Ischial ramus, 126, 511
Ischial spine(s), 123, 126, 200, 510, 511, 556
   gender differences in, 128
Ischial tuberosity, 121, 122, 126, 510, 511, 556
   female, 218, 221, 224
   male, 201, 202, 211, 212, 214
Ischioanal fossa, 196, 197, 201–202
   female, 221
   male, 201, 202, 213
Ischiocavernosus muscles
   female, 223
   male, 215
Ischiococcygeus muscle, 217, 225, 231, 232
Ischiofemoral ligament, 556
Ischiopubic ramus, 121, 122, 125, 126, 511
   female, 218
   male, 211
Ischiorectal fossa, 196, 197, 201–202
Ischium, 117, 123, 126, 507, 511
   ramus of, 126, 511
IVC (inferior vena cava), 89, 92, 93, 186, 188, 189

J

Jejunal artery, 178, 179
Jejunum, 153, 162, 163, 173–174
Jugular bulb, 310, 327
Jugular foramen, 261, 262, 322, 326, 327
Jugular notch, 54, 58, 61
Jugular tubercle, 262
Jugular vein
   anterior, 285
   external, 275, 285, 286, 294
   internal, 288, 289, 310
      left, 108

K

Kidneys, 153, 183, 186, 189, 190, 248
Knee joint, 554, 558, 564

L

L4 nerve, 243
L5 nerve, 243
Labia majora, 219, 220, 236
Labia minora, 219, 220, 236
Labial artery
   anterior, 225
   posterior, 225
Labial nerve(s)
   anterior, 225
   posterior, 225
Labial vein
   anterior, 225
   posterior, 225
Labyrinthine artery, 314, 315
Lacrimal artery, 332, 334
Lacrimal bone, 258, 259, 264
Lacrimal gland, 332–335
Lacrimal nerve, 332, 351
Lacrimal vein, 332
Lactiferous ducts, 60
Lacunar ligament, 145
Lambdoid suture, 259, 260, 305
Laminae, 6
   inspection of removed, 41
   thoracic, 51
Laminectomy, 40
Large intestine, 147, 175–176, 248
Laryngeal artery, superior, 290, 298, 370
Laryngeal cartilages, 393
Laryngeal cavity, 393
Laryngeal joints, 393
Laryngeal muscles, 393, 395
   intrinsic, 400, 402
Laryngeal nerves, 393
   external, 291, 298, 370, 396
   internal, 291, 298, 370, 396, 399
   recurrent, 299, 370, 396, 399
      left, 86, 104, 299, 370
      right, 104, 298, 299
   superior, 291, 370, 396, 399
Laryngeal prominence, 272, 298, 397
Laryngeal skeleton, 397
Laryngeal vein, superior, 298, 370
Laryngopharynx, 371, 399
Larynx, 371, 393–402, 416
   dissection overview of, 394
   external surface of, 396–397
   internal features of, 398–402
Lateral apertures, 316
Lateral arcuate ligaments, 192, 193
Lateral circumflex femoral artery, 534, 535, 541

Lateral collateral digital ligaments
  of foot, 560
  of hand, 497
Lateral collateral ligament, 558
Lateral condyle, 508, 512, 513, 558
Lateral cricoarytenoid muscle, 395, 402
Lateral crus, of superficial inguinal ring, 138
Lateral cuneiform, 561
Lateral cutaneous nerves
  of abdomen, 136
  of arm, 459
  of forearm, 440, 457, 475
  of thigh, 520, 526, 527, 530
Lateral cutaneous neurovascular bundles, 63
Lateral epicondyle
  of femur, 512
  of humerus, 427, 430, 431, 495
Lateral femoral cutaneous nerves, 194, 195, 521
Lateral glossoepiglottic folds, 392
Lateral longitudinal arch, of foot, 561
Lateral malleolus, 508, 513, 544
Lateral meniscus, 558
Lateral nasal artery, alar branch of, 383
Lateral nasal cavity, vasculature of, 383–384
Lateral nasal wall, 381–382
Lateral pectoral nerve, 66, 67, 451, 459
Lateral plantar artery, 549–552
  cutaneous branches of, 549
Lateral plantar nerve, 540, 549–552
  cutaneous branches of, 549
Lateral plantar vein, 550–552
Lateral pterygoid muscle, 342, 357, 360, 365, 367
  removal of, 366
Lateral pterygoid plate, 265, 266, 362
Lateral rectus muscle, 333–335
Lateral sacral arteries, 239–242
Lateral sulcus, 313
Lateral supracondylar line, 512
Lateral supraepicondylar ridge, 430
Lateral sural nerve, 520
Lateral thoracic artery, 452
Lateral thoracic vein, 136
Lateral umbilical folds, 144
Lateral ventricles, 316
Latissimus dorsi muscle, 12, 17, 20, 420, 443, 446
Least splanchnic nerves, 109
Left adrenal vein, 188
Left atrioventricular valve, 99–101
Left atrium, 84, 92, 93, 99, 114
  auricle of, 91
Left brachiocephalic vein, 106
Left colic artery, 180
Left colic flexure, 162
Left colic lymph nodes, 180
Left common carotid artery, 110, 111, 297
Left coronary artery, 92, 93, 100, 101, 114
Left crus, 192
Left gastric artery, 158, 159, 161, 168, 169
Left gastric vein, 181
Left gastro-omental artery, 158, 159, 161, 164, 169
Left gastro-omental vein, 159, 164
Left gonadal artery, 189
Left gonadal vein, 188, 229
Left hepatic artery, 160
Left hepatic duct, 168
Left intercostal veins, 107
Left internal jugular vein, 108
Left (obtuse) marginal artery, 92, 93
Left ovarian vein, 188, 229
Left phrenic nerve, 78
Left pulmonary artery, 80, 81, 86, 88
Left pulmonary veins, 80, 81, 90
Left recurrent laryngeal nerve, 86, 104, 370
Left renal vein, 188, 189
Left subclavian artery, 110, 111, 297
Left subclavian vein, 108
Left suprarenal vein, 188
Left testicular vein, 188, 229
Left triangular ligament, 165, 166
Left vagus nerve, 86, 104, 298, 299
Left ventricle, 84, 91, 100, 114
Leg, 537–545
  dissection overview of, 538
  innervation of, 537
    popliteal fossa, 540
  lateral compartment of, 544
  muscles of, 537
    anterior compartment, 544
    anterior region, 504, 537
    anterolateral, 544
    lateral region, 505, 537
    popliteal fossa, 539
    posterior region, 505, 537, 542–543
  popliteal fossa of, 539
    muscles of, 539
    nerves of, 540
    vessels of, 541
  vasculature of, 537
    arteries, 545
    popliteal fossa, 541
Lens, 337
Lesser curvature, of stomach, 151, 156

Lesser occipital nerve, 270, 275, 282
Lesser omentum, 147, 151–152, 166
Lesser palatine artery, 384, 385
Lesser palatine foramen, 261
Lesser palatine nerve, 377, 384–386
Lesser palatine vein, 385
Lesser petrosal nerve, groove and hiatus for, 263
Lesser sac, 152, 166
Lesser sciatic foramen, 121
Lesser sciatic notch, 121, 123–126, 510, 511
Lesser splanchnic nerves, 109
Lesser trochanter, 508, 512
Lesser tubercle, 427, 430, 446
Levator anguli oris muscle, 356
Levator ani muscle, 202, 216, 221, 224, 231
Levator costarum muscles, 26, 32
Levator labii superioris alaeque nasi muscle, 341, 356
Levator labii superioris muscle, 341, 356
Levator palpebrae superioris muscle, 332, 333
Levator scapulae muscle, 12, 21, 269, 276, 420, 443
Levator veli palatini muscle, 372, 376, 388
Ligamentum arteriosum, 86, 91
Ligamentum flavum, 41
Ligamentum teres hepatis, 144
Linea alba, 136, 137, 140–142
Linea aspera, 508, 512
Linea semilunaris, 137
Linea terminalis, 120, 510
Lingual artery, 290, 292, 367, 390
  deep, 390
Lingual frenulum, 390
Lingual nerve, 365, 367, 390
Lingual tonsils, 392
Lingual vein, 367
Lingula
  of lung, 80, 81
  of mandible, 364
Lip, frenulum of, 372
Liver, 147, 153, 165–167, 248
  bare area of, 166
  caudate lobe of, 159, 167
  inferior (visceral) surface of, 165, 167
  left lobe of, 159, 165, 167
  peritoneal attachments of, 147
  porta hepatis of, 168
  quadrate lobe of, 167
  right lobe of, 159, 165, 167
  round ligament of, 165, 167
Lobule, of ear, 406
Long ciliary artery, 334

Long ciliary nerve, 334
Long ciliary vein, 334
Long plantar ligament, 553, 559, 560
Long thoracic nerve, 447, 453
Longissimus capitis muscle, 25, 35
Longissimus cervicis muscle, 25
Longissimus muscle, 25, 28, 29
Longissimus thoracis muscle, 25
Longitudinal arch, of foot, 561
Longitudinal ligament
  inferior, 345
  posterior, 345
  superior, 345
Longus capitis muscle, 343, 347, 348
Longus colli muscle, 297, 343, 348
Lower limb
  arteries of, 563–564
  gluteal region of, 516, 517, 522–523
  joints of, 554–561, 564
  lymphatic system of, 507, 564
    superficial, 521
  muscles of, 502–506, 562–563
  nerves of, 563
    cutaneous, 520
  osteology of, 507–515, 562
  skin removal from, 518
  superficial structures of, 516–521
    cutaneous nerves, 520
    lymph nodes, 521
    veins, 519
  veins of, 564
    superficial, 519
Lower subscapular nerve, 453
Lumbar arteries, 187
Lumbar para-aortic lymph nodes, 238
Lumbar plexus, 194, 524, 526–529, 563
Lumbar spinal enlargement, 43
Lumbar triangle, 17
Lumbar vein, 188
Lumbar vertebrae, 5, 7
Lumbar vessels, 16
Lumbosacral plexus of nerves, 526
Lumbosacral trunk, 195, 243, 526, 528
Lumbrical muscles
  of foot, 506, 550, 551
  of hand, 424, 486, 489
Lunate, 433, 434, 496
Lung(s), 114
  base of
    left, 80, 81
    right, 82, 83
  dissection overview of, 74
  left, 73, 74, 80–81, 114
  removal from thoracic cavity of, 79

Lung(s) *(Continued)*
  right, 73, 74, 82–83, 114
  root of
    left, 81
    right, 73, 83
Lymph nodes
  appendicular, 179
  cecal, 179
  colic
    left, 180
    middle, 179
    right, 179
  ileocolic, 179
  iliac, 186, 238
  inferior mesenteric, 180
  lumbar para-aortic, 238
  paracolic, 179, 180
  preaortic, 180, 186, 238
  sigmoid, 180
  superior rectal, 180

M

Main pancreatic duct, 172
Major calyx, 190
Major duodenal papilla, 172
Malleolus
  lateral, 508, 513, 544
  medial, 508, 513
Malleus, 405, 408
Mammary gland, 60
Mandible, 254, 256, 258, 259, 389
  alveolar process of, 258, 259
  angle of, 258, 259
  body of, 258, 259
  coronoid process of, 259, 364
  inferior border of, 272
  lingula of, 364
  ramus of, 258, 259, 362, 364
Mandibular branches, of facial nerve, 355
Mandibular condyle, neck of, 364
Mandibular division, of trigeminal nerve, 322, 324
  accessory meningeal branch of, 322
  branches of, 377
Mandibular foramen, 364
Mandibular fossa, 261
Mandibular molar teeth, 390
Mandibular nerve, 322, 324
  accessory meningeal branch of, 322
Manubrium, 54, 110, 297
  jugular notch of, 272

Marginal artery (of Drummond), 179, 180
  left (obtuse), 92, 93
  right (acute), 92, 93
Masseter artery, 363
Masseter muscle, 342, 354, 357, 360
Masseter nerve, 363
Masseter vein, 363
Mastication, muscles of, 342, 357, 360, 362
Mastoid air cells, 405
Mastoid antrum, 408
Mastoid notch, 260, 261
Mastoid process, 9, 259, 261, 272
Maxilla, 254, 256, 258, 259, 261, 264
  frontal process of, 258
  zygomatic process of, 258
Maxillary artery, 290, 365, 367
  branches of, 362
Maxillary division, of trigeminal nerve, 322, 324
Maxillary nerve, 322–324
Maxillary sinuses, 378, 387
  opening to, 382
Meatus
  inferior, 378, 381
  internal acoustic, 262, 322, 326, 327, 408
  middle, 378, 381
  superior, 381
Medial arcuate ligaments, 192, 193
Medial circumflex femoral artery, 522, 523, 534, 535
Medial collateral digital ligaments
  of foot, 560
  of hand, 497
Medial collateral ligament, 558
Medial condyle, 508, 512, 513, 558
Medial crus, of superficial inguinal ring, 138
Medial cuneiform, 560, 561
Medial cutaneous nerve
  of arm, 440, 451, 459, 475
  of forearm, 440, 441, 451, 459
  of thigh, 520
Medial epicondyle
  of femur, 512
  of humerus, 427, 430, 431, 444, 495
Medial glossoepiglottic folds, 392
Medial longitudinal arch, of foot, 561
Medial malleolus, 508, 513
Medial meniscus, 558
Medial pectoral nerve, 66, 67, 451, 459
Medial plantar artery, 549–552
Medial plantar nerve, 540, 549–552
Medial plantar vein, 550–552
Medial pterygoid muscle, 342, 357, 360, 365

Medial rectus muscle, 333, 335
Medial supracondylar line, 512
Medial supraepicondylar ridge, 430
Medial sural nerve, 520
Medial umbilical folds, 144
Medial umbilical ligament
  female, 241
  male, 239
Median aperture, 316
Median arcuate ligament, 192, 193
Median cubital vein, 439, 440
Median nerve, 450, 459, 475, 481, 483
  palmar branch of, 480
  palmar cutaneous branch of, 440, 475
  recurrent branch of, 483
Median raphe, 369
Median sacral artery, 187
Median umbilical fold, 144
Mediastinal parietal pleura, 75–77
Mediastinum(a), 102–112
  anterior, 84, 102
  arteries of, 102
  dissection overview of, 103
  lymphatic system of, 108
  middle, 75, 84, 102
    removal of heart from, 89–90
  muscles of, 102
  nerves of, 102
  posterior, 102, 104
    nerves in, 109
  superior, 102, 110–112
    trachea and related structure in, 105
  veins of, 102
    azygos, 106–107
Medulla oblongata, 313, 327
Membranous urethra, 234, 235
Meningeal artery
  accessory, 367
  middle, 322, 324, 325, 367
    branches of, 307, 308
    groove for, 263, 305
  posterior, 327
Meningeal vein, middle, 322, 324
  branches of, 307
Meninges
  cranial, 301, 308, 417
    dissection overview of, 302
  spinal, 37, 42, 45
Meniscus
  lateral, 558
  medial, 558
Mental foramen, 258, 259, 351
Mental nerve, 353
Mental protuberance, 258, 272

Mental tubercle, 258
Mentalis muscle, 341, 356
Mesenteric artery
  inferior, 157, 180, 187
  superior, 157, 177, 178, 187
Mesenteric lymph nodes
  inferior, 180
  superior, 179
Mesenteric plexus, superior, 177
Mesenteric vein
  inferior, 181
  superior, 177, 181
Mesentery, 163, 173
Mesocolon, 147
  sigmoid, 154, 155
  transverse, 150, 162, 163, 173
Mesosalpinx, 230
Mesovarium, 230
Metacarpal arteries, palmar, 487
Metacarpal bones, 427, 433, 434, 496
Metacarpal ligaments, palmar, 496, 497
Metacarpophalangeal (MP) joint(s), 489
Metacarpophalangeal (MP) joint capsule, 497
Metacarpophalangeal (MP) ligaments, 497
Metatarsal(s), 514, 515, 560, 561
Metatarsal arteries
  dorsal, 545
  plantar, 552
Metatarsal ligaments
  deep transverse, 560
  plantar, 560
Metatarsophalangeal joint(s), 560
Metatarsophalangeal joint capsules, 560
Midaxillary line, 13
Middle adrenal artery, 187, 191
Middle cardiac vein, 94
Middle cerebral artery, 314, 315
Middle cervical ganglia, 370
Middle clinoid process, 263
Middle colic artery, 178, 179
Middle colic lymph node, 179
Middle collateral artery, 461, 462, 465, 473
Middle concha, 381, 383
Middle cranial fossa, 263, 312, 320, 322–325
Middle ear, 403, 405, 407–410
Middle ethmoidal air cells, 382
Middle lobe, of right lung, 82, 83
Middle meatus, 378, 381
Middle mediastinum, 75, 84, 102
  removal of heart from, 89–90

Middle meningeal artery, 322, 324, 325, 367
   branches of, 307, 308
   groove for, 263, 305
Middle meningeal vein, 322, 324
   branches of, 307
Middle nasal concha, 378
Middle pharyngeal constrictor muscle, 361, 369, 391, 399
Middle rectal artery, 239–242
Middle sacral artery, 187
Middle sacral vein, 188
Middle scalene muscle, 276, 277, 343, 348
Middle superior alveolar artery, 387
Middle superior alveolar nerve, 387
Middle superior alveolar vein, 387
Middle suprarenal artery, 187, 191
Middle thyroid vein, 298
Midgut, 170
   dissection overview of, 171
   duodenum in, 170, 172
   ileum in, 173–174
   jejunum in, 173–174
   large intestine in, 175
   superior mesenteric artery to, 177–179
Minor calyces, 190
Minor duodenal papilla, 172
Mitral valve, 99–101
Moderator band, 98
Mons pubis, 219, 236
MP. *See* Metacarpophalangeal (MP).
Multifidus muscle, 26, 31, 32
Muscular triangle, 278, 292
Musculocutaneous nerve, 450, 457, 459, 475
Musculophrenic artery, 72, 112
Musculophrenic vessels, 143
Mylohyoid muscle, 281, 293, 295, 389–391
Mylohyoid nerve, 295, 367
Myocardium, 87, 98

N

Nasal aperture, posterior, 261
Nasal arteries
   external, 383
   lateral, alar branch of, 383
   posterior inferior lateral, 384
   posterior lateral, 384
   posterior superior lateral, 384
   septal branch from, 383
Nasal bone, 258, 259, 381
Nasal cavity, 258, 371, 379
   arteries of, 373
   dissection overview of, 375
   lateral, vasculature of, 383–384
   nerves of, 373
   osteology of, 373
   structure of, 373
Nasal concha, 258
   inferior, 378
   middle, 378
   superior, 381, 383
Nasal crest, 258
Nasal nerve
   external, 334, 351
   posterior inferior lateral, 384
   posterior superior lateral, 384
Nasal septum, 379, 380, 384
Nasal spine
   anterior, 258
   posterior, 261
Nasal wall, lateral, 381–382
Nasalis muscle, 356
Nasion, 258
Nasociliary nerve, 334
Nasolacrimal duct, 264
   opening of, 381
Nasopalatine nerve, 377, 380, 384
   palatine branches of, 380, 385
Nasopharyngeal tonsils, 371
Nasopharynx, 358, 371
Navicular, 514, 515, 559, 561
Neck
   anterior triangle of, 278–299
      arteries of, 278
      borders of, 283
      cervical plexus in, 282
      dissection overview of, 280
      glands of, 298–299
      lymphatics of, 279
      muscles of, 278, 281, 292
      overview of, 283
      recurrent laryngeal nerves in, 299
      superficial structures of, 284–285
      veins of, 278
   arteries of, 414–415
   carotid triangle of, 278, 286–291
   fascia/membranes of, 417
   glands of, 415–416
   joints of, 412
   ligaments of, 412
   lymphatics of, 415
   muscles of, 412–413
   muscular triangle of, 278, 292
   nerves of, 413–414

Neck *(Continued)*
   occipital triangle of, 274, 275
   osteology of, 254, 411–412
   posterior triangle of, 267–277
      arteries of, 267
      borders of, 274
      cervical fascia in, 267, 271
      cervical plexus in, 270
      contents of, 275–277
      dissection overview of, 268
      muscles of, 267, 269, 274
      nerves of, 267
      osteology of, 267
      veins of, 267
   root of, 296–297
   submandibular triangle of, 278, 294–295
   submental triangle of, 278, 293
   superficial aspect of, 273
   supraclavicular triangle of, 274, 275
   surface anatomy of, 272
   veins of, 415
Nipple, 58, 60, 61
Nodal branch, 92
Nodules, of aortic valve, 100
Nuchal line
   inferior, 260, 261
   superior, 9, 260, 261

O

Oblique arytenoid muscle, 395, 400, 402
Oblique fissure, of lung
   left, 80, 81
   right, 82, 83
Oblique line, 258
Oblique muscle
   external, 17, 131, 133, 137, 138, 140
   inferior, 335
   internal, 131, 133, 140
   superior, 332–334, 335
Oblique pericardial sinus, 88, 90
Obliquus capitis inferior muscle, 27, 35, 36
Obliquus capitis superior muscle, 27, 35, 36
Obturator artery, 225, 239, 241, 534
Obturator canal, 231, 510
Obturator externus muscle, 503, 522, 532, 533
Obturator fascia, 201, 202
Obturator foramen, 121–123, 508, 510
Obturator groove, 124–126, 511
Obturator internus muscle, 201, 202, 214, 221, 231, 232, 504, 522, 523
Obturator membrane, 510

Obturator nerve, 194, 195, 243, 526–528, 533
   anterior division of, 533
   cutaneous branch of, 520
   posterior division of, 533
Obtuse marginal artery, 92, 93
Occipital artery, 36, 275, 276, 290
Occipital bone, 9, 256, 259–262, 305, 326
   basal part of, 261
   removal of wedge of, 306
   squamous part of, 260
Occipital condyle, 261
Occipital crest
   external, 260, 261
   internal, 262
Occipital dural sinus, groove for, 306
Occipital lobe, 313
Occipital nerve
   greater, 33, 34, 36, 275
   lesser, 270, 275, 282
Occipital pole, 313
Occipital protuberance
   external, 9, 13, 17, 260, 261
   internal, 262, 326
Occipital sinus, 310
Occipital triangle, 274, 275
Occipitalis muscle, 303
Occipitofrontalis muscle, facial belly of, 341, 356
Occipitomastoid suture, 259, 260
Oculomotor nerve, 314, 323, 324, 328
   inferior division of, 333
   superior division of, 333
Odontoid process, 7
Olecranon fossa, 427, 430, 431
Olecranon process, of ulna, 427, 432
Olfactory bulbs, 312
Olfactory nerve, 312, 328
Olfactory tracts, 312
Omental appendices, 176
Omental bursa, 152
Omental foramen, 151, 152
Omentum
   greater, 147, 149–150, 159, 161, 162
   lesser, 147, 151–152, 166
Omohyoid muscle, 269, 274, 276, 281, 285, 292
   innervation of, 270, 282
Ophthalmic artery, 314, 315, 323, 334
Ophthalmic nerve, 323, 324
Ophthalmic vein, 310, 334
Opponens digiti minimi muscle, 424, 485
Opponens pollicis muscle, 423, 484
Optic canal, 263, 264, 322, 324

Optic chiasm, 312, 332
Optic nerve, 312, 314, 328, 333
Oral cavity, 371, 375
    tongue in, 389–392
Orbicularis oculi muscle, 341, 356
Orbicularis oris muscle, 341, 356
Orbit, 264, 329–337, 416
    anterior approach to, 335
    dissection overview of, 330
    eyeball (globe) of, 329, 336–337
    glands of, 329
    muscles of, 329
    nerves of, 329
    osteology of, 329
    superior approach to, 331–334
    vessels of, 329
Orbital fissure
    inferior, 264
    superior, 263, 264, 322, 324
Orbital plates, 321
Oropharynx, 371, 372
Os coxae, 117, 123, 196, 245, 507, 510, 562
Ossicles, 405, 408
Osteology, of back, 3–9, 44
Ovarian arteries, 187, 229
Ovarian ligament, 155, 229, 230, 236
Ovarian vein
    left, 188, 229
    right, 188, 229
Ovary(ies), 155, 229, 230, 236
    suspensory ligament of, 155, 229, 230

P

Palate, 374, 375, 388
    hard, 261, 372, 379, 380
    soft, 372, 379
        muscles of, 376
Palatine aponeurosis, 388
Palatine artery
    greater, 383–385
        terminal part of, 383
    lesser, 384, 385
Palatine bone, 254, 256–257, 261, 264, 388
    pyramidal process of, 261
Palatine branches
    of nasopalatine nerve, 380, 385
    of sphenopalatine artery, 380
Palatine canal, 386
    contents of, 385
    nerve to, 386

Palatine foramen
    greater, 261
    lesser, 261
Palatine nerves, 385, 386
    greater, 377, 384–386
    lesser, 377, 384–386
Palatine tonsils, 372, 388, 392
Palatine vein
    greater, 385
    lesser, 385
Palatoglossal arch, 372, 388, 392
Palatoglossus muscle, 372, 376, 388, 390, 391
Palatopharyngeal arch, 372, 388, 392
Palatopharyngeus muscle, 361, 372, 376
Palm
    adductor compartment of, 479, 487
    central compartment of, 479, 486
    hypothenar compartment of, 479, 485
    nerves of, 483
    thenar compartment of, 479, 484
    vessels of, 482
Palmar aponeurosis, 468, 480
    transverse fibers of, 468
Palmar branch
    of median nerve, 480
    of ulnar nerve, 480
Palmar carpal ligament, 481
Palmar carpometacarpal ligaments, 497
Palmar cutaneous branch
    of median nerve, 440, 475
    of ulnar nerve, 440
Palmar digital arteries
    common, 482
    proper, 482
Palmar digital nerves
    common, 483
    proper, 483
Palmar interossei muscles, 424, 487
Palmar metacarpal arteries, 487
Palmar metacarpal ligaments, 496, 497
Palmar radiocarpal ligaments, 496
Palmar ulnocarpal ligament, 496
Palmaris brevis muscle, 423, 480
Palmaris longus muscle, 422, 468
Palmaris longus tendon, 480, 481
Pampiniform plexus, of veins, 208–210
Pancreas, 153, 168, 170, 172, 248
Pancreatic duct
    accessory, 172
    main, 172
Pancreaticoduodenal ampulla, 172

Pancreaticoduodenal arteries
    anterior
        inferior, 177
        superior, 160, 169, 177
    inferior, 178
    posterior
        inferior, 177
        superior, 160, 177
    superior, 158, 160
Papillary muscle(s), 98
    anterior, 98, 100
    posterior, 98, 100
    septal, 98
Paracolic lymph nodes, 179, 180
Paranasal sinuses, 378
Pararectal fossae, 154, 155
Parathyroid glands, 299
Paraumbilical veins, 136
Paravesical fossae, 154, 155
Parietal bone, 253, 257, 259, 260, 305
Parietal lobe, 313
Parietal pericardium, 78, 87
Parietal peritoneum, 133, 140–142, 144
Parietal pleura, 71, 75
    cervical, 75, 76
    costal, 75–77, 107, 109
    diaphragmatic, 75, 76
    mediastinal, 75–77
Parietomastoid suture, 259
Parotid duct, 354, 365
Parotid gland, 275, 354, 355, 363
Parotid region, 339, 354–355
Patella, 507, 508, 513, 531, 562
Patellar ligament, 531
Patellar surface, 508
Pecten pubis, 120, 125
Pectinate muscles, 96, 99
Pectineal ligament, 145
Pectineal line, 124–126, 508, 511
Pectineus muscle, 502, 530–533
Pectoral artery, 452
Pectoral branch, 67, 68
Pectoral nerve
    lateral, 66, 67, 451, 459
    medial, 66, 67, 451, 459
Pectoralis major muscle, 57, 60, 63, 64, 420, 446
Pectoralis minor muscle, 57, 66, 420, 446
Pedicle, 6
    thoracic, 51
Pelvic aperture
    inferior, 122
    superior, 120

Pelvic autonomics, 244
Pelvic bone, 123–126, 511
Pelvic diaphragm, 201, 202, 214, 226, 231–232
Pelvic inlet, 119–121
    gender differences in, 128
Pelvic nerve, 244
Pelvic organs
    female, 226, 236–237
    male, 226, 234–235
Pelvic outlet, 122
Pelvic peritoneum
    female, 155, 230
    male, 154
Pelvic splanchnic nerves, 244
Pelvic structures, 226
Pelvic walls, 121
Pelvis, 226–244, 562
    arteries of, 246
    bony, 510–511
    dissection overview of, 227
    female
        muscles of, 231, 232
        organs of, 226, 236–237
        overview of, 229
        peritoneum of, 230
        structures of, 226
        vasculature of, 226, 238, 241–242
    gender differences in, 128
    hemisection of, 233
    ligaments of, 248
    lymphatics of, 247
    male
        organs of, 226, 234–235
        overview of, 228
        structures of, 226
        vasculature of, 226, 238–240
    muscles of, 226, 231–232, 245–246
    nerves of, 226, 243–244, 247
    osteology of, 117, 120–128, 226, 245, 510–511
    overview of, 228–229, 245–249
    veins of, 246–247
Penile fascia
    deep, 213
    superficial, 213
Penile raphe, 212
Penis, 249
    bulb of, 214–216
    crus of, 214–216
    shaft of, 212, 213
    suspensory ligament of, 208, 209, 215, 234
Perforating artery, 523

Index   577

Perforating branches, 534
  anterior, 112
  of deep artery of thigh, 535
Pericardial cavity, 87
Pericardial sac, 78, 84, 87, 90, 114
  heart in, 86
  opening of, 87
  posterior surface of, 104
Pericardial sinus(es), 88
  oblique, 88, 90
  transverse, 88, 90
Pericardial space, 87
Pericardiophrenic vessels, 78
Pericardium
  parietal, 78, 87
  visceral, 87
Pericranium, 303
Perineal artery, 217, 225
Perineal body, 201, 202
  female, 224
  male, 201, 202, 215, 216
Perineal membrane, 223, 224
Perineal muscle
  deep transverse
    female, 224
    male, 216
  superficial transverse
    female, 224
    male, 215, 216
Perineal nerve, 217
  deep, 217, 225
  superficial, 225
Perineal space
  deep
    female, 203, 205, 221, 224, 236
    male, 203, 205, 214, 215, 234
  superficial
    female, 203, 205, 221, 223
    male, 203, 205, 214–215
Perineal vein
  female, 225
  male, 217
Perineum
  female, 219, 221
  overview of, 249
Periorbita, 331, 332
Perirenal fat, 189
Peritoneal cavity, 149–152
Peritoneum, 147, 154, 155, 248
  dissection overview of, 148
  parietal, 133, 140–142, 144, 150
  pelvic
    female, 155, 230
    male, 154

Peritoneum (Continued)
  urogenital, 249
  visceral, 150
Petrosal nerve
  greater, 325, 386, 408, 409
    groove and hiatus for, 263, 322
  lesser, groove and hiatus for, 263
Petrosal sinuses
  inferior, 310, 323, 327
    groove for, 262
  superior, 310, 323, 327
Phalanges
  of foot, 514, 515, 560
  of hand, 427, 433, 434
Pharyngeal artery, ascending, 290
Pharyngeal constrictor muscles, 361, 369
  inferior, 361, 369, 370
  middle, 361, 369, 391, 399
  superior, 361, 369, 372, 399
Pharyngeal recess, 399
Pharyngeal tubercle, 261
Pharyngobasilar fascia, 369
Pharynx, 299, 358, 369–372, 415
  dissection overview of, 359
  laryngo-, 371, 399
  muscles of, 361
  naso-, 358, 371
  oro-, 372
  posterior and lateral aspects of, 370
  posterior approach to, 369
Phrenic arteries, inferior, 187, 191
Phrenic nerve(s), 78, 270, 277, 282, 297
Phrenic vein, inferior, 188
Phrenicocolic ligament, 175
Pia mater, 307, 308
  spinal, 42
Pinna, 405
Piriform aperture, 258
Piriform fossa, 399
Piriformis muscle, 200, 231, 232, 504, 522, 523
Pisiform bone, 433, 434, 482, 483, 485, 496
Pituitary gland, 323
  stalk of, 324
Plantar aponeurosis, 549
Plantar artery
  deep, 552
  lateral, 549–552
    cutaneous branches of, 549
  medial, 549–552
Plantar calcaneonavicular ligament, 553, 559, 560
Plantar compartment, of foot, muscles of, 506

Plantar digital arteries, proper, 552
Plantar digital nerves
  common, 552
  proper, 552
Plantar interosseous muscles, 506, 553
Plantar ligaments, 560
  long, 553, 559, 560
Plantar metatarsal arteries, 552
Plantar metatarsal ligaments, 560
Plantar nerves
  lateral, 540, 549–552
    cutaneous branches of, 549
  medial, 540, 549–552
Plantar tarsometatarsal ligaments, 560
Plantar vein
  lateral, 550–552
  medial, 550–552
Plantaris muscle, 505, 542
Plantaris tendon, 542
Platysma muscle, 269, 273, 341, 356
Pleura, visceral, 75–77
Pleural cavity, 76
Pleural recesses, 73, 76–77
Pleural spaces, 73, 75–77
Pons, 313
Pontine arteries, 314, 315
Popliteal artery, 534, 535, 539–541, 545
Popliteal fossa, 539
  muscles of, 539
  nerves of, 540
  vessels of, 541
Popliteal vein, 539
Popliteus muscle, 505, 540, 543, 545
Porta hepatis, 151, 168
Portal triad(s)
  extrahepatic, 168
  intrahepatic, 167
Portal vein, 168, 170, 181, 247
Postcentral gyrus, 313
Posterior abdominal wall, 183–195
  abdominal aorta, 183, 186, 187
  adrenal glands, 189, 191
  arteries of, 183
  diaphragm, 183, 186, 192
  dissection overview of, 184
  inferior vena cava, 183, 186, 188
  kidneys, 183, 186, 189–190
  lymphatics of, 183
  muscles of, 183, 185, 193
  nerves of, 183, 194–195
  overview of, 186
  veins of, 183
Posterior auricular artery, 290
Posterior auricular vein, 285

Posterior cerebral arteries, 314, 315
Posterior chamber, of eye, 337
Posterior circumflex humeral artery, 445, 452, 465
Posterior clinoid process, 263, 322
Posterior communicating artery, 314, 315
Posterior cranial fossa, 262, 320, 326–327
Posterior cricoarytenoid muscle, 395, 400, 402
Posterior cruciate ligament, 558
Posterior cutaneous nerve
  of arm, 441
  of forearm, 441
  of thigh, 520, 523, 526
Posterior cutaneous neurovascular bundles, 10, 16
Posterior descending artery, 92
Posterior ethmoidal air cells, 382
Posterior ethmoidal artery, 334, 383
  septal branch of, 383
Posterior ethmoidal nerve, 334, 380
Posterior ethmoidal vein, 334
Posterior gluteal line, 511
Posterior inferior cerebellar arteries, 314, 315
Posterior inferior iliac spine, 124–126, 508, 511
Posterior inferior lateral nasal artery, 384
Posterior inferior lateral nasal nerve, 384
Posterior inferior pancreaticoduodenal artery, 177
Posterior intercostal arteries, 16, 111, 112
Posterior intercostal veins, 108
Posterior interosseous artery, 462, 473
Posterior interventricular artery, 92, 93
Posterior interventricular groove, 91
Posterior labial artery, 225
Posterior labial nerves, 225
Posterior labial vein, 225
Posterior lateral nasal arteries, 384
Posterior longitudinal ligament, 345
Posterior mediastinum, 102, 104
  nerves in, 109
Posterior meningeal artery, 327
Posterior nasal aperture, 261
Posterior nasal spine, 261
Posterior papillary muscle, 98, 100
Posterior rami, 16
Posterior roots, spinal, 42
Posterior sacral foramina, 127
Posterior scalene muscle, 277, 343, 348
Posterior scapular region, 443–445
Posterior scrotal artery, 217

Posterior scrotal nerves, 208, 217
Posterior scrotal vein, 217
Posterior scrotal vessels, 208
Posterior superior alveolar artery, 387
Posterior superior alveolar foramina, 265
Posterior superior alveolar nerve, 367, 377, 387
Posterior superior alveolar vein, 387
Posterior superior iliac spine, 124–126, 508, 511
Posterior superior lateral nasal artery, 384
Posterior superior lateral nasal nerve, 384
Posterior superior pancreaticoduodenal arteries, 160, 177
Posterior talofibular ligament, 559
Posterior tibial artery, 540, 541, 545, 551
  medial calcaneal branches of, 549
Posterior tibial vein, 551
Posterior ulnar recurrent artery, 461, 462, 465, 473, 474
Posterior vagal trunk, 104
Preaortic lymph nodes, 180, 186, 238
Precentral gyrus, 313
Pretracheal fascia, 271
Prevertebral fascia, 271, 346, 348
Prevertebral muscles, 343, 348
Prevertebral region, 343, 348
Princeps pollicis artery, 482, 487
Procerus muscle, 341, 356
Pronator quadratus muscle, 422, 470
Pronator teres muscle, 421, 468
Proper digital arteries
  of foot, 549
  of hand, 480
Proper digital nerves
  of foot, 549
  of hand, 480
Proper digital veins
  of foot, 549
  of hand, 480
Proper hepatic artery, 158, 160, 168, 169
Proper hepatic vein, 159
Proper palmar digital arteries, 482
Proper palmar digital nerves, 483
Proper plantar digital arteries, 552
Proper plantar digital nerves, 552
Prostate gland, 154, 214, 234, 235
Prostatic plexus of veins, 234, 235
Prostatic urethra, 234
Psoas major muscle, 185, 192–195, 502
  transection of, 529
Psoas minor muscle, 185, 193, 502
Psoas muscle, 530
Pterion, 259

Pterygoid canal
  nerve of, 385, 386
  opening of, 261
Pterygoid fossa, 261
Pterygoid hamulus, 388
Pterygoid muscle
  lateral, 342, 357, 360, 365, 367
    removal of, 366
  medial, 342, 357, 360, 365
Pterygoid plate, lateral, 265, 266
Pterygoid plexus, of veins, 310, 365
Pterygoid process
  lateral plate of, 261
  medial plate of, 261
Pterygomaxillary fissure, 265, 266
Pterygopalatine fossa, 265–266, 377
Pterygopalatine ganglion, 384–387
Pubic arch, gender differences in, 128
Pubic crest, 120, 124–126, 133, 511
Pubic ramus
  inferior, 124–126, 508, 511
  superior, 124–126, 508, 511
Pubic symphysis, 119, 120, 122, 123
  female, 218, 236
  male, 211, 234, 235
Pubic tubercle, 120–122, 125, 510, 511
Pubis, 117, 123, 125, 511, 556
Pubococcygeus muscle, 231, 232
Pubofemoral ligament, 556
Puborectalis muscle, 231, 232
Pubovesical ligament, 237
Pudendal artery, 200, 528
  external
    female, 225
    male, 217
  internal, 201, 202, 243
    female, 225, 241, 242
    male, 217, 239, 240
Pudendal canal, 201, 202
Pudendal nerve, 200–202, 243, 526, 528
  branches of
    female, 225
    male, 217
  female, 225
  male, 217
Pudendal vein, 200
  external
    female, 225
    male, 217
  internal, 201, 202
    female, 225
    male, 217

Pulmonary arteries, 78
  left, 80, 81, 86, 88
  right, 82, 83
Pulmonary ligament
  left, 80, 81
  right, 82, 83
Pulmonary surface, of heart, 91
Pulmonary trunk, 86, 89, 110
Pulmonary valve, 98, 101
Pulmonary veins, 89–93, 99
  left, 80, 81, 90
  right, 82, 83
Pupil, 337
Pyloric sphincter, 156
Pylorus, 156, 172
Pyramidalis muscle, 131, 137

Q

Quadrangular membrane, 401
Quadrangular space, 444, 445, 464
Quadratus femoris muscle, 504, 522, 523
Quadratus lumborum muscle, 185, 192–195
Quadratus plantae muscle, 506, 551
Quadriceps femoris muscles, 502, 531

R

Radial artery, 461, 462, 482, 488
  distal portion of, 474
  proximal portion of, 462, 473
  superficial branch of, 482, 488
  superficial palmar branch of, 482
Radial collateral artery, 461, 462, 465, 473
Radial collateral ligament, 495, 496
Radial fossa, 430
Radial groove, 427, 430
Radial nerve, 444, 450, 453, 460, 464, 476
  deep branch of, 475, 476
  superficial branch of, 440, 441, 475, 476, 488
Radial notch, 432
Radial recurrent artery, 461, 462, 465, 473, 474
Radial tuberosity, 427, 432, 495
Radiocarpal joint, 496
Radiocarpal ligaments, palmar, 496
Radius, 425, 427, 432, 434
  head of, 427, 432
  neck of, 432
  overview of, 498
  styloid process of, 427, 432

Rami communicantes, gray and white, 107, 109
Raphe, median, 369
Rectal artery
  inferior, 201, 202, 217, 225
  middle, 239–242
  superior, 180
Rectal nerve, inferior, 201, 202, 217, 225
Rectal sheath, 137
Rectal vein
  inferior, 201, 202
    female, 225
    male, 217
  superior, 181
Rectouterine pouch, 155
Rectovesical pouch, 154
Rectum, 153–155, 176, 201, 202
  transection of, 182
Rectus abdominis muscle, 131, 140–142, 245
  epigastric vessels in, 143
Rectus capitis anterior muscle, 343, 347, 348
Rectus capitis lateralis muscle, 343, 347, 348
Rectus capitis posterior major muscle, 27, 35, 36
Rectus capitis posterior minor muscle, 27, 35, 36
Rectus femoris muscle, 502, 531
Rectus muscle
  lateral, 333–335
  medial, 333, 335
  superior, 333, 335
Rectus sheath, 140–143
Recurrent laryngeal nerves, 299, 370, 396, 399
  left, 86, 104, 299, 370
  right, 104, 298, 299
Recurrent median nerve, 483
Renal arteries, 157, 169, 187
Renal columns, 190
Renal cortex, 190
Renal medulla, 190
Renal papillae, 190
Renal pelvis, 190
Renal pyramids, 190
Renal vein
  left, 188, 189
  right, 188, 189
Reproductive system
  female, 226, 236–237
  male, 226, 234–235
Retina, 337
  central artery and vein of, 334, 337

Retromammary space, 60
Retromandibular vein, 285, 354
Retropharyngeal space, 346, 348
Rhomboid major muscle, 12, 21, 420, 443
Rhomboid minor muscle, 12, 21, 420, 443
Rib(s), 3, 44, 49, 52
    floating, 54
    number 12, 119
Rib articulations, 53
Rib cage, 54, 71
Right adrenal vein, 188
Right atrioventricular valve, 96, 98, 101
Right atrium, 84, 91–94, 98, 114
    incisions of, 95
    internal structures of, 96
Right brachiocephalic vein, 106
Right colic artery, 178, 179
Right colic flexure, 162, 175
Right colic lymph nodes, 179
Right common carotid artery, 110, 111
Right coronary artery, 92, 93, 101, 114
Right crus, 192
Right gastric artery, 158–160, 169
Right gastric vein, 181
Right gastro-omental artery, 158, 160, 169
Right gonadal artery, 189
Right gonadal vein, 188, 189, 229
Right hepatic artery, 160
Right hepatic duct, 168
Right hepatic flexure, 175
Right intercostal veins, 106
Right (acute) marginal artery, 92, 93
Right ovarian vein, 188, 229
Right phrenic nerve, 78
Right pulmonary artery, 82, 83
Right pulmonary veins, 82, 83
Right recurrent laryngeal nerve, 104
Right renal vein, 188, 189
Right subclavian artery, 110, 111
Right suprarenal vein, 188
Right testicular vein, 188, 229
Right triangular ligament, 165, 166
Right vagus nerve, 86, 104, 298, 299
Right ventricle, 84, 91, 114
    incisions of, 97
    internal structures of, 98
Rima glottis, 398
Risorius muscle, 341, 356
Rotator cuff, 493
Rotatores muscles, 26, 31, 32
Round ligament, 159
    of femur, 557
    of liver, 165, 167
    of uterus, 138, 144, 146, 229, 230

S

S1 nerve, 243
S2 nerve, 243
S3 nerve, 243
S4 nerve, 243
S5 nerve, 243
SA (sinuatrial) branch, of right coronary artery, 92
SA (sinuatrial) node, 96
Saccule, of larynx, 401
Sacral arteries
    lateral
        female, 241, 242
        male, 239, 240
    median, 187
    middle, 187
Sacral canal, 127
Sacral cornua, 127
Sacral foramina
    anterior, 127
    posterior, 127
Sacral hiatus, 127
Sacral plexus, 516, 524, 526, 528, 563
Sacral promontory, 120
Sacral vein, middle, 188
Sacrococcygeal ligament, anterior, 231, 232
Sacroiliac joint, 120
Sacrospinous ligament, 121, 200, 239–242
Sacrotuberous ligament, 121, 122, 199–202
Sacrum, 5, 8, 13, 117, 119, 122, 127
    ala of, 120, 127
    promontory of, 127
Saddle joint, 497
Sagittal sinus
    inferior, 310
    superior, 306–308, 310
        groove for, 305
Sagittal suture, 260, 305
Salpingopharyngeal fold, 371, 372, 382
Salpingopharyngeus muscle, 361, 372, 388
Saphenous nerve, 519, 520, 533, 535
Saphenous vein
    great, 519, 520
    small, 519, 520
Sartorius muscle, 502, 530, 531, 533, 535
Scalene muscles, 269, 276, 277, 343, 348
    anterior, 276, 277, 343, 348
    middle, 276, 277, 343, 348
    posterior, 277, 343, 348
Scalp, 303
    aponeurosis of, 303
    dissection overview of, 302
    layers of, 300, 303

Scaphoid, 433, 434, 496
Scaphoid fossa, 261, 406
Scapula, 9, 54, 425, 427, 429
    acromion of, 13, 54, 58, 61, 272, 427, 429, 493
    inferior angle of, 427
    lateral border of, 429
    medial (vertebral) margin of, 427, 429
    overview of, 498
    spine of, 427, 429
Scapular artery
    circumflex, 445, 452
    dorsal, 21, 444, 449
Scapular nerve, dorsal, 21, 444, 447, 449
Scapular notch, greater, 429
Scapular region, posterior, 443–445
Scarpa's fascia, 133, 135
Sciatic foramen
    greater, 121
    lesser, 121
Sciatic nerve, 200, 243, 523, 526, 540
Sciatic notch
    greater, 121, 123, 508, 510
    lesser, 121, 123–126, 510, 511
Sclera, 335, 337
Scrotal artery
    anterior, 217
    posterior, 217
Scrotal fascia, superficial, 208, 209
Scrotal nerves
    anterior, 208
    posterior, 208, 217
Scrotal sac, 207
Scrotal septum, 208, 209
Scrotal vein
    anterior, 217
    posterior, 217
Scrotal vessels
    anterior, 208
    posterior, 208
Scrotum, 201, 202, 212, 249
    layers of, 132, 206, 208
    overview of, 207
Sella turcica, 320, 322
Semicircular canals, 405, 408
Semimembranosus muscle, 504, 536, 539, 542
Seminal vesicles, 234, 235
Seminiferous tubules, 210
Semispinalis capitis muscle, 26, 28, 34
Semispinalis cervicis muscle, 26
Semispinalis muscle, 22, 26, 31, 32
Semispinalis thoracis muscle, 26
Semitendinosus muscle, 504, 536, 539, 542

Septal cartilage, 379
Septal papillary muscle, 98
Septomarginal trabecula, 98
Septum penis, 213
Serratus anterior muscle, 57, 63, 64, 420, 446, 447
Serratus posterior inferior muscle, 12, 22
Serratus posterior superior muscle, 12, 21, 22, 28
Sesamoid bones, 560
Short ciliary artery, 333
Short ciliary nerve, 333, 334
Short ciliary vein, 333
Short gastric arteries, 158, 161, 169
Short gastric vessels, 164
Shoulder, 490–494, 500
    anterior region of, 446
    muscles of, 435, 498
        deltoid, 442
    posterior scapular region of, 443–445
Sigmoid arteries, 180
Sigmoid colon, 153, 176
Sigmoid lymph nodes, 180
Sigmoid mesocolon, 154, 155
Sigmoid sinuses, 310, 327
    groove for, 262
Sinuatrial (SA) branch, of right coronary artery, 92
Sinuatrial (SA) node, 96
Sinus(es), paranasal, 378
Sinus venarum, 96
Skull, 9
    anterior and posterior cranial fossae of, 262, 317
    anterior view of, 258
    base of, 317–327
        anterior cranial fossa in, 317
        dissection overview for, 319
        dural venous sinuses in, 318
        middle cranial fossa in, 317
        posterior cranial fossa in, 317
    foramina of, 256–257
    inferior view of, 261
    lateral view of, 259
    middle cranial fossae of, 263, 317
    orbit of, 264
    osteology of, 253–254, 256–266
    posterior view of, 260
    pterygopalatine fossa of, 265–266
Small cardiac vein, 94
Small intestine, 147, 248
Small saphenous vein, 519, 520
Soft palate, 372, 379
    muscles of, 376

Soleal line, 508, 513
Soleus muscle, 505, 540, 542–545
Spermatic cord, 138, 146, 208, 249
    contents of, 209
    layers of, 206
    overview of, 207
Spermatic fascia
    external, 208
    internal, 208
Sphenoethmoidal recess, 381, 382
Sphenoid air sinus, 371, 382, 387
Sphenoid bone, 253, 256, 257, 261–266, 321, 322
    body of, 261, 262
    greater wing of, 259, 261, 263, 264, 320
    lateral pterygoid plate of, 265, 266, 362
    lesser wing of, 262, 264, 320, 321
Sphenoid sinus, 378, 379, 384, 399
Sphenomandibular ligament, 365, 368
Sphenopalatine artery, 367, 380, 383, 384
    lateral branches of, 383
    palatine branches of, 380
    septal branch of, 383
Sphenopalatine foramen, 381
Sphenopalatine vein, 380
Sphenoparietal sinuses, 323
Sphenoparietal suture, 259
Sphenosquamous suture, 259
Sphincter urethrovaginalis, 224
Spinal accessory nerve, 19, 275, 287, 328, 370
    spinal roots of, 327
Spinal artery, anterior, 314, 315
Spinal canal, 42–43
Spinal cord, 37–43, 45
    central canal of, 316
    venous plexus of, 327
Spinal nerves, 37, 43, 243, 247
Spinal root ganglia, 42, 43
Spinalis cervicis muscle, 25
Spinalis muscle, 25, 28, 29
Spinalis thoracis muscle, 25
Spinoglenoid notch, 429
Spinous process, 6, 7
    of C7, 13
    thoracic, 51
Splanchnic nerves
    greater, 107, 109
    least, 109
    lesser, 109
    pelvic, 244
Spleen, 153, 158, 164
Splenic artery, 158, 159, 161, 164, 168, 169
Splenic vein, 164, 181

Splenius capitis muscle, 21, 22, 25, 28, 34, 269, 276
Splenius cervicis muscle, 22, 25, 28, 34
Splenorenal ligament, 164
Spongy urethra, 213, 215, 216, 234, 235
"Spring" ligament, plantar, 553, 559, 560
Squamous suture, 259
Stapedius muscle, 405
Stapes, 405, 408
Stellate ganglion, 370
Sternal angle, 54
Sternal body, 58, 61
Sternoclavicular joint, 54, 58, 61, 72, 492
Sternoclavicular ligament, 492
Sternocleidomastoid muscle, 269, 272, 274–277, 281, 286
Sternocostal head, 446
Sternocostal surface, of heart, 91
Sternohyoid muscle, 281, 292, 296
    innervation of, 270, 282
Sternothyroid muscle, 281, 292, 296
    innervation of, 270, 282
Sternum, 49, 53, 54, 55, 119
Stomach, 147, 150, 153, 156
    greater curvature of, 149, 150, 156
    lesser curvature of, 151, 156
    nerves of, 159
Straight sinus, 310
Styloglossus muscle, 376, 390, 391
Stylohyoid muscle, 281, 295, 369, 370, 391
Styloid process
    of radius, 427, 432
    of temporal bone, 259, 261, 362, 368
Stylomandibular ligament, 368
Stylomastoid foramen, 261
Stylopharyngeus muscle, 361, 369, 370, 372, 391
Subacromial bursa, 442, 494
Subarachnoid space
    cranial, 307, 308
    spinal, 42
Subclavian artery, 112, 448, 452
    left, 110, 111, 297
    right, 110, 111
Subclavian vein, 86, 296
    left, 108
Subclavian vessels, 55, 72
Subclavius muscle, 57, 66, 67, 420, 446
Subcostal nerve, 136, 194, 195, 526, 527
Subcutaneum, 271
Subdural space
    cranial, 307, 308
    spinal, 42
Sublingual artery, 390

Sublingual caruncle, 390
Sublingual gland, 390
Submandibular duct, 390
Submandibular ganglion, 390
Submandibular gland, 294, 390
Submandibular lymph nodes, 285, 289, 294
Submental lymph nodes, 285, 289, 293
Submental triangle, 278, 293
Submental vein, 293
Suboccipital muscles, 27, 35, 36, 44
Suboccipital nerve, 36
Suboccipital region, 23
Suboccipital triangle, 23, 33–36
Subphrenic recess, 165, 166
Subscapular artery, 452
Subscapular bursa, 493, 494
Subscapular fossa, 427, 429
Subscapular nerve
    inferior, 461
    lower, 453
    superior, 461
    upper, 453
Subscapularis muscle, 421, 443, 446
Subscapularis tendon, 493, 494
Sulcus terminalis, 96, 392
Superciliary arch, 258
Superficial auricular nerve, 355
Superficial cervical fascia, 271
Superficial cervical lymph nodes, 285, 289
Superficial circumflex iliac vein, 136, 519
Superficial clitoral fascia, 222
Superficial dorsal vein
    female, 222
    male, 213
Superficial epigastric vein, 136, 519
Superficial fascia
    of anterior chest wall, 63
    of anterolateral abdominal wall, 133, 135
Superficial fibular nerve, 520, 540, 545
Superficial inguinal lymph nodes, 521
Superficial inguinal ring, 129, 137, 138, 145, 146
Superficial palmar arch, 482
Superficial palmar branch, of radial artery, 482
Superficial penile fascia, 213
Superficial perineal nerve, 225
Superficial perineal space
    female, 203, 205, 221, 223
    male, 203, 205, 214–215
Superficial radial nerve, 440, 441, 475, 476
Superficial scrotal fascia, 208, 209
Superficial temporal artery, 290, 354, 365, 367

Superficial temporal vein, 354
Superficial transverse perineal muscle
    female, 223, 224
    male, 215, 216
Superior adrenal artery, 187, 191
Superior articular process, 6
    of sacrum, 127
    thoracic, 51, 53
Superior cerebellar arteries, 314, 315
Superior cervical ganglia, 370
Superior concha, 381, 383
Superior costal facet, thoracic, 51, 53
Superior epigastric artery, 72, 112
Superior epigastric vessels, 143
Superior extensor retinaculum, 544
Superior gemellus muscle, 504, 522, 523
Superior gluteal artery, 225, 239–243, 523, 528
Superior gluteal nerve, 243, 523, 526, 528
Superior gluteal vein, 523
Superior horn, of thyroid cartilage, 397
Superior hypogastric plexus, 244
Superior laryngeal artery, 30, 290, 298
Superior laryngeal nerve, 291, 370, 396, 399
    internal, 298
Superior laryngeal vein, 298, 370
Superior lateral cutaneous nerve, of arm, 441
Superior lateral genicular artery, 535, 541
Superior lobe, of lung
    left, 80, 81
    right, 82, 83
Superior longitudinal ligament, 345
Superior meatus, 381
Superior medial genicular artery, 535, 541
Superior mediastinum, 102, 110–112
Superior mesenteric artery, 157, 177, 178, 187
Superior mesenteric ganglia, 177
Superior mesenteric lymph nodes, 179
Superior mesenteric plexus, 177
Superior mesenteric vein, 177, 181
Superior nuchal line, 9, 260, 261
Superior oblique muscle, 332–334, 335
Superior orbital fissure, 263, 264, 322, 324
Superior pancreaticoduodenal artery, 158, 160
Superior pelvic aperture, 120
Superior petrosal sinuses, 310, 323, 327
Superior pharyngeal constrictor muscle, 361, 369, 372, 399
Superior pubic ramus, 124–126, 508, 511
Superior rectal artery, 180

Superior rectal lymph nodes, 180
Superior rectal vein, 181
Superior rectus muscle, 333, 335
Superior sagittal sinus, 306–308, 310
   groove for, 305
Superior subscapular nerve, 461
Superior suprarenal artery, 187, 191
Superior thoracic artery, 68, 112, 452
Superior thyroid artery, 290, 298
Superior thyroid vein, 298
Superior ulnar collateral artery, 461, 462, 465, 473
Superior vena cava (SVC), 86, 89, 91–93
Superior vertebral notch, 6
Superior vesical arteries, 239–242
Supinator crest, 432
Supinator muscle, 423, 472
Supraclavicular nerves, 270, 273, 282
Supraclavicular triangle, 274, 275
Supracondylar line
   lateral, 512
   medial, 512
Supraepicondylar ridge
   lateral, 430
   medial, 430
Supraglenoid tubercle, 429
Suprahyoid muscles, 281
Supraorbital artery, 332, 334, 335
Supraorbital foramen, 351
Supraorbital nerve, 332, 335, 351
Supraorbital notch, 258
Supraorbital vein, 332, 335
Suprarenal arteries
   inferior, 187, 191
   middle, 187, 191
   superior, 187, 191
Suprarenal glands, 153, 186, 189, 191
Suprarenal vein
   left, 188
   right, 188
Suprascapular artery, 277, 297, 445
Suprascapular ligament, 444
Suprascapular nerve, 444, 445, 447, 449, 464
Suprascapular notch, 429, 444
Suprascapularis muscle, 442
Supraspinatus muscle, 421, 443, 463, 464
Supraspinatus tendon, 493, 494
Supraspinous fossa, 427, 429
Supraspinous ligaments, 39
Supratrochlear artery, 334
Supratrochlear nerve, 332, 351
Supraventricular crest, 98
Supreme thoracic artery, 68, 112, 452

Sural nerve, 520
   lateral, 520
   medial, 520
Suspensory ligament(s)
   of axilla, 66
   of breast, 60
   of duodenum, 163, 192
   of ovary, 155, 229, 230
   of penis, 208, 209, 215, 234, 235
Sustentaculum tali, 560
Sutural bones, 305
Suture(s), 263
   coronal, 259
   lambdoid, 259, 260
   occipitomastoid, 259, 260
   parietomastoid, 259
   sagittal, 260
   sphenoparietal, 259
   sphenosquamous, 259
   squamous, 259
SVC (superior vena cava), 86, 89, 91–93
Sympathetic chain, 194, 195, 244, 346
Sympathetic ganglion, 107, 109, 194, 195, 528
Sympathetic nerve fibers
   to male external genitalia, 208
   to viscera, 244
Sympathetic trunk, 243, 370, 528

T

Taenia coli muscles, 162, 175, 176
Talocalcaneonavicular joint, 559
Talofibular ligaments
   anterior, 559
   posterior, 559
Talus, 514, 515, 559, 561
Tarsal bones, 514, 515
Tarsometatarsal ligaments
   dorsal, 559
   plantar, 560
Tectorial membrane, 345
Tegmen tympani, 263
   removal of, 407
Temporal arteries
   deep, 365, 367
   superficial, 290, 354, 365, 367
Temporal bone, 9, 253, 256, 259–263, 322, 326
   mastoid part of, 259
   petrous part of, 262, 322
   squamous part of, 259
   tympanic part of, 259
   zygomatic process of, 259

Temporal branch, of facial nerve, 355
Temporal lobe, 313
Temporal nerves, deep, 365, 367
Temporal pole, 313
Temporal vein, superficial, 354
Temporalis muscle, 342, 357, 360, 364
Temporomandibular joint, 362, 366, 368
Tendinous arch, of obturator internus muscle, 231, 232
Tendinous intersections, of anterior abdominal wall, 137
Tensor fascia lata muscle, 502, 531
Tensor tympani muscle, 405, 408
Tensor veli palatini muscle, 372, 376, 381, 388
Tensor veli palatini tendon, 372
Tentorium cerebelli, 309, 310, 327
Teres major muscle, 421, 443, 446
Teres minor muscle, 421, 443
Teres minor tendon, 494
Testicular arteries, 187, 208–210, 229
Testicular vein
   left, 188, 229
   right, 188, 229
Testicular vessels, 145, 154, 228
Testis, 132, 209, 210, 249
Thenar compartment, of hand, 479, 484
Thenar eminence, 480
Thenar muscles, 423, 480, 482–484
Thigh, 524–536
   anteromedial region of
     muscles of, 531–532
     nerves of, 533
     vessels of, 534–535
   deep artery of, 534, 535
   dissection overview of, 525
   femoral triangle of, 530
   muscles of, 524
     anterior region, 502
     anteromedial region, 531–532
     gluteal and posterior regions, 503–504
     medial region, 502–503
     posterior region, 524
   nerves of, 524, 526–529
     anteromedial, 533
     intermediate cutaneous, 520
     lateral cutaneous, 520, 527, 530
     medial cutaneous, 520
     posterior cutaneous, 520, 523, 526
   posterior region of, muscles of, 536
   vasculature of, 524
     anteromedial, 534–535
Third ventricle, 316

Thoracic aorta, 55, 111, 112
Thoracic artery
   internal, 112, 143, 297
   lateral, 452
   superior (supreme), 68, 112, 452
Thoracic duct, 108, 296
Thoracic nerve, long, 447, 453
Thoracic rib cage, 54
Thoracic situs, 73–78
Thoracic sympathetic trunks, 107, 109
Thoracic vein
   internal, 136
   lateral, 136
Thoracic vertebrae, 5, 7, 51
Thoracic vessels, internal, 70, 72
Thoracoacromial artery, 67, 68, 452
Thoracoacromial trunk, 67, 68
Thoracodorsal artery, 452
Thoracodorsal nerve, 453, 460
Thoracoepigastric vein, 136
Thoracolumbar fascia, 17
Thorax
   anterior wall of. See Anterior chest wall.
   dissection overview of, 50
   lymphatic system in, 108
   muscles of, 113
   nerves of, 113–114
   osteology of, 49–54, 113
   overview of, 113–114
   vessels of, 113
Thumb, saddle joint of, 497
Thymus gland, 86
Thyroarytenoid muscle, 395, 402
Thyrocervical trunk, 276, 290, 297
Thyrohyoid membrane, 291, 298, 396, 397
Thyrohyoid muscle, 281, 291, 292, 396
   innervation of, 270
Thyroid artery
   inferior, 290, 297, 298
   superior, 290, 298
Thyroid cartilage, 284, 397, 399, 400
   inferior horn of, 399
Thyroid gland, 284, 290, 298
Thyroid vein
   inferior, 298
   middle, 298
   superior, 298
Tibia, 507, 508, 513, 562
Tibial artery
   anterior, 540, 545
     recurrent branch of, 541
   posterior, 540, 541, 545, 551
     medial calcaneal branches of, 549
Tibial collateral ligament, 558

Tibial nerve, 539, 540, 541, 545, 551
  medial calcaneal branches of, 549
Tibial tuberosity, 508, 513
Tibial vein, posterior, 551
Tibialis anterior muscle, 504, 544
Tibialis anterior tendon, 540, 545, 553, 560
Tibialis posterior muscle, 505, 543
Tibialis posterior tendon, 540, 545, 553, 560
Tibiotalar joint, 559
Toe, great, 515
Tongue, 389–392, 399, 416
  muscles of, 376, 389, 391
  oral part of, 392
  pharyngeal part of, 392
Tonsils
  lingual, 392
  nasopharyngeal, 371
  palatine, 372, 388, 392
Torus tubarius, 371, 382
Trabeculae carneae, 98, 100
Trachea, 105, 284, 297, 299
Tracheal rings, 105
  first, 298
Tracheobronchial lymph nodes, 108
  left, 81
  right, 83
Tragus, 406
Transversalis fascia, 140–142, 144
Transverse acetabular ligament, 557
Transverse arch, of foot, 561
Transverse arytenoid muscle, 395, 400, 402
Transverse cervical artery, 276, 277, 290, 297
  deep branch of, 21, 276, 445
  superficial branch of, 19, 276
Transverse cervical ligament, 237
Transverse cervical nerve, 270, 275, 282
Transverse colon, 153, 162, 175, 176
Transverse costal facet, thoracic, 51, 53
Transverse dural sinuses, grooves for, 306
Transverse facial artery, 354
Transverse facial vein, 354
Transverse foramen, 7
Transverse humeral ligament, 457, 493
Transverse ligament, of atlas, 345
Transverse mesocolon, 150, 162, 163, 173
Transverse pericardial sinus, 88, 90
Transverse process, 6, 7
  of atlas, 348
  thoracic, 51
Transverse sinuses, 310
  groove for, 262
Transversospinalis group, 26–27, 29, 30, 31
Transversus abdominis muscle, 131, 133, 140, 142

Transversus thoracis muscle, 57, 72
Trapezium, 433, 434, 496
Trapezius muscle, 12, 17, 18–19, 33, 269, 274–276, 420
Trapezoid bones, 433, 434, 496
Trapezoid ligament, 493
Trapezoid line, 428
Triangle of auscultation, 17
Triangular ligament
  left, 165, 166
  right, 165, 166
Triceps brachii muscle, 421, 443, 463
  lateral head of, 444, 445, 464
  long head of, 444, 445, 464
Tricuspid valve, 96, 98, 101
Trigeminal ganglion, 324
Trigeminal impression, 263
Trigeminal nerves, 323, 328, 351–353
  mandibular division of, 322, 324
    branches of, 377
      accessory meningeal, 322
  maxillary division of, 322, 324
  ophthalmic division of, 324
Trigone
  female, 236
  male, 234
Triquetrum, 433, 434, 496
Trochanter
  greater, 508, 512, 523
  lesser, 508, 512
Trochlea, 332–335, 430
Trochlear nerve, 312, 323, 324, 328, 332
Trochlear notch, 432
True vocal cords, 398
Tubercle
  greater, 427, 430
  lesser, 427, 430
  of trapezium, 433, 434
Tuberculum sellae, 263
Tunica albuginea
  female, 222
  male, 208–210, 213
Tunica vaginalis, 132, 209, 210
Tympanic artery, anterior, 367
Tympanic membrane, 405, 408, 410

U

UG. *See* Urogenital (UG).
Ulna, 425, 427, 432, 434
  coronoid process of, 427, 432, 457
  olecranon process of, 427, 432
  overview of, 498

Ulnar artery, 461, 462, 482, 487
  deep branch of, 482
  distal portion of, 474
  proximal portion of, 462, 473
Ulnar collateral artery
  inferior, 461, 462, 473
  superior, 461, 462, 465, 473
Ulnar collateral ligament, 495, 496
Ulnar nerve, 450, 451, 459, 475, 483, 487
  deep branch of, 483, 487
  dorsal branch of, 441
  palmar branch of, 480
  palmar cutaneous branch of, 440
  superficial branch of, 483
Ulnar notch, 432
Ulnar recurrent artery
  anterior, 461, 462, 473, 474
  posterior, 461, 462, 465, 473, 474
Ulnocarpal ligament, palmar, 496
Umbilical artery
  female, 225, 241, 242
  male, 239, 240
  obliterated, 132, 144, 239–242
Umbilical folds
  lateral, 144
  medial, 144
  median, 144
Umbilical ligament, medial, 239
Umbilicus, 133, 135, 144
Uncinate process, 382
Upper limb
  fascia of, 435, 500
  innervation of, 435–436, 499–500
  joints of, 490–497, 500
  muscles of, 420–424, 435, 498–499
  osteology of, 425–434, 498
  overview of, 498–500
  skin removal from, 438
  superficial structures of, 435–441
  vasculature of, 436, 499
Upper subscapular nerve, 453
Urachus, 132, 144
Ureters, 186, 189, 190, 228
  female, 236
  male, 234
Urethra
  female, 219, 223, 224, 236
  male, 234, 249
    membranous, 234, 235
    prostatic, 234
    spongy, 213, 215, 216, 234, 235
Urethral orifice, external, 219
Urethral sphincter, male, 235
Urethrovaginal sphincter, 224

Urinary bladder, 154, 228, 248
  female, 236
  male, 234
Urogenital (UG) diaphragm
  female, 221, 223, 224
  male, 214–216, 234, 235
Urogenital (UG) peritoneum, 249
Urogenital (UG) triangle, 203–225
  female, 203, 218–225
    branches of pudendal artery and nerve in, 225
    deep perineal space in, 203, 205, 224
    dissection of, 220
      overview of, 204
    external genitalia in, 203, 219, 222
    overview of, 218
    perineum in, 219, 221
    shaft of clitoris in, 222
    superficial perineal space in, 203, 205, 221, 223
  male, 203, 207–217
    branches of pudendal artery and nerve in, 217
    deep perineal space in, 203, 205, 215
    dissection of, 212
      overview of, 204
    external genitalia in, 203, 207–213
    overview of, 211
    scrotum in, 206–208
    shaft of penis in, 213
    spermatic cord in, 207, 209
    superficial perineal space in, 203, 205, 214–215
    testis in, 210
    perineum in, 214
Uterine artery, 225, 230, 241, 242
Uterine cavity, 236
Uterine tubes, 155, 229, 230, 236
Uterine venous plexus, 230
Uterosacral ligament, 237
Uterus, 236, 248–249
  body of, 236
  fundus of, 236
  isthmus of, 236
  round ligament of, 138, 144, 146, 229, 230
Uvula, 372, 388

V

Vagal ganglion, inferior, 370
Vagal trunk
  anterior, 104
  posterior, 104

Vagina, 155, 219, 221, 236
  anterior fornix of, 236
  lateral fornices of, 236
  posterior fornix of, 236
Vaginal artery, 241
Vaginal orifice, 219, 223
Vagus nerve(s), 104, 289, 328, 370
  inferior ganglion of, 370
  left, 86, 104, 298, 299
  right, 86, 104, 298, 299
Vallate papillae, 392
Vallecula, 392
Vasa recta, 178
Vastus intermedius muscle, 502, 531
Vastus lateralis muscle, 502, 531
Vastus medialis muscle, 502, 531
Vena cava
  inferior, 89, 92, 93, 186, 188, 189
  superior, 86, 89, 91–93
Vena caval hiatus, 192
Venae comitantes, 461, 534
Ventral rami, 447
Ventricles
  of brain, 301, 316
  cardiac
    left, 84, 91, 100, 114
    right, 84, 91, 114
      incisions of, 97
      internal structures of, 98
  of larynx, 401
Ventricular system, 301, 316

Vermiform appendix, 153, 175
Vertebrae, 5
  cervical, 5, 7
  lumbar, 5, 7
  thoracic, 5, 7, 51
  typical, 6
Vertebral arch, 6
  thoracic, 51
Vertebral arteries, 36, 297, 311, 314, 327
Vertebral body(ies), 6, 7
  in posterior mediastinum, 104
  thoracic, 51, 53
Vertebral canal, 5, 6
  thoracic, 51
Vertebral column, 3, 5, 44, 113
  removal of head and neck viscera from, 347
Vertebral foramen, 6, 7
  thoracic, 51
Vertebral ligaments, 37, 39, 44
Vertebral notch
  inferior, 6
  superior, 6
Vertebral prominens, 13
Vertebral structures, 3, 44, 49, 113
Vesical arteries
  inferior, 239, 240
  superior, 239, 240
Vesicouterine pouch, 155
Vestibular folds, of larynx, 398, 401

Vestibular glands, greater, 222, 223
Vestibular ligament, 401
Vestibule
  of ear, 405, 408
  of larynx, 401
  nasal, 381
  of vagina, 219
    bulb of, 221, 223, 224
Vestibulocochlear nerve, 312, 325, 328, 405, 408
Vidian nerve, 377, 386
Visceral pericardium, 87
Visceral peritoneum, 150
Visceral pleura, 75–77
Visceral plexus, 244
Visceral surface, of liver, 165, 167
Vitreous body, 337
Vocal cords
  false, 398
  true, 398
Vocal folds, 401
Vocal ligaments, 398, 401
Vocalis muscle, 395
Vomer, 257, 261, 380

W

White rami communicantes, 107, 109
Windpipe, 105, 284, 297, 299
Wrist joint, 490–492, 496, 500

X

Xiphoid process, 54, 58, 61, 119, 133

Z

Zonular fibers, 337
Zygapophyseal joint, 6
Zygomatic arch, 354, 364
Zygomatic bone, 257–259, 264–266
  temporal process of, 259
Zygomatic branches, of facial nerve, 355
Zygomatic process
  of frontal bone, 258
  of maxilla, 258
  of temporal bone, 259
Zygomaticofacial foramen, 259, 265
Zygomaticofacial nerve, 352
Zygomaticotemporal foramen, 265, 266
Zygomaticotemporal nerve, 352
Zygomaticus major muscle, 341, 356
Zygomaticus minor muscle, 341, 356